Artificial Intelligence in Image-Based Screening, Diagnostics, and Clinical Care

Artificial Intelligence in Image-Based Screening, Diagnostics, and Clinical Care

Guest Editors

Sameer Antani
Zhiyun Xue
Sivaramakrishnan Rajaraman

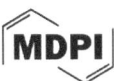

Basel • Beijing • Wuhan • Barcelona • Belgrade • Novi Sad • Cluj • Manchester

Guest Editors

Sameer Antani	Zhiyun Xue	Sivaramakrishnan Rajaraman
Division of Intramural	Division of Intramural	Division of Intramural
Research (DIR)	Research (DIR)	Research (DIR)
National Library of Medicine	National Library of Medicine	National Library of Medicine
National Institutes of Health	National Institutes of Health	National Institutes of Health
Bethesda	Bethesda	Bethesda
USA	USA	USA

Editorial Office
MDPI AG
Grosspeteranlage 5
4052 Basel, Switzerland

This is a reprint of the Special Issue, published open access by the journal *Diagnostics* (ISSN 2075-4418), freely accessible at: https://www.mdpi.com/journal/diagnostics/special_issues/056W2N8F7D.

For citation purposes, cite each article independently as indicated on the article page online and as indicated below:

Lastname, A.A.; Lastname, B.B. Article Title. *Journal Name* **Year**, *Volume Number*, Page Range.

ISBN 978-3-7258-3501-0 (Hbk)
ISBN 978-3-7258-3502-7 (PDF)
https://doi.org/10.3390/books978-3-7258-3502-7

© 2025 by the authors. Articles in this book are Open Access and distributed under the Creative Commons Attribution (CC BY) license. The book as a whole is distributed by MDPI under the terms and conditions of the Creative Commons Attribution-NonCommercial-NoDerivs (CC BY-NC-ND) license (https://creativecommons.org/licenses/by-nc-nd/4.0/).

Contents

About the Editors vii

Preface ix

Sivaramakrishnan Rajaraman, Zhiyun Xue and Sameer Antani
Editorial on Special Issue "Artificial Intelligence in Image-Based Screening, Diagnostics, and Clinical Care"
Reprinted from: *Diagnostics* 2024, 14, 1984, https://doi.org/10.3390/diagnostics14171984 1

Prasanth Ganesan, Ruibin Feng, Brototo Deb, Fleur V. Y. Tjong, Albert J. Rogers, Samuel Ruipérez-Campillo, et al.
Novel Domain Knowledge-Encoding Algorithm Enables Label-Efficient Deep Learning for Cardiac CT Segmentation to Guide Atrial Fibrillation Treatment in a Pilot Dataset
Reprinted from: *Diagnostics* 2024, 14, 1538, https://doi.org/10.3390/diagnostics14141538 6

Manjur Kolhar, Raisa Nazir Ahmed Kazi, Hitesh Mohapatra and Ahmed M Al Rajeh
AI-Driven Real-Time Classification of ECG Signals for Cardiac Monitoring Using i-AlexNet Architecture
Reprinted from: *Diagnostics* 2024, 14, 1344, https://doi.org/10.3390/diagnostics14131344 20

Yangqin Feng, Jordan Sim Zheng Ting, Xinxing Xu, Chew Bee Kun, Edward Ong Tien En, Hendra Irawan Tan Wee Jun, et al.
Deep Neural Network Augments Performance of Junior Residents in Diagnosing COVID-19 Pneumonia on Chest Radiographs
Reprinted from: *Diagnostics* 2023, 13, 1397, https://doi.org/10.3390/diagnostics13081397 38

Abdul Rahaman Wahab Sait and Ashit Kumar Dutta
Developing a Deep-Learning-Based Coronary Artery Disease Detection Technique Using Computer Tomography Images
Reprinted from: *Diagnostics* 2023, 13, 1312, https://doi.org/10.3390/diagnostics13071312 50

Dana Li, Lea Marie Pehrson, Rasmus Bonnevie, Marco Fraccaro, Jakob Thrane, Lea Tøttrup, et al.
Performance and Agreement When Annotating Chest X-ray Text Reports—A Preliminary Step in the Development of a Deep Learning-Based Prioritization and Detection System
Reprinted from: *Diagnostics* 2023, 13, 1070, https://doi.org/10.3390/diagnostics13061070 64

Zhiyun Xue, Feng Yang, Sivaramakrishnan Rajaraman, Ghada Zamzmi and Sameer Antani
Cross Dataset Analysis of Domain Shift in CXR Lung Region Detection
Reprinted from: *Diagnostics* 2023, 13, 1068, https://doi.org/10.3390/diagnostics13061068 88

Sivaramakrishnan Rajaraman, Feng Yang, Ghada Zamzmi, Zhiyun Xue and Sameer Antani
Assessing the Impact of Image Resolution on Deep Learning for TB Lesion Segmentation on Frontal Chest X-rays
Reprinted from: *Diagnostics* 2023, 13, 747, https://doi.org/10.3390/diagnostics13040747 106

Chadi Barakat, Marcel Aach, Andreas Schuppert, Sigurður Brynjólfsson, Sebastian Fritsch, and Morris Riedel
Analysis of Chest X-ray for COVID-19 Diagnosis as a Use Case for an HPC-Enabled Data Analysis and Machine Learning Platform for Medical Diagnosis Support
Reprinted from: *Diagnostics* 2023, 13, 391, https://doi.org/10.3390/diagnostics13030391 124

Dana Li, Lea Marie Pehrson, Lea Tøttrup, Marco Fraccaro, Rasmus Bonnevie, Jakob Thrane, et al.
Inter- and Intra-Observer Agreement When Using a Diagnostic Labeling Scheme for Annotating Findings on Chest X-rays—An Early Step in the Development of a Deep Learning-Based Decision Support System
Reprinted from: *Diagnostics* **2022**, *12*, 3112, https://doi.org/10.3390/diagnostics12123112 . . . . **139**

Elena Stamate, Alin-Ionut Piraianu, Oana Roxana Ciobotaru, Rodica Crassas, Oana Duca, Ana Fulga, et al.
Revolutionizing Cardiology through Artificial Intelligence—Big Data from Proactive Prevention to Precise Diagnostics and Cutting-Edge Treatment—A Comprehensive Review of the Past 5 Years
Reprinted from: *Diagnostics* **2024**, *14*, 1103, https://doi.org/10.3390/diagnostics14111103 . . . . **154**

Dilber Uzun Ozsahin, Cemre Ozgocmen, Ozlem Balcioglu, Ilker Ozsahin and Berna Uzun
Diagnostic AI and Cardiac Diseases
Reprinted from: *Diagnostics* **2022**, *12*, 2901, https://doi.org/10.3390/diagnostics12122901 . . . . **218**

Alina Cornelia Pacurari, Sanket Bhattarai, Abdullah Muhammad, Claudiu Avram, Alexandru Ovidiu Mederle, Ovidiu Rosca, et al.
Diagnostic Accuracy of Machine Learning AI Architectures in Detection and Classification of Lung Cancer: A Systematic Review
Reprinted from: *Diagnostics* **2023**, *13*, 2145, https://doi.org/10.3390/diagnostics13132145 . . . . **234**

About the Editors

Sameer Antani

Dr. Sameer Antani is a Principal Investigator (Tenure-Track) in the Division of Intramural Research (DIR) of the National Library of Medicine (NLM) at the National Institutes of Health (NIH). He is a Fellow of the American Institute for Medical and Biological Engineering (AIMBE), a Fellow of the Institute of Electrical and Electronics Engineers (IEEE), and a Senior Member of the SPIE. His research focuses on developing novel algorithms in medical imaging, as well as on multimodal machine learning (ML) and artificial intelligence (AI). He also works on ML/AI for resource-limited and global health settings and on characterizing data and innovations in ML/AI algorithm design to enable reliable AI predictions for disease screening, diagnostics, risk prediction, and treatment. His scientific contributions and research leadership have been recognized through several awards, including the NLM Board of Regents Awards and NIH Director's Awards.

Zhiyun Xue

Dr. Zhiyun (Jaylene) Xue is a Staff Scientist in the Division of Intramural Research (DIR) of the National Library of Medicine (NLM), National Institutes of Health (NIH). She has been working on several medical imaging informatics projects. By applying her knowledge and expertise in the fields of machine learning (ML), image processing, and computer vision to analyze biomedical images in different modalities, Dr. Xue directs her R&D efforts toward advancing biomedical informatics and data science research, assisting clinicians at the point-of-care, improving public health, and addressing the needs of underserved populations.

Sivaramakrishnan Rajaraman

Dr. Sivaramakrishnan Rajaraman is working as a research scientist in the Division of Intramural Research (DIR) at the National Library of Medicine (NLM), National Institutes of Health (NIH). He is involved in projects that apply computational sciences and engineering techniques to advance life science applications, utilizing medical images to aid healthcare professionals in low-cost decision-making for POC screening and diagnostics. As a versatile researcher, he has expertise in artificial intelligence, machine learning, data science, biomedical image analysis, and computer vision. Dr. Rajaraman serves on the Editorial Boards of the journals including *PLOS Digital Health*, *PeerJ*, and *PLOS ONE*. He is a Life Member of the Society of Photo-optical Instrumentation Engineers (SPIE) and a Senior Member of the Institute of Electrical and Electronics Engineers (IEEE) and the IEEE Engineering in Medicine & Biology Society (EMBS).

Preface

This Special Issue "Artificial Intelligence in Image-Based Screening, Diagnostics, and Clinical Care", highlights transformative advancements in AI-driven medical imaging. By addressing challenges like limited datasets and noisy data, the featured works showcase innovative methodologies that enhance diagnostic precision, facilitate early detection, and improve patient outcomes. The compilation includes original research and reviews exploring cutting-edge AI applications for screening, diagnostics, and clinical workflows.

Sameer Antani, Zhiyun Xue, and Sivaramakrishnan Rajaraman
Guest Editors

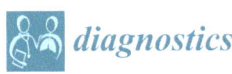

Editorial

Editorial on Special Issue "Artificial Intelligence in Image-Based Screening, Diagnostics, and Clinical Care"

Sivaramakrishnan Rajaraman, Zhiyun Xue and Sameer Antani *

Computational Health Research Branch, National Library of Medicine, National Institutes of Health, Bethesda, MD 20894, USA; sivaramakrishnan.rajaraman@nih.gov (S.R.); zhiyun.xue@nih.gov (Z.X.)
* Correspondence: sameer.antani@nih.gov

Citation: Rajaraman, S.; Xue, Z.; Antani, S. Editorial on Special Issue "Artificial Intelligence in Image-Based Screening, Diagnostics, and Clinical Care". *Diagnostics* **2024**, *14*, 1984. https://doi.org/10.3390/diagnostics14171984

Received: 20 August 2024
Accepted: 4 September 2024
Published: 7 September 2024

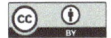

Copyright: © 2024 by the authors. Licensee MDPI, Basel, Switzerland. This article is an open access article distributed under the terms and conditions of the Creative Commons Attribution (CC BY) license (https:// creativecommons.org/licenses/by/ 4.0/).

1. Introduction

In an era of rapid advancements in artificial intelligence (AI) technologies, particularly in medical imaging and natural language processing, strategic efforts to leverage AI's capabilities in analyzing complex medical data and integrating it into clinical workflows have emerged as a key driver of innovation in healthcare. As the global healthcare landscape shifts towards precision medicine, the incorporation of AI into image-based screening, diagnostics, and clinical care is becoming increasingly crucial, offering significant opportunities to enhance patient outcomes and improve healthcare delivery. Advancements in AI, particularly in deep learning (DL) [1], a subset of machine learning (ML), have significantly advanced medical imaging, and accurate analyses. These developments represent a paradigm shift, where AI not only automates processes but also enhances precision in diagnostics, allowing for personalized interventions tailored to individual patient needs. However, integrating AI into clinical workflow presents several challenges that must be carefully addressed. The effectiveness and generalizability of AI-driven solutions can be adversely affected by the data quality, imbalance, and limited availability of well-annotated training data [2]. The imbalance in datasets [3] refers to pathological cases in various grades of severity that are significantly smaller compared to healthy controls. These factors complicate the development of robust, reliable, bias-free, and generalizable models and limit their use in real-world clinical environments.

As Guest Editors of the Special Issue "Artificial Intelligence in Image-Based Screening, Diagnostics, and Clinical Care", we present a collection of research findings addressing some of these challenges, showcasing cutting-edge advancements in AI applications in healthcare. This Special Issue not only highlights technological progress but also explores the practical implications of AI in clinical practice, offering insights that are critical for the ongoing evolution of the field. We believe that the contributions within this Special Issue will serve as a catalyst for future research and encourage the broader medical and scientific communities to fully explore AI's potential in transforming patient care.

2. Highlights of the Special Issue

2.1. Overview of Published Research

This Special Issue "Artificial Intelligence in Image-Based Screening, Diagnostics, and Clinical Care" offers a comprehensive collection of 12 research studies that explore various AI methodologies, each contributing to the advancement of precision medicine and the improvement of clinical care.

2.2. AI in Cardiac Diagnostics

Cardiac diagnostics are crucial areas where AI has demonstrated significant impact, particularly in enhancing the accuracy and efficiency of clinical workflows. The study "Novel Domain Knowledge-Encoding Algorithm Enables Label-Efficient Deep Learning for Cardiac CT Segmentation to Guide Atrial Fibrillation Treatment in a Pilot Dataset" [4] addresses a critical challenge in AI-driven medical imaging: the need for large, labeled datasets. The authors propose a novel methodology that encodes domain-specific cardiac geometry knowledge to automate the labeling process, thereby reducing the dependency on extensive training data. This innovative approach achieved high segmentation accuracy in cardiac CT images with minimal training data, highlighting the potential for AI to improve personalized treatment strategies, such as cardiac ablation for atrial fibrillation, where precise segmentation of cardiac structures is essential.

Complementing this, the study "AI-Driven Real-Time Classification of ECG Signals for Cardiac Monitoring Using i-AlexNet Architecture" [5] focuses on the application of AI in real-time cardiac monitoring. The authors developed a new model called the *i-AlexNet* model, a modified version of the classic AlexNet [6] architecture, which excels in classifying ECG signals with remarkable accuracy. With a classification accuracy of 98.8%, this study not only underscores the robustness of AI in cardiac monitoring but also highlights its potential to revolutionize real-time, data-driven healthcare solutions.

AI's ability to accurately classify normal and anomalous ECG signals in real time can greatly assist clinicians in making timely and accurate decisions, ultimately improving patient outcomes. The review article "Revolutionizing Cardiology through Artificial Intelligence—Big Data from Proactive Prevention to Precise Diagnostics and Cutting-Edge Treatment—A Comprehensive Review of the Past 5 Years" [7] discusses findings from multiple studies, exploring how AI is being integrated into various branches of cardiology, including imaging, electrophysiology, and interventional procedures. This comprehensive review not only highlights the rapid advancements in AI technologies and their potential to revolutionize cardiovascular care but also addresses the ethical and legal challenges associated with their implementation.

The study "Diagnostic AI and Cardiac Diseases" [8] further explores the diagnostic applications of AI for cardiac conditions. The authors review AI-driven tools for detecting various cardiac diseases, emphasizing the importance of AI as a support system for clinical decision making. By categorizing the reviewed studies according to specific cardiac conditions, the article provides a structured overview of how AI is enhancing diagnostic accuracy and improving patient outcomes.

The study "Developing a Deep-Learning-Based Coronary Artery Disease Detection Technique Using Computer Tomography Images" [9] presents an advanced DL model for coronary artery disease (CAD) detection. By utilizing YOLOV7 [10] for feature extraction and optimizing the hyperparameters of the UNet++ model, the authors created a CAD detection system that surpasses current methods, highlighting AI's potential for fine-tuning across different medical imaging applications, including oncology.

2.3. AI in Chest X-ray (CXR) Analysis

Chest X-ray (CXR) image analysis represents another critical area where AI is making significant strides, particularly in the context of detecting infectious diseases and chronic conditions. A significant portion of the Special Issue is dedicated to the application of AI in CXR analysis. The study "Deep Neural Network Augments Performance of Junior Residents in Diagnosing COVID-19 Pneumonia on Chest Radiographs" [11] demonstrates how AI can enhance clinical decision making, especially for less experienced practitioners. The authors developed a DL network capable of distinguishing COVID-19 pneumonia from other types of pneumonia, significantly improving the diagnostic accuracy of junior residents. This research underscores AI's potential as an educational tool, bridging the experience gap and improving the overall quality of care in high-pressure situations.

In addressing domain-specific challenges, the study "Cross Dataset Analysis of Domain Shift in CXR Lung Region Detection" [12] investigates the impact of domain shift, a phenomenon where differences in data sources can affect AI model performance. By analyzing five CXR datasets from different sources, the authors provide insights into how to mitigate domain shifts and enhance the robustness of AI models in diverse clinical environments. This study contributes to the broader goal of developing AI models that can be generalized across various settings, a key concern for the real-world deployment of AI in healthcare.

The study titled "Assessing the Impact of Image Resolution on Deep Learning for TB Lesion Segmentation on Frontal Chest X-rays" [13] investigates the influence of image resolution on the effectiveness of DL models in segmenting lesions consistent with tuberculosis (TB) in CXRs. An Inception-V3 encoder-based UNet [14] model was systematically evaluated in this segmentation task using image-mask pairs across various spatial resolutions, identifying the optimal resolution for accurate TB lesion segmentation. This research is particularly relevant for developing AI models that are both computationally efficient and diagnostically accurate, especially in resource-limited settings where high-resolution imaging may not be feasible.

Expanding on the application of AI in CXR analysis, the study "Analysis of Chest X-ray for COVID-19 Diagnosis as a Use Case for an HPC-Enabled Data Analysis and Machine Learning Platform for Medical Diagnosis Support" [15] demonstrates how high-performance computing (HPC) can accelerate the development of AI tools for real-time clinical applications. By leveraging an HPC platform, the authors re-trained the COVID-Net [16] model, optimizing its performance through large-scale hyperparameter tuning. This study highlights the importance of computational resources in AI development, particularly in responding to global health crises like the COVID-19 pandemic.

The article titled "Performance and Agreement When Annotating Chest X-ray Text Reports—A Preliminary Step in the Development of a Deep Learning-Based Prioritization and Detection System" [17] addresses the crucial issue of consistency in data annotation. The study investigates how different annotators, ranging from radiologists to medical students, interpret and label CXR radiological reports. The findings reveal notable variability in annotation quality, which directly impacts the development of reliable AI-based decision support systems. By emphasizing the importance of consistent and accurate annotations, this research contributes to the ongoing discourse on the role of human expertise in training AI models, particularly in fields where sub-specialization is common. Additionally, the article "Inter- and Intra-Observer Agreement When Using a Diagnostic Labeling Scheme for Annotating Findings on Chest X-rays" [18] explores the variability in annotation consistency among radiologists, a key factor in the successful deployment of AI systems. The study evaluates how experience levels affect annotation consistency, providing valuable insights into the challenges of standardizing data for AI training. The findings suggest that descriptive labels, as opposed to interpretive ones, may increase agreement among radiologists, thereby improving the reliability of AI-based decision support systems.

2.4. AI in Oncology: Lung Cancer Detection

Oncology, particularly lung cancer detection, is another focal point of this Special Issue, where AI's potential to enhance early detection and treatment outcomes is thoroughly explored. The study "Diagnostic Accuracy of Machine Learning AI Architectures in Detection and Classification of Lung Cancer: A Systematic Review" [19] provides a comprehensive assessment of various ML/DL architectures used in lung cancer detection. The review analyzes multiple studies, highlighting the sensitivity, specificity, and overall accuracy of these models in distinguishing between malignant and benign lung lesions. This systematic review underscores the potential of AI to significantly improve early detection and classification of lung cancer, a critical factor in improving patient prognosis. The study also emphasizes the need for further research to optimize and validate AI algorithms, ensuring their clinical relevance and applicability in routine practice.

2.5. Innovative Approaches

The studies featured in this Special Issue collectively demonstrate innovative approaches to addressing the challenges associated with limited and imperfect medical data. For instance, the methods proposed in [4] demonstrate a notable advancement in reducing the dependency on large datasets by incorporating domain knowledge directly into the

AI training process. This method not only enhances model efficiency but also opens new avenues for AI applications in areas where data scarcity is a limiting factor. The integration of HPC, as seen in [15], represents a forward-looking approach to accelerating AI development, making it possible to deploy highly optimized models in real-time clinical settings. This innovation is particularly relevant in the context of global health emergencies, where rapid and accurate diagnostics are paramount. Moreover, studies [17,18] on exploring the annotation consistency in CXR labeling highlight the human factors that must be considered in AI development. The review articles on AI in cardiology [7,8] and lung cancer detection [19] further illustrate the broad applicability of AI across different medical fields. By discussing recent advancements and identifying areas for future research, these reviews offer a roadmap for the continued integration of AI into clinical practice.

3. Conclusions

3.1. Summary of Key Points

In this Special Issue on "Artificial Intelligence in Image-Based Screening, Diagnostics, and Clinical Care", we have examined the diverse and transformative role of AI across a wide range of medical applications. The 12 research studies featured in this issue have highlighted the potential of AI to enhance precision medicine, improve diagnostic accuracy, and streamline clinical workflows.

3.2. Call to Action

As we look to the future, the medical and scientific communities must continue to explore and expand the possibilities of AI in healthcare. The advancements discussed in this Special Issue are just the beginning. There remains a wealth of untapped potential in AI technologies, particularly in the areas of multi-modal data integration, explainable AI, and bias mitigation. Future research must not only focus on pushing the boundaries of what AI can achieve but also on ensuring that these technologies are developed and deployed in ways that are ethical, equitable, and centered around patient care. Collaboration across disciplines will be key to achieving these goals. AI researchers, clinicians, data scientists, ethicists, and policymakers must work together to create AI systems that are not only optimal but also aligned with the needs and values of the healthcare community. By fostering a collaborative and interdisciplinary approach, we can ensure that AI continues to evolve as a tool that enhances, rather than replaces, the expertise and judgment of human clinicians.

The studies included here represent a significant contribution to the field of AI in medical data analysis, but there is much more to be done. By engaging with this Special Issue and contributing to this field, you become part of a growing community dedicated to exploring the frontiers of AI in healthcare. Together, we can push the boundaries of what is possible, improving patient outcomes and making high-quality healthcare more accessible to people around the world.

Author Contributions: Conceptualization, S.R., Z.X. and S.A.; Data curation, S.R.; Formal analysis, S.R. and S.A.; Funding acquisition, S.A.; Investigation, S.A.; Methodology, S.R., Z.X. and S.A.; Project administration, S.A.; Resources, S.A.; Software, S.R.; Supervision, S.A.; Validation, S.R., Z.X. and S.A.; Visualization, S.R.; Writing—original draft, S.R.; Writing—review and editing, S.R., Z.X. and S.A. All authors have read and agreed to the published version of the manuscript.

Funding: This research was supported by the Intramural Research Program of the National Library of Medicine (NLM) at the National Institutes of Health (NIH).

Conflicts of Interest: The authors declare no conflicts of interest.

References

1. Esteva, A.; Robicquet, A.; Ramsundar, B.; Kuleshov, V.; DePristo, M.; Chou, K.; Cui, C.; Corrado, G.; Thrun, S.; Dean, J. A Guide to Deep Learning in Healthcare. *Nat. Med.* **2019**, *25*, 24–29. [CrossRef] [PubMed]
2. Rajaraman, S.; Zamzmi, G.; Yang, F.; Xue, Z.; Antani, S.K. Data Characterization for Reliable AI in Medicine. In *Recent Trends in Image Processing and Pattern Recognition*; Springer: Berlin/Heidelberg, Germany, 2023; Volume 1704, pp. 3–11. [CrossRef]
3. Ganesan, P.; Rajaraman, S.; Long, R.; Ghoraani, B.; Antani, S. Assessment of Data Augmentation Strategies Toward Performance Improvement of Abnormality Classification in Chest Radiographs. In Proceedings of the Annual International Conference of the IEEE Engineering in Medicine and Biology Society, EMBS, Berlin, Germany, 23–27 July 2019.
4. Ganesan, P.; Feng, R.; Deb, B.; Tjong, F.V.Y.; Rogers, A.J.; Ruipérez-Campillo, S.; Somani, S.; Clopton, P.; Baykaner, T.; Rodrigo, M.; et al. Novel Domain Knowledge-Encoding Algorithm Enables Label-Efficient Deep Learning for Cardiac CT Segmentation to Guide Atrial Fibrillation Treatment in a Pilot Dataset. *Diagnostics* **2024**, *14*, 1538. [CrossRef] [PubMed]
5. Kolhar, M.; Kazi, R.N.A.; Mohapatra, H.; Al Rajeh, A.M. AI-Driven Real-Time Classification of ECG Signals for Cardiac Monitoring Using i-AlexNet Architecture. *Diagnostics* **2024**, *14*, 1344. [CrossRef] [PubMed]
6. Lecun, Y.; Bengio, Y.; Hinton, G. Deep Learning. *Nature* **2015**, *521*, 436–444. [CrossRef] [PubMed]
7. Stamate, E.; Piraianu, A.-I.; Ciobotaru, O.R.; Crassas, R.; Duca, O.; Fulga, A.; Grigore, I.; Vintila, V.; Fulga, I.; Ciobotaru, O.C. Revolutionizing Cardiology through Artificial Intelligence—Big Data from Proactive Prevention to Precise Diagnostics and Cutting-Edge Treatment—A Comprehensive Review of the Past 5 Years. *Diagnostics* **2024**, *14*, 1103. [CrossRef] [PubMed]
8. Uzun Ozsahin, D.; Ozgocmen, C.; Balcioglu, O.; Ozsahin, I.; Uzun, B. Diagnostic AI and Cardiac Diseases. *Diagnostics* **2022**, *12*, 2901. [CrossRef] [PubMed]
9. Wahab Sait, A.R.; Dutta, A.K. Developing a Deep-Learning-Based Coronary Artery Disease Detection Technique Using Computer Tomography Images. *Diagnostics* **2023**, *13*, 1312. [CrossRef] [PubMed]
10. Ragab, M.G.; Abdulkadir, S.J.; Muneer, A.; Alqushaibi, A.; Sumiea, E.H.; Qureshi, R.; Al-Selwi, S.M.; Alhussian, H. A Comprehensive Systematic Review of YOLO for Medical Object Detection (2018 to 2023). *IEEE Access* **2024**, *12*, 57815–57836. [CrossRef]
11. Feng, Y.; Sim Zheng Ting, J.; Xu, X.; Bee Kun, C.; Ong Tien En, E.; Irawan Tan Wee Jun, H.; Ting, Y.; Lei, X.; Chen, W.-X.; Wang, Y.; et al. Deep Neural Network Augments Performance of Junior Residents in Diagnosing COVID-19 Pneumonia on Chest Radiographs. *Diagnostics* **2023**, *13*, 1397. [CrossRef] [PubMed]
12. Xue, Z.; Yang, F.; Rajaraman, S.; Zamzmi, G.; Antani, S. Cross Dataset Analysis of Domain Shift in CXR Lung Region Detection. *Diagnostics* **2023**, *13*, 1068. [CrossRef] [PubMed]
13. Rajaraman, S.; Yang, F.; Zamzmi, G.; Xue, Z.; Antani, S. Assessing the Impact of Image Resolution on Deep Learning for TB Lesion Segmentation on Frontal Chest X-rays. *Diagnostics* **2023**, *13*, 747. [CrossRef] [PubMed]
14. Ronneberger, O.; Fischer, P.; Brox, T. U-Net: Convolutional Networks for Biomedical Image Segmentation. In *Lecture Notes in Computer Science (Including Subseries Lecture Notes in Artificial Intelligence and Lecture Notes in Bioinformatics)*; Springer: Berlin/Heidelberg, Germany, 2015.
15. Barakat, C.; Aach, M.; Schuppert, A.; Brynjólfsson, S.; Fritsch, S.; Riedel, M. Analysis of Chest X-ray for COVID-19 Diagnosis as a Use Case for an HPC-Enabled Data Analysis and Machine Learning Platform for Medical Diagnosis Support. *Diagnostics* **2023**, *13*, 391. [CrossRef] [PubMed]
16. Wang, L.; Lin, Z.Q.; Wong, A. COVID-Net: A Tailored Deep Convolutional Neural Network Design for Detection of COVID-19 Cases from Chest X-ray Images. *Sci. Rep.* **2020**, *10*, 19549. [CrossRef] [PubMed]
17. Li, D.; Pehrson, L.M.; Bonnevie, R.; Fraccaro, M.; Thrane, J.; Tøttrup, L.; Lauridsen, C.A.; Butt Balaganeshan, S.; Jankovic, J.; Andersen, T.T.; et al. Performance and Agreement When Annotating Chest X-ray Text Reports—A Preliminary Step in the Development of a Deep Learning-Based Prioritization and Detection System. *Diagnostics* **2023**, *13*, 1070. [CrossRef] [PubMed]
18. Li, D.; Pehrson, L.M.; Tøttrup, L.; Fraccaro, M.; Bonnevie, R.; Thrane, J.; Sørensen, P.J.; Rykkje, A.; Andersen, T.T.; Steglich-Arnholm, H.; et al. Inter- and Intra-Observer Agreement When Using a Diagnostic Labeling Scheme for Annotating Findings on Chest X-rays—An Early Step in the Development of a Deep Learning-Based Decision Support System. *Diagnostics* **2022**, *12*, 3112. [CrossRef] [PubMed]
19. Pacurari, A.C.; Bhattarai, S.; Muhammad, A.; Avram, C.; Mederle, A.O.; Rosca, O.; Bratosin, F.; Bogdan, I.; Fericean, R.M.; Biris, M.; et al. Diagnostic Accuracy of Machine Learning AI Architectures in Detection and Classification of Lung Cancer: A Systematic Review. *Diagnostics* **2023**, *13*, 2145. [CrossRef] [PubMed]

Disclaimer/Publisher's Note: The statements, opinions and data contained in all publications are solely those of the individual author(s) and contributor(s) and not of MDPI and/or the editor(s). MDPI and/or the editor(s) disclaim responsibility for any injury to people or property resulting from any ideas, methods, instructions or products referred to in the content.

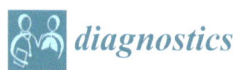

Article

Novel Domain Knowledge-Encoding Algorithm Enables Label-Efficient Deep Learning for Cardiac CT Segmentation to Guide Atrial Fibrillation Treatment in a Pilot Dataset

Prasanth Ganesan [1,†], Ruibin Feng [1,†], Brototo Deb [1], Fleur V. Y. Tjong [1,2], Albert J. Rogers [1], Samuel Ruipérez-Campillo [1,3], Sulaiman Somani [1], Paul Clopton [1], Tina Baykaner [1], Miguel Rodrigo [1,4], James Zou [5], Francois Haddad [1], Matei Zaharia [6] and Sanjiv M. Narayan [1,*]

1. Department of Medicine and Stanford Cardiovascular Institute (CVI), Stanford University, Stanford, CA 94305, USA; prash030@stanford.edu (P.G.); ruibin@stanford.edu (R.F.)
2. Heart Center, Department of Clinical and Experimental Cardiology, Amsterdam UMC, University of Amsterdam, 1105 AZ Amsterdam, The Netherlands
3. Department of Computer Science, ETH Zurich, 8092 Zurich, Switzerland
4. CoMMLab, Universitat de València, 46100 Valencia, Spain
5. Department of Biomedical Data Science, Stanford University, Stanford, CA 94305, USA
6. Department of Computer Science, University of California Berkeley, Berkeley, CA 94720, USA
* Correspondence: sanjiv1@stanford.edu
† These authors contributed equally to this work.

Citation: Ganesan, P.; Feng, R.; Deb, B.; Tjong, F.V.Y.; Rogers, A.J.; Ruipérez-Campillo, S.; Somani, S.; Clopton, P.; Baykaner, T.; Rodrigo, M.; et al. Novel Domain Knowledge-Encoding Algorithm Enables Label-Efficient Deep Learning for Cardiac CT Segmentation to Guide Atrial Fibrillation Treatment in a Pilot Dataset. *Diagnostics* **2024**, *14*, 1538. https://doi.org/10.3390/diagnostics14141538

Academic Editor: Ali Gholamrezanezhad

Received: 15 May 2024
Revised: 7 July 2024
Accepted: 10 July 2024
Published: 17 July 2024

Copyright: © 2024 by the authors. Licensee MDPI, Basel, Switzerland. This article is an open access article distributed under the terms and conditions of the Creative Commons Attribution (CC BY) license (https://creativecommons.org/licenses/by/4.0/).

Abstract: Background: Segmenting computed tomography (CT) is crucial in various clinical applications, such as tailoring personalized cardiac ablation for managing cardiac arrhythmias. Automating segmentation through machine learning (ML) is hindered by the necessity for large, labeled training data, which can be challenging to obtain. This article proposes a novel approach for automated, robust labeling using domain knowledge to achieve high-performance segmentation by ML from a small training set. The approach, the domain knowledge-encoding (DOKEN) algorithm, reduces the reliance on large training datasets by encoding cardiac geometry while automatically labeling the training set. The method was validated in a hold-out dataset of CT results from an atrial fibrillation (AF) ablation study. **Methods:** The DOKEN algorithm parses left atrial (LA) structures, extracts "anatomical knowledge" by leveraging digital LA models (available publicly), and then applies this knowledge to achieve high ML segmentation performance with a small number of training samples. The DOKEN-labeled training set was used to train a nnU-Net deep neural network (DNN) model for segmenting cardiac CT in $N = 20$ patients. Subsequently, the method was tested in a hold-out set with $N = 100$ patients (five times larger than training set) who underwent AF ablation. **Results:** The DOKEN algorithm integrated with the nn-Unet model achieved high segmentation performance with few training samples, with a training to test ratio of 1:5. The Dice score of the DOKEN-enhanced model was 96.7% (IQR: 95.3% to 97.7%), with a median error in surface distance of boundaries of 1.51 mm (IQR: 0.72 to 3.12) and a mean centroid–boundary distance of 1.16 mm (95% CI: −4.57 to 6.89), similar to expert results ($r = 0.99$; $p < 0.001$). In digital hearts, the novel DOKEN approach segmented the LA structures with a mean difference for the centroid–boundary distances of −0.27 mm (95% CI: −3.87 to 3.33; $r = 0.99$; $p < 0.0001$). **Conclusions:** The proposed novel domain knowledge-encoding algorithm was able to perform the segmentation of six substructures of the LA, reducing the need for large training data sets. The combination of domain knowledge encoding and a machine learning approach could reduce the dependence of ML on large training datasets and could potentially be applied to AF ablation procedures and extended in the future to other imaging, 3D printing, and data science applications.

Keywords: cardiac CT segmentation; machine learning; domain knowledge encoding; atrial fibrillation; ablation

1. Introduction

The segmentation of cardiac computed tomography (CT) images has historically been performed by semi-automated algorithms such as graph-cuts [1], region growing [2] with manual seed inputs, and other traditional image-processing methods. Deep neural networks (DNN) showed superior performance to traditional image processing even for complex tasks such as segmenting a person of interest in an image of a crowded street [3] or classifying complex diseases from radiology scans [4,5]. However, DNN models require a large amount of training data, which, in the context of cardiac CT segmentation, is challenging to obtain. Several publicly available medical datasets include <100 cases [6–8] due to technical, privacy, and regulatory concerns. Since deep learning typically reserves the majority of cases for training, models are thus often tested on <40 cases [8], which may limit generalizability [9,10].

This begs the question as to whether high DNN performance can be obtained when the number of training samples is smaller than that of test-set samples. The focus of this work is to explore the idea of achieving high DNN segmentation performance in cardiac CT images from a small number of training samples. A DNN was applied to raw CT images to segment the left atrium (LA) body and other LA substructures: four pulmonary veins (PVs) and one LA appendage (LAA), which are central to treating patients with atrial fibrillation (AF). Although this paper focuses on a label-efficient segmentation approach of the six LA substructures for AF application, the approach can theoretically be extended to segment other chambers of the heart as well.

This article proposes a novel approach called the domain knowledge-encoding (DOKEN) algorithm, which extracts "anatomical knowledge" by leveraging digital LA models (available publicly) and then applies this knowledge to achieve high DNN segmentation performance with small number of training samples. The DOKEN algorithm essentially pre-processes the training samples before inputting them for DNN training. The pre-processing involves automatic labeling to obtain robust ground-truth labels of LA substructures. The performance of the DOKEN-labeled DNN model was tested in a hold-out dataset >5 times larger than the training set.

The purpose of this study is to test the hypothesis that ML models could be trained using very small datasets if combined with some domain knowledge of the task at hand. This method of training using conceptual domain knowledge principles rather than massive training data [11,12] is analogous to how humans can learn from small data [12]. Lake et al. used this approach to generate handwritten characters with human-level performance from one exemplar by parsing characters into simple primitives that were composited to create new characters [13]. However, for medical image analysis, such domain knowledge has rarely been used to reduce training sizes for DNN [14,15]. In the following sections, we describe the methods, results, discussion and conclusions.

2. Methods

Figure 1 outlines the method. (1) The proposed DOKEN algorithm encoded domain knowledge of the LA body and other anatomies; (2) the algorithm was used to train a nnU-Net DNN to segment cardiac CT images using only a small training set; and (3) the trained DNN was tested in a large hold-out set.

2.1. Dataset for Training and Testing

The CT dataset used in this study consists of $N = 120$ patients who had undergone AF ablation between October 2014 and July 2019 and had cardiac CT scans. All patients signed informed consent at Stanford Health Care. We split this dataset randomly into $N = 20$ for DNN model training (Training Set), with $N = 100$ patients as a hold-out test set (Test Set). Note that the number of samples in the training set is 5 times smaller than the test set samples, which is one of the key contributions of this study. Separately, for developing the DOKEN algorithm, $N = 6$ publicly available 3D digital heart models built using Gaussian process morphable models [16] was used.

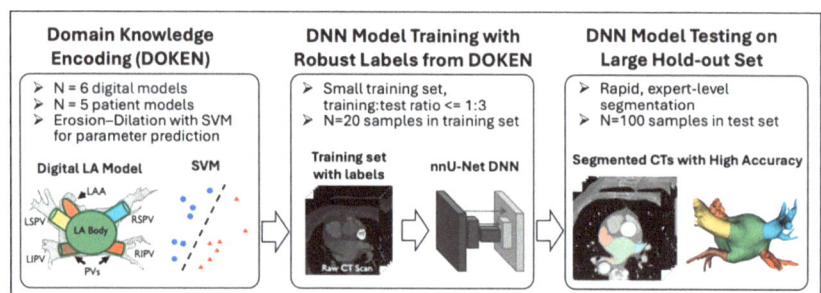

Figure 1. Method overview: proposed domain knowledge-encoding algorithm used to label CT images for efficient DNN training on a training set significantly smaller than the test set. LA: left atrium, LSPV: left superior pulmonary vein, LIPV: left inferior pulmonary vein, RSPV: right superior pulmonary. Each color represents an LA sub-structure.

2.2. Domain Knowledge-Encoding (DOKEN) Algorithm

The goal of the DOKEN algorithm is to automatically generate robust ground-truth labels of LA substructures for DNN training. The algorithm consists of the following two steps:

I. Segmentation of digital LA models: $N = 6$ digital LA models (publicly available) were segmented based on an iterative erosion–dilation (ED) process (Figure 2).

II. Tuning ED parameter using patient LA models: The iterative ED process requires optimal iteration number as a parameter, which decides the accurate segmentation of the LA body and other substructures. To determine this parameter, 5 manually segmented LA models were used to train support vector machines (SVMs) to predict the optimal iteration in the ED process.

The two steps are used to develop the DOKEN algorithm, and once its developed, it takes training images as input and generates ground-truth labels as output. The two development steps are detailed below.

I. Segmentation of digital LA models

We reasoned that heart structures can be geometrically parsed by separating the convex LA body from the concave whole heart. Three-dimensional voxel erosion, dilation [17], and subtraction were used for this purpose.

To segment PV and LAA from the digital heart, a binary erosion operation was used, which can be defined as $A \ominus B = \{x \in E^N \mid x + b \in A \text{ for every } b \in B\}$. Then, in order to recover the original dimension of LA, binary dilation was applied, defined as $A \oplus B = \{x \in E^N \mid c = a + b \text{ for some } a \in A \text{ and } b \in B\}$, where A and B are sets in N-space (E^N) with elements a and b. In our case, A is the heart model and B is a structuring element, which is a $3 \times 3 \times 3$ cube where the center and its 6 neighbors are set to 1 and the remaining elements are 0s.

First, the digital shells were segmented by the application of erosion to concave junctions between PVs and LAA with the LA (Figure 2(A1)). The PVs and LAA are smaller and consist of more 1-connected voxels than the LA body and thus erode more rapidly. However, it is non-trivial to iteratively erode just the PVs and LAA to leave the residual convex LA. To do so, an *Erosion Index* was proposed to monitor the progression of erosion:

$$Erosion\ Index = \frac{V(Convex(E_i)) - V(E_i)}{V(E_i)},$$

where E_i is the 3D model after the ith erosion, $Convex(\cdot)$ is the convex hull, and $V(\cdot)$ returns the volume of a 3D shape. The erosion index approaches 0 as the shape becomes convex. The index data are preprocessed with a Savitzky–Golay filter and fitted with a polynomial function. The global minimum of the fitting function is calculated to determine the number of iterations for erosion (Figure 2B).

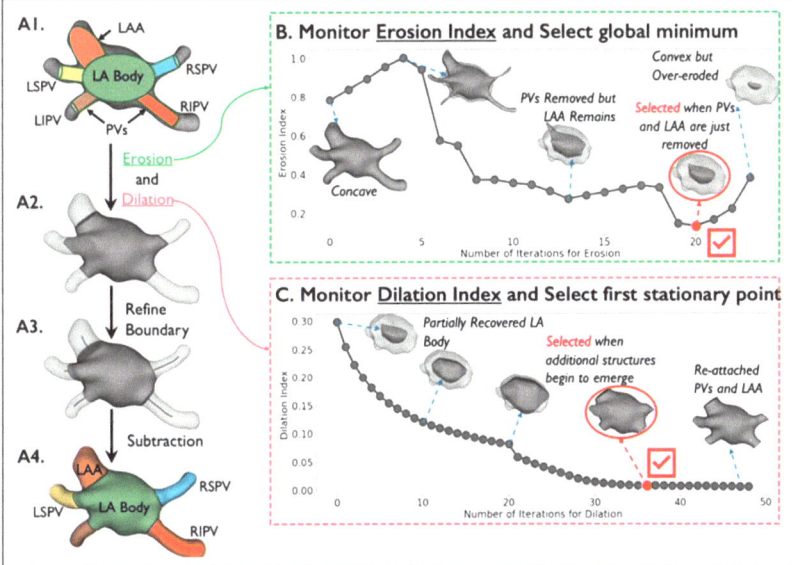

Figure 2. Segmentation of digital LA models by erosion–dilation: Detailed description of the first step of the DOKEN algorithm. (**A1**–**A4**) The pipeline of our DOKEN algorithm. (**B**,**C**) Iterative variations of the erosion and dilation indices along with variations in LA model corresponding to iterations. The ED parameters from this step are then learned by an SVM for labeling clinical data.

Because erosion may remove outer layers of the LA, a dilation operation was applied to recover its original dimension (Figure 2(A2)) by paving voxels on the contour and stopping just before the PVs and LAA are re-attached (Figure 2(A3)), which is monitored by the proposed *Dilation Index* by measuring the number of added voxels after each dilation:

$$Dilation\ Index = \frac{V(D_{i+1}) - V(D_i)}{V(D_i)},$$

where D_i is the 3D shell after the ith dilation and $V(\cdot)$ returns the volume of a 3D shape. Similarly, we processed the index data using a Savitzky–Golay filter then fitted them with a polynomial function. The first stationary point of the fitting function determines the number of dilation iterations (Figure 2C).

After the left atrium body is isolated after erosion and dilation, the boundaries between the LA body and the PVs and LAA were refined by calculating centerlines from the LA centroid to the centroid of each segmented structure. This approach has been used to extract and segment the aorta and great vessels [6,18,19]. Below is a step-by-step algorithm of boundary refinement and centerline calculation:

1. Extrapolate a Voronoi diagram [20] from the shell (Figure 2(A1)) to all internal points to create a maximal sphere centered at that point.
2. Calculate the centroid of the LA body and the centroid of each virtually dissected substructure (4 PVs and LAA).
3. For each substructure centroid, create a centerline automatically by minimizing the integral of the radius of maximal inscribed spheres along the path that connects the substructure centroid to the LA body centroid.
4. Replace the boundary between the left atrium and each substructure by a plane orthogonal to the corresponding centerline and close to the original boundary generated by the ED process (Figure 2(A4)).

II. Tuning the ED parameter using patient LA models

The parameters for the ED process, i.e., the optimal number of iterations, that are suitable for digital models may not apply to clinical data due to heterogeneities such as anatomy variability and imaging artifacts present in the clinical data. The parameters were made suitable for clinical data using a support vector machine (SVM) to predict the parameter value for input clinical CT. Two SVMs (one for each parameter) were trained with manually annotated seed samples ($N = 5$) to predict the optimal number of erosion and dilation iterations. The ED process with parameters predicted by SVMs forms the DOKEN algorithm and will be used to generate robust labels for training the DNN model.

2.3. Training the DNN for CT Segmentation from a Small Training Set

DOKEN was applied to $N = 20$ training data to label the different LA structures in each sample. This was used as ground truth for training the DNN.

We implemented nnU-Net (Figure 3)—a DNN model which has been widely used in 23 public datasets [21]. To train the nnU-Net model, first, each input CT scan was z-score normalized by subtracting its mean, followed by division by its standard deviation. Then the images were re-sampled using third-order spline interpolation. The target voxel spacing was set as the median spacing of the training samples. To improve the generalizability, a set of data augmentation techniques were randomly applied on the fly during training, including rotations, flipping, scaling, Gaussian noise and blur, and random changes in brightness, contrast, and gamma. During the training process, the batch size was set to 2 due to the GPU memory limitation, and the DL model was trained for 1000 epochs. Stochastic gradient descent [22] was used to optimize the model. The initial learning rate and Nesterov momentum were set to 0.01 and 0.99, respectively. The sum of cross-entropy and Dice loss were used as training loss. Figure 4 shows the convergence of training loss, validation loss, and validation accuracy (measured by Dice) during training.

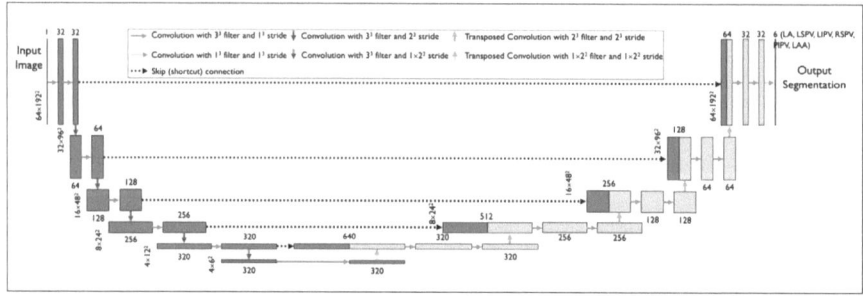

Figure 3. DNN model architecture: nn-Unet was applied to segment raw cardiac CT images. The model was trained using a DOKEN-labeled training set (small size) and was tested on a large hold-out test set.

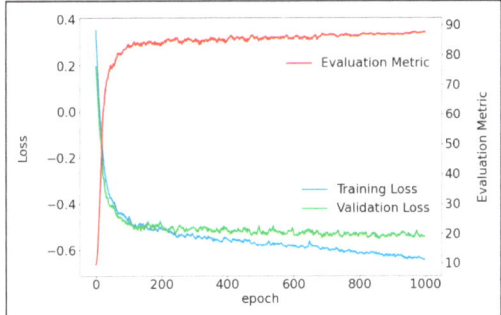

Figure 4. Convergence of training loss, validation loss, and the Dice validation accuracy.

2.4. Experimental Setting for Performance Evaluation

The DOKEN algorithm's ability was empirically evaluated to parse cardiac geometry and the DNN model's ability to segment cardiac structures from CT images. The large test set (N = 100) was used to manually annotate the ground-truth labels for the 6 substructures by a panel of clinical experts. The manual annotation was performed using a commercially available software tool (EnSite Verismo Segmentation Tool v.2.0.1; Abbott/St Jude Medical, Inc., St. Paul, MN, USA) to manually segment a shell containing the LA body with 4 PVs and the LAA. This whole shell was further parsed ("refined") into its 6 substructures using 3D Slicer [23], manually. The parsing performance of the DOKEN algorithm was measured by centroid–boundary distances against manual annotations. The CT segmentation performance of the DNN model was measured by Dice scores, average surface distance, and centroid–boundary distances, also against manual annotations.

2.5. Performance Evaluation

A newly designed metric, the centroid–boundary distance, was used along with two standard metrics for segmentation tasks [6–8,24–27]—Dice similarity coefficient and average surface distance—to evaluate the model's accuracy in capturing the 2D LA-PV/LAA boundaries, the global 3D structures, and the local 3D shapes and contours, respectively. Mathematically, the centroid–boundary distance is calculated as the average of all the distances from the centroid of the heart to points on the LA-PV/LAA boundary. The Dice similarity score measures spatial overlap between the model prediction and the ground truth, while 0 indicates no overlap and 1 indicates complete overlap, which can be mathematically expressed as

$$Dice\ Similarity\ Score = \frac{2 \times True\ Positive}{2 \times True\ Positive + False\ Positive + False\ Negative}.$$

The average surface distance is calculated as the average of all the distances from points on the boundary from model prediction to the ground-truth boundary. The success rate of the *DOKEN* algorithm was also calculated, where success was defined as an intersect over union (IoU) between the algorithm prediction and expert manual annotation larger than 0.5. This metric has been widely used for detection tasks [28].

2.6. Statistical Analysis

Continuous data are expressed by mean ± SD and categorical data by percentages. The distance and Dice scores were summarized as medians and interquartile range (IQR). Pearson correlation's test was used to assess the similarity of LA volumes and the LA sphericity index estimated from model prediction and ground truth. The Student's t-test, Chi-square test, or McNemar's test was applied as appropriate. $p < 0.05$ was considered significant.

3. Results

3.1. DOKEN Algorithm Can Robustly Parse Cardiac Geometry

In digital hearts, the novel DOKEN approach separated the PVs and LAA from the left atrial bodies (Figure 5A) with a mean difference for the centroid–boundary distances of -0.27 mm (95% CI: -3.87 to 3.33; r = 0.99; $p < 0.0001$; Figure 5B). Randomly, five shells of seed data was selected from the $N = 5$ digital atria for tuning, with LA sizes from 71 to 140 mL that cover a broad range of patients [29].

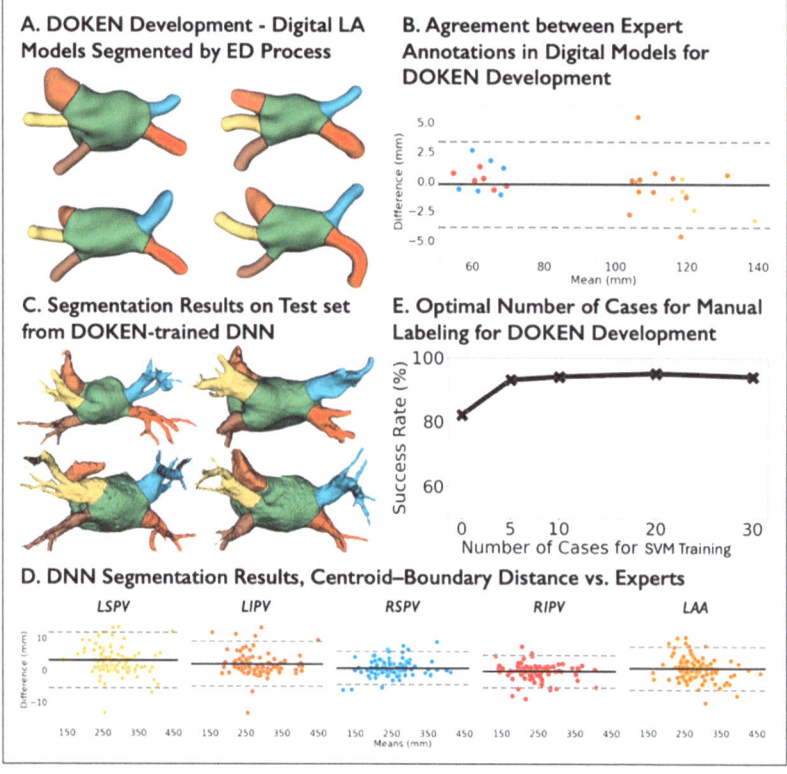

Figure 5. Evaluation of the DOKEN algorithm and the DNN performance for CT image segmentation. (**A**) Examples of digital LA models segmented by the DOKEN algorithm. (**B**) Bland–Altman plot of centroid–boundary distance of $N = 6$ digital LA models segmented by DOKEN compared to experts. (**C**) Examples of patient LA models segmented by the DOKEN algorithm. (**D**) Bland–Altman plot of centroid–boundary distance of $N = 100$ patient LA models in the test set segmented by DOKEN compared to experts. (**E**) Success rate of DOKEN algorithm with different seed cases for SVM training. Refer to panel D for color codes for the plot in panel B.

In the test set ($N = 100$), the performance of the tuned DOKEN algorithm was compared to expert annotations. Figure 5C presents example results on the test set. The DOKEN method produced a mean difference and limits of agreement for the centroid–boundary distance of 1.46 mm (95% CI: −5.58 to 8.49; r = 0.99; $p < 0.0001$; Figure 5D). The success rate of the algorithm's parsing when adding more seed data for tuning was assessed. As shown in Figure 5E, the success rate increased from 67% (no tuning) to 94% by tuning with $N = 5$ shells of seed data ($p = 0.034$; McNemar's test) and then showed only modest changes (consistency) when tuning in 10–30 shells (92–94%), justifying the selection of seed number.

3.2. DNN Trained by DOKEN-Labeled Samples Can Accurately Segment CT

Figure 6 shows comparisons between DNN prediction (left) and manually labeled (right) atria from select samples representing the 25th, 50th, and 75th percentile accuracy in the hold-out set ($N = 100$). The Dice score was 96.7% (IQR: 95.3% to 97.7%, Figure 7A), with a median error in surface distance of boundaries of 1.51 mm (IQR: 0.72 to 3.12, Figure 7B) and a mean centroid–boundary distance of 1.16 mm (95% CI: −4.57 to 6.89, Figure 7C), again similar to expert results (r = 0.99; $p < 0.001$, Figure 7D).

Thus, this approach enabled a >10-fold reduction in the relative ratio of training to test cases, inverting the ratio of training:test cases to less than 1:5 from a typical ratio of >3:1.

3.3. Analysis of Anatomical Variants

As previously noted, real CT data have more heterogeneity than digital models, such as variation in patient anatomies. Some anatomies could, in fact, be outliers, i.e., their shape does not follow the typical configuration identified in clinical studies. As no pre-screening was performed to eliminate such anatomy variants, it was analyzed if and how variation in anatomies would affect the method's performance.

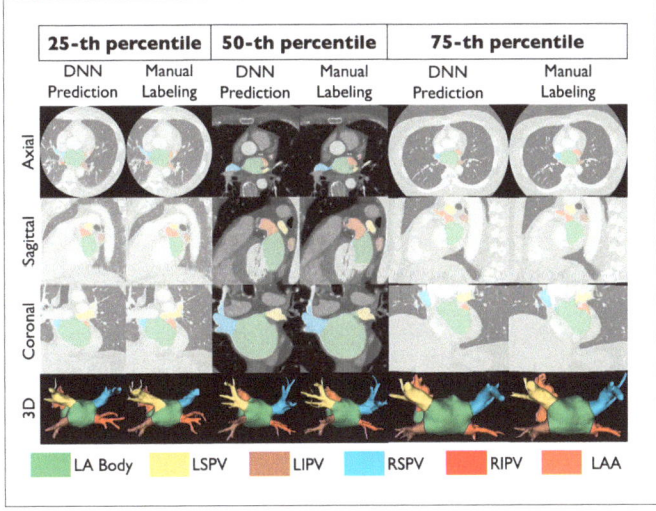

Figure 6. Example results showing DNN segmentation and manual annotation by experts.

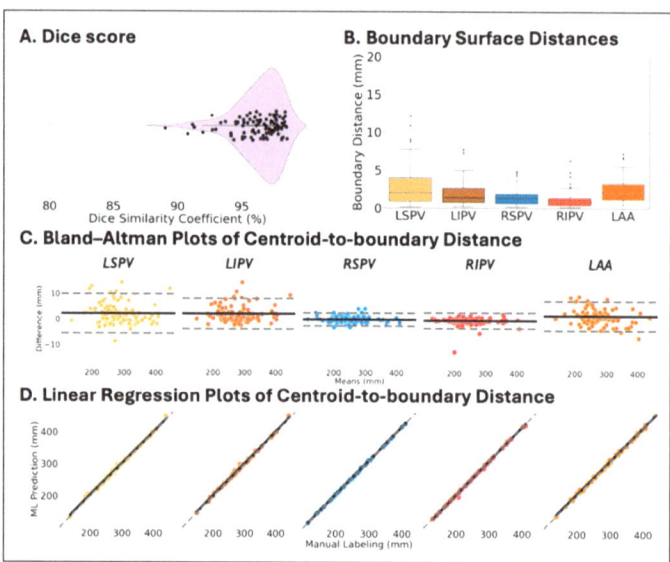

Figure 7. Accuracy of CT image segmentation between DNN prediction and expert labeling in the test set ($N = 100$). (**A**) Violin plot of mean Dice score. (**B**) Box plot of the surface distance of boundaries of 4 PVs and LAA. (**C**,**D**) Bland–Altman and linear regression plots of centroid–boundary distance of 4 PVs and LAA.

Overall, 100% cases with four PV ostia (the most common anatomic configuration, representing 66 cases) were parsed with boundary distances of 1.26 mm (95% CI: −5.15 to 7.68; r = 0.99; $p < 0.0001$). Three main outlier variants were identified (Figure 8): (1) common left PV ostia ($N = 12$), which was successfully parsed despite a lack of specific training on such cases; (2) LAA occlusion by a closure device ($N = 3$), where residual LAA stumps proximal to the occlusion device were correctly identified despite a lack of specific training in such cases; and (3) supplemental PVs or ostial-branch PV, where the DOKEN algorithm was able to segment 19/25 cases.

In summary, 28/34 of identified variants were successfully parsed with anatomic agreement within 1.95 mm (95% CI: −6.34 to 10.25), which again was in line with expert annotations (r = 0.99; $p < 0.0001$), despite lack of specific training for variants. In the remaining six cases, errors arose mostly from missing PVs or branches relative to the four-PV digital model, which could be addressed by geometric models that adapt to a range of PVs.

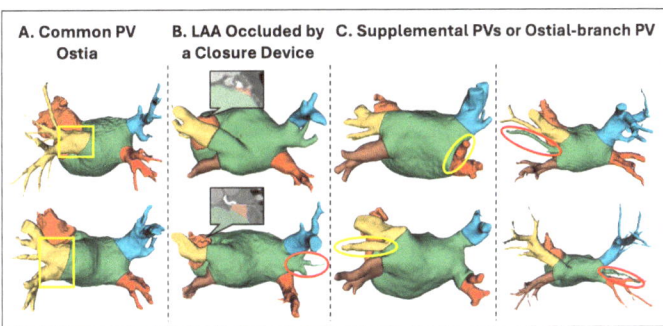

Figure 8. Robust segmentation performance of anatomical variants by the DOKEN algorithm. Three main variants were identified: (**A**) common left PV ostia ($N = 12$), (**B**) LAA occlusion by a closure device ($N = 3$), and (**C**) supplemental PVs or ostial-branch PV ($N = 25$). DOKEN successfully parsed 28/34 of the identified variants (boxed/circled in yellow). However, it missed some extra PVs or branches in the remaining cases (circled in red).

4. Discussion

Domain knowledge encoding of atrial geometry was able to accelerate a DNN for the segmentation of CT images and enable its training on very small datasets. In this study, the training-to-testing ratio was <1 training to 5 test, which indicates a far lower need for training than the conventional published ratios of >3:1 for ML [8,24,26]. This approach was then tested in a hold-out test set, in which the model accelerated segmentation while maintaining similar accuracy to experts. This novel approach could broaden the ease of access and accuracy of AF ablation. More broadly, this approach has analogies to natural intelligence, which has the potential to reduce the need for large, annotated datasets to train ML and could be applied for diverse applications in imaging as well as 3D printing. A simple post-processing step involving a 3D smoothing operation such as a Taubin filter [30] could extend the proposed work for 3D printing applications (illustrated in Supplemental Figure S1).

4.1. DNN Segmentation of Cardiac CT Images

Cardiac CT is increasing used [24,26,31] to guide ablation for AF and to predict clinical endpoints such as the risk of AF recurrence [32,33]. However, the segmentation of these large 70–200 MB datasets manually by experts takes tens of minutes [6–8,24] and 4.4–10 min even with latest commercial software such as the CARTO Segmentation Module version 6 (Biosense Webster, Irvine, CA, USA) [34,35]. The present approach greatly accelerates these reports while retaining high accuracy for routine and variant anatomy while achieving competitive accuracy (93.5–96.7%) with previous work (e.g., 91–97% [25] and 93.4% [24]). This study involved a dataset of $N = 120$ patients at a single center. The future extension of this work should expand the study cohort with data from multiple institutions, and the labeling should be further refined using a fusion of annotations from multiple experts and addressing discrepancies by an adjudication committee. One such example is demonstrated in our previous work [36], where we used an independent external dataset to test the performance of the algorithm.

The approach also circumvents the limitation that most CT studies that segmented the LA often did not specifically segment the PVs and LAA [24,26]. Similarly, software tools such as SimVascular (v.2023, https://github.com/SimVascular, accessed on 14 May 2024) provide automatic segmentation, which uses an ML model (CNN) that was trained using a public dataset MM-WHS [7], which only focuses on labels for the chambers but not specifically for the complex substructures such as narrow veins (PVs) and the anisotropic-shaped LAA, which are critical for AF ablation. The DOKEN algorithm, on the other hand, offers a scalable solution to segment complex structures in large medical databases. Further, the DOKEN algorithm's goal is focused on segmenting intricate cardiac structures and is not intended to be an alternative for advanced tools like SimVascular, which can perform high-fidelity simulations.

Another limitation is the size of publicly available labeled datasets, which are often small, typically provide test cohorts of <40 cases [6–8], and may create overfitted ML models that generalize poorly [37]. The DOKEN algorithm enabled training from smaller datasets, inverting the typical ratio of training:test cases and reducing the relative size of training to test cases by 10-fold. This "inversed training–test ratio" paradigm has recently been applied in domains outside medicine such as for Amazon co-purchasing product predictions [38]. Other cardiac imaging applications include the segmentation of magnetic resonance imaging (MRI) data to boost ML by reducing the need for large training data sets.

4.2. Challenges in Machine Learning

LeCun et al. and others have stated that difficulties in obtaining large training datasets are among the greatest challenges to machine learning [39]. Obtaining such data is particularly challenging in medicine [40], healthcare [41], and biosciences [42] due to privacy and regulatory requirements. The mathematical encoding of domain knowledge, which emulates some features of natural intelligence, may be a useful approach to address such limitations.

Domain knowledge can be applied in diverse ways. Databases and anatomic atlases have long been used for image segmentation [43,44] but do not encode knowledge principles in a fashion that could be generalized by learning algorithms. Indeed, Trutti et al. [44] pointed out that atlases may identify only a fraction of important structures (7% of 455 subcortical nuclei in the brain), and it is not clear how such "flat" data could be used to identify variants, as we demonstrated. Encoding anatomical knowledge also de-emphasizes low-level details while maintaining high-level abstract information, which may be central to human cognition [12]. The extent of detail required for mathematically encoding is unclear and should be defined for separate applications. Domain knowledge encoding need not be restricted to anatomy and could be applied to processes such as cellular metabolism and physician diagnostic patterns or reports [15].

Alternative approaches are being studied to circumvent large training datasets. Synthetic data may be generated in large quantities to mitigate a lack of actual training data [45], but while they may appear very realistic, they may lack diversity or even introduce bias due to the overfitting [46]. Data augmentation is a widely used approach to training ML on altered versions of the input data to increase the size of the training set [47] but does not capture variations in larger real data [48].

5. Conclusions

The novel domain knowledge-encoding algorithm was able to perform the segmentation of six substructures of the LA, reducing the need for large training data sets. The training set had as few as 20 samples, and the hold-out test set included hundreds of patients. The combination of domain knowledge encoding and machine learning approaches could reduce the dependence of ML on large training datasets and could potentially be applied to AF ablation procedures and extended in the future to other imaging, 3D printing, and data science applications.

Supplementary Materials: The following supporting information can be downloaded at: https://www.mdpi.com/article/10.3390/diagnostics14141538/s1, Figure S1: Demonstration of a potential application of our DOKEN algorithm in 3D printing.

Author Contributions: Conceptualization, P.G., R.F., B.D., F.V.Y.T., J.Z., M.Z. and S.M.N.; Methodology, R.F., J.Z., M.Z. and S.M.N.; Software, R.F.; Validation, P.C. and T.B.; Formal analysis, R.F. and P.C.; Investigation, B.D., F.V.Y.T., A.J.R., S.R.-C., S.S., P.C., M.R., J.Z., F.H., M.Z. and S.M.N.; Data curation, P.G., B.D., F.V.Y.T. and S.M.N.; Writing—original draft, P.G. and R.F.; Writing—review & editing, P.G., R.F., B.D., F.V.Y.T., A.J.R., S.S., T.B., M.R., J.Z., F.H. and S.M.N.; Supervision, J.Z., M.Z. and S.M.N.; Project administration, S.M.N.; Funding acquisition, S.M.N. All authors have read and agreed to the published version of the manuscript.

Funding: This research was funded by grants from the National Institutes of Health under award numbers R01 HL149134 and R01 HL83359.

Institutional Review Board Statement: The study was conducted in accordance with the Declaration of Helsinki, and approved by the review board of Stanford University Human Subjects Protection Committee (NCT02997254, 2016).

Informed Consent Statement: Written informed consent was obtained from all participants involved in the study.

Data Availability Statement: The code and networks with trained weights will be released upon acceptance. The 3D digital heart models are publicly available at https://zenodo.org/record/4309958#.YdlOJRPMJqs, accessed on 14 May 2024. The CT dataset used in the study is not currently permitted for public release due to the sensitive nature of patient data.

Acknowledgments: Narayan reports grant support from the National Institutes of Health (R01 HL149 134 and R01 HL83359) and from the Laurie C. McGrath Foundation, consulting from Uptodate Inc., and TDK Inc., intellectual property owned by University of California Regents and Stanford University. Tjong: Consulting honoraria to institution from Abbott, Boston Scientific, Daiichi Sankyo; no personal gain. Rogers: grants from NIH (F32HL144101), NIH LRP, and Stanford SSPS. Clopton: consulting at the American College of Cardiology. Rodrigo: equity interests in Corify Health Care. Ganesan reports intellectual property owned by Florida Atlantic University and NIH. All other authors have reported that they have no relationships relevant to the contents of this paper to disclose.

Conflicts of Interest: SN reports grant support from the National Institutes of Health (R01 HL149134 and R01 HL83359), consulting from Uptodate Inc., and TDK Inc., intellectual property owned by University of California Regents and Stanford University. FT: Consulting honoraria to institution from Abbott, Boston Scientific, Daiichi Sankyo; no personal gain. AR: grants from NIH (F32HL144101), NIH LRP, and Stanford SSPS. PC: consulting at American College of Cardiology. MR: equity interests in Corify Health Care. The remaining authors declare that the research was conducted in the absence of any commercial or financial relationships that could be construed as a potential conflict of interest.

References

1. Boykov, Y.; Funka-Lea, G. Graph cuts and efficient ND image segmentation. *Int. J. Comput. Vis.* **2006**, *70*, 109–131. [CrossRef]
2. Preetha, M.M.S.J.; Suresh, L.P.; Bosco, M.J. Image segmentation using seeded region growing. In Proceedings of the 2012 International Conference on Computing, Electronics and Electrical Technologies (ICCEET), Nagercoil, India, 21–22 March 2012; IEEE: Piscataway, NJ, USA, 2012; pp. 576–583.
3. Rodriguez, M.D.; Shah, M. Detecting and segmenting humans in crowded scenes. In Proceedings of the 15th ACM international conference on Multimedia, Augsburg, Germany, 24–29 September 2007; pp. 353–356.
4. Rajaraman, S.; Siegelman, J.; Alderson, P.O.; Folio, L.S.; Folio, L.R.; Antani, S.K. Iteratively pruned deep learning ensembles for COVID-19 detection in chest X-rays. *IEEE Access* **2020**, *8*, 115041–115050. [CrossRef] [PubMed]
5. Ganesan, P.; Rajaraman, S.; Long, R.; Ghoraani, B.; Antani, S. Assessment of data augmentation strategies toward performance improvement of abnormality classification in chest radiographs. In Proceedings of the 2019 41st Annual International Conference of the IEEE Engineering in Medicine and Biology Society (EMBC), Berlin, Germany, 23–27 July 2019; IEEE: Piscataway, NJ, USA; pp. 841–844.
6. Tobon-Gomez, C.; Geers, A.J.; Peters, J.; Weese, J.; Pinto, K.; Karim, R.; Ammar, M.; Daoudi, A.; Margeta, J.; Sandoval, Z.; et al. Benchmark for algorithms segmenting the left atrium from 3D CT and MRI datasets. *IEEE Trans. Med. Imaging* **2015**, *34*, 1460–1473. [CrossRef] [PubMed]
7. Zhuang, X.; Li, L.; Payer, C.; Štern, D.; Urschler, M.; Heinrich, M.P.; Oster, J.; Wang, C.; Smedby, Ö.; Bian, C.; et al. Evaluation of algorithms for multi-modality whole heart segmentation: An open-access grand challenge. *Med. Image Anal.* **2019**, *58*, 101537. [CrossRef] [PubMed]

8. Xu, X.; Wang, T.; Zhuang, J.; Yuan, H.; Huang, M.; Cen, J.; Jia, Q.; Dong, Y.; Shi, Y. Imagechd: A 3d computed tomography image dataset for classification of congenital heart disease. In Proceedings of the International Conference on Medical Image Computing and Computer-Assisted Intervention, Lima, Peru, 4–8 October 2020; Springer: Berlin/Heidelberg, Germany; pp. 77–87.
9. Gianfrancesco, M.A.; Tamang, S.; Yazdany, J.; Schmajuk, G. Potential biases in machine learning algorithms using electronic health record data. *JAMA Intern. Med.* **2018**, *178*, 1544–1547. [CrossRef] [PubMed]
10. Futoma, J.; Simons, M.; Panch, T.; Doshi-Velez, F.; Celi, L.A. The myth of generalisability in clinical research and machine learning in health care. *Lancet Digit. Health* **2020**, *2*, e489–e492. [CrossRef] [PubMed]
11. Markman, E.M. *Categorization and Naming in Children: Problems of Induction*; Mit Press: Cambridge, MA, USA, 1989.
12. Van Gerven, M. Computational foundations of natural intelligence. *Front. Comput. Neurosci.* **2017**, *11*, 112. [CrossRef]
13. Lake, B.M.; Salakhutdinov, R.; Tenenbaum, J.B. Human-level concept learning through probabilistic program induction. *Science* **2015**, *350*, 1332–1338. [CrossRef] [PubMed]
14. Liu, L.; Wolterink, J.M.; Brune, C.; Veldhuis, R.N. Anatomy-aided deep learning for medical image segmentation: A review. *Phys. Med. Biol.* **2021**, *66*, 11TR01. [CrossRef]
15. Xie, X.; Niu, J.; Liu, X.; Chen, Z.; Tang, S.; Yu, S. A survey on incorporating domain knowledge into deep learning for medical image analysis. *Med. Image Anal.* **2021**, *69*, 101985. [CrossRef]
16. Nagel, C.; Schuler, S.; Dössel, O.; Loewe, A. A bi-atrial statistical shape model for large-scale in silico studies of human atria: Model development and application to ECG simulations. *Med. Image Anal.* **2021**, *74*, 102210. [CrossRef] [PubMed]
17. Soille, P. *Erosion and Dilation, Morphological Image Analysis*; Springer: Berlin, Germany, 2004.
18. Krissian, K.; Carreira, J.M.; Esclarin, J.; Maynar, M. Semi-automatic segmentation and detection of aorta dissection wall in MDCT angiography. *Med. Image Anal.* **2014**, *18*, 83–102. [CrossRef] [PubMed]
19. Razeghi, O.; Sim, I.; Roney, C.H.; Karim, R.; Chubb, H.; Whitaker, J.; O'Neill, L.; Mukherjee, R.; Wright, M.; O'neill, M.; et al. Fully automatic atrial fibrosis assessment using a multilabel convolutional neural network. *Circ. Cardiovasc. Imaging* **2020**, *13*, e011512. [CrossRef] [PubMed]
20. Piccinelli, M.; Veneziani, A.; Steinman, D.A.; Remuzzi, A.; Antiga, L. A framework for geometric analysis of vascular structures: Application to cerebral aneurysms. *IEEE Trans. Med. Imaging* **2009**, *28*, 1141–1155. [CrossRef] [PubMed]
21. Isensee, F.; Jaeger, P.F.; Kohl, S.A.; Petersen, J.; Maier-Hein, K.H. nnU-Net: A self-configuring method for deep learning-based biomedical image segmentation. *Nat. Methods* **2021**, *18*, 203–211. [CrossRef] [PubMed]
22. Ketkar, N. Stochastic gradient descent. In *Deep Learning with Python*; Springer: Berlin/Heidelberg, Germany, 2017; pp. 113–132.
23. Fedorov, A.; Beichel, R.; Kalpathy-Cramer, J.; Finet, J.; Fillion-Robin, J.C.; Pujol, S.; Bauer, C.; Jennings, D.; Fennessy, F.; Sonka, M.; et al. 3D Slicer as an image computing platform for the Quantitative Imaging Network. *Magn. Reson. Imaging* **2012**, *30*, 1323–1341. [CrossRef] [PubMed]
24. Baskaran, L.; Maliakal, G.; Al'Aref, S.J.; Singh, G.; Xu, Z.; Michalak, K.; Dolan, K.; Gianni, U.; van Rosendael, A.; van den Hoogen, I.; et al. Identification and quantification of cardiovascular structures from CCTA: An end-to-end, rapid, pixel-wise, deep-learning method. *Cardiovasc. Imaging* **2020**, *13*, 1163–1171.
25. Xu, H.; Niederer, S.A.; Williams, S.E.; Newby, D.E.; Williams, M.C.; Young, A.A. Whole Heart Anatomical Refinement from CCTA Using Extrapolation and Parcellation. In Proceedings of the International Conference on Functional Imaging and Modeling of the Heart, Stanford, CA, USA, 21–25 June 2021; Springer: Berlin/Heidelberg, Germany, 2021; pp. 63–70.
26. Chen, H.H.; Liu, C.M.; Chang, S.L.; Chang, P.Y.C.; Chen, W.S.; Pan, Y.M.; Fang, S.T.; Zhan, S.Q.; Chuang, C.M.; Lin, Y.J.; et al. Automated extraction of left atrial volumes from two-dimensional computer tomography images using a deep learning technique. *Int. J. Cardiol.* **2020**, *316*, 272–278. [CrossRef] [PubMed]
27. Xie, W.; Yao, Z.; Ji, E.; Qiu, H.; Chen, Z.; Guo, H.; Zhuang, J.; Jia, Q.; Huang, M. Artificial intelligence–based computed tomography processing framework for surgical telementoring of congenital heart disease. *ACM J. Emerg. Technol. Comput. Syst. (JETC)* **2021**, *17*, 1–24. [CrossRef]
28. Lin, T.Y.; Maire, M.; Belongie, S.; Hays, J.; Perona, P.; Ramanan, D.; Dollár, P.; Zitnick, C.L. Microsoft coco: Common objects in context. In Proceedings of the European Conference on Computer Vision, Zurich, Switzerland, 6–12 September 2014; Springer: Berlin/Heidelberg, Germany, 2014; pp. 740–755.
29. Sangsriwong, M.; Cismaru, G.; Puiu, M.; Simu, G.; Istratoaie, S.; Muresan, L.; Gusetu, G.; Cismaru, A.; Pop, D.; Zdrenghea, D.; et al. Formula to estimate left atrial volume using antero-posterior diameter in patients with catheter ablation of atrial fibrillation. *Medicine* **2021**, *100*, e26513. [CrossRef]
30. Taubin, G. Curve and surface smoothing without shrinkage. In Proceedings of the IEEE International Conference on Computer Vision, Cambridge, MA, USA, 20–23 June 1995; IEEE: Piscataway, NJ, USA, 1995; pp. 852–857.
31. Chen, C.; Qin, C.; Qiu, H.; Tarroni, G.; Duan, J.; Bai, W.; Rueckert, D. Deep learning for cardiac image segmentation: A review. *Front. Cardiovasc. Med.* **2020**, *7*, 25. [CrossRef] [PubMed]
32. Nakamori, S.; Ngo, L.H.; Tugal, D.; Manning, W.J.; Nezafat, R. Incremental value of left atrial geometric remodeling in predicting late atrial fibrillation recurrence after pulmonary vein isolation: A cardiovascular magnetic resonance study. *J. Am. Heart Assoc.* **2018**, *7*, e009793. [CrossRef] [PubMed]

33. Firouznia, M.; Feeny, A.K.; LaBarbera, M.A.; McHale, M.; Cantlay, C.; Kalfas, N.; Schoenhagen, P.; Saliba, W.; Tchou, P.; Barnard, J.; et al. Machine learning–derived fractal features of shape and texture of the left atrium and pulmonary veins from cardiac computed tomography scans are associated with risk of recurrence of atrial fibrillation postablation. *Circ. Arrhythmia Electrophysiol.* **2021**, *14*, e009265. [CrossRef] [PubMed]
34. Tovia-Brodie, O.; Belhassen, B.; Glick, A.; Shmilovich, H.; Aviram, G.; Rosso, R.; Michowitz, Y. Use of new imaging CARTO® segmentation module software to facilitate ablation of ventricular arrhythmias. *J. Cardiovasc. Electrophysiol.* **2017**, *28*, 240–248. [CrossRef]
35. Tops, L.F.; Bax, J.J.; Zeppenfeld, K.; Jongbloed, M.R.; Lamb, H.J.; van der Wall, E.E.; Schalij, M.J. Fusion of multislice computed tomography imaging with three-dimensional electroanatomic mapping to guide radiofrequency catheter ablation procedures. *Heart Rhythm.* **2005**, *2*, 1076–1081. [CrossRef]
36. Feng, R.; Deb, B.; Ganesan, P.; Tjong, F.V.; Rogers, A.J.; Ruipérez-Campillo, S.; Somani, S.; Clopton, P.; Baykaner, T.; Rodrigo, M.; et al. Segmenting computed tomograms for cardiac ablation using machine learning leveraged by domain knowledge encoding. *Front. Cardiovasc. Med.* **2023**, *10*, 1189293. [CrossRef]
37. Ng, A.Y. Preventing "overfitting" of cross-validation data. In Proceedings of the Fourteenth International Conference on Machine Learning (ICML), Nashville, TN, USA, 8–12 July 1997; Volume 97, pp. 245–253.
38. Hu, W.; Fey, M.; Zitnik, M.; Dong, Y.; Ren, H.; Liu, B.; Catasta, M.; Leskovec, J. Open graph benchmark: Datasets for machine learning on graphs. *Adv. Neural Inf. Process. Syst.* **2020**, *33*, 22118–22133.
39. LeCun, Y.; Bengio, Y.; Hinton, G. Deep learning. *Nature* **2015**, *521*, 436–444. [CrossRef]
40. Topol, E.J. High-performance medicine: The convergence of human and artificial intelligence. *Nat. Med.* **2019**, *25*, 44–56. [CrossRef]
41. Esteva, A.; Robicquet, A.; Ramsundar, B.; Kuleshov, V.; DePristo, M.; Chou, K.; Cui, C.; Corrado, G.; Thrun, S.; Dean, J. A guide to deep learning in healthcare. *Nat. Med.* **2019**, *25*, 24–29. [CrossRef]
42. Sapoval, N.; Aghazadeh, A.; Nute, M.G.; Antunes, D.A.; Balaji, A.; Baraniuk, R.; Barberan, C.J.; Dannenfelser, R.; Dun, C.; Edrisi, M.; et al. Current progress and open challenges for applying deep learning across the biosciences. *Nat. Commun.* **2022**, *13*, 1728. [CrossRef] [PubMed]
43. Vakalopoulou, M.; Chassagnon, G.; Bus, N.; Marini, R.; Zacharaki, E.I.; Revel, M.P.; Paragios, N. Atlasnet: Multi-atlas non-linear deep networks for medical image segmentation. In Proceedings of the International Conference on Medical Image Computing and Computer-Assisted Intervention, Granada, Spain, 16–20 September 2018; Springer: Berlin/Heidelberg, Germany, 2018; pp. 658–666.
44. Trutti, A.C.; Fontanesi, L.; Mulder, M.J.; Bazin, P.-L.; Hommel, B.; Forstmann, B.U. A probabilistic atlas of the human ventral tegmental area (VTA) based on 7 Tesla MRI data. *Brain Struct. Funct.* **2021**, *226*, 1155–1167. [CrossRef] [PubMed]
45. Chen, R.J.; Lu, M.Y.; Chen, T.Y.; Williamson, D.F.; Mahmood, F. Synthetic data in machine learning for medicine and healthcare. *Nat. Biomed. Eng.* **2021**, *5*, 493–497. [CrossRef] [PubMed]
46. Bhanot, K.; Qi, M.; Erickson, J.S.; Guyon, I.; Bennett, K.P. The problem of fairness in synthetic healthcare data. *Entropy* **2021**, *23*, 1165. [CrossRef]
47. Shorten, C.; Khoshgoftaar, T.M. A survey on image data augmentation for deep learning. *J. Big Data* **2019**, *6*, 60. [CrossRef]
48. Shen, J.; Dudley, J.; Kristensson, P.O. The imaginative generative adversarial network: Automatic data augmentation for dynamic skeleton-based hand gesture and human action recognition. In Proceedings of the 2021 16th IEEE International Conference on Automatic Face and Gesture Recognition (FG 2021), Jodhpur, India, 15–18 December 2021; IEEE: Piscataway, NJ, USA, 2021; pp. 1–8.

Disclaimer/Publisher's Note: The statements, opinions and data contained in all publications are solely those of the individual author(s) and contributor(s) and not of MDPI and/or the editor(s). MDPI and/or the editor(s) disclaim responsibility for any injury to people or property resulting from any ideas, methods, instructions or products referred to in the content.

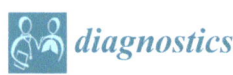

Article

AI-Driven Real-Time Classification of ECG Signals for Cardiac Monitoring Using i-AlexNet Architecture

Manjur Kolhar [1,*], Raisa Nazir Ahmed Kazi [2], Hitesh Mohapatra [3,*] and Ahmed M Al Rajeh [2]

1. Department Health Informatics, College of Applied Medical Sciences, King Faisal University, Al Hofuf 61421, Saudi Arabia
2. College of Applied Medical Sciences, King Faisal University, Al Hofuf 61421, Saudi Arabia; rnahmed@kfu.edu.sa (R.N.A.K.); amalrajeh@kfu.edu.sa (A.M.A.R.)
3. School of Computer Engineering, Kalinga Institute of Industrial Technology (Deemed to Be University), Bhubaneswar 751024, Odisha, India
* Correspondence: mkolhar@kfu.edu.sa (M.K.); hiteshmahapatra@gmail.com (H.M.)

Abstract: The healthcare industry has evolved with the advent of artificial intelligence (AI), which uses advanced computational methods and algorithms, leading to quicker inspection, forecasting, evaluation and treatment. In the context of healthcare, artificial intelligence (AI) uses sophisticated computational methods to evaluate, decipher and draw conclusions from patient data. AI has the potential to revolutionize the healthcare industry in several ways, including better managerial effectiveness, individualized treatment regimens and diagnostic improvements. In this research, the ECG signals are preprocessed for noise elimination and heartbeat segmentation. Multi-feature extraction is employed to extract features from preprocessed data, and an optimization technique is used to choose the most feasible features. The i-AlexNet classifier, which is an improved version of the AlexNet model, is used to classify between normal and anomalous signals. For experimental evaluation, the proposed approach is applied to PTB and MIT_BIH databases, and it is observed that the suggested method achieves a higher accuracy of 98.8% compared to other works in the literature.

Keywords: artificial intelligence; ECG signals; optimization; AlexNet; performance

Citation: Kolhar, M.; Kazi, R.N.A.; Mohapatra, H.; Al Rajeh, A.M. AI-Driven Real-Time Classification of ECG Signals for Cardiac Monitoring Using i-AlexNet Architecture. *Diagnostics* **2024**, *14*, 1344. https://doi.org/10.3390/diagnostics14131344

Academic Editor: Dechang Chen

Received: 28 April 2024
Revised: 6 June 2024
Accepted: 14 June 2024
Published: 25 June 2024

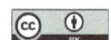

Copyright: © 2024 by the authors. Licensee MDPI, Basel, Switzerland. This article is an open access article distributed under the terms and conditions of the Creative Commons Attribution (CC BY) license (https://creativecommons.org/licenses/by/4.0/).

1. Introduction

Cardiovascular disorders are the primary cause of death worldwide, and ECG signals are routinely utilized to detect them [1]. Furthermore, the American Cardiovascular Society states that early diagnosis of these conditions is critical to the well-being of patients [2]. The major method for keeping an eye on heart activity is a diagnostic electrocardiogram (ECG). It is only effective for a certain period, and ongoing patient care is still necessary beyond therapeutic sessions. Traditionally, practitioners have employed portable ECG monitors to record heart activity for extended periods of time in order to conduct additional research. One electrically powered portable device used to capture and preserve long-term ECG readings was presented in [3]. But these gadgets are unable to provide feedback on the patient's medical condition in real time, and cardiac specialists have to spend a lot of time and resources analyzing data collected over time.

AI has emerged as a tool for developing computer-aided systems that can differentiate between healthy individuals and those with illnesses based on specific symptoms [4]. AI research and development combines principles with computer science to create systems that can learn from datasets and existing knowledge, continuously enhancing their capabilities [5]. This interdisciplinary field encompasses machine learning (ML) and Deep Learning (DL) [6]. Machine learning facilitates the creation of data-driven models adept at classification, regression and clustering tasks. Traditional ML techniques like regression, Random Forest, support vector machine and K nearest neighbors necessitate feature engineering, where experts in the field extract relevant features from raw data to build effective and interpretable models.

Deep Learning, a branch within ML, employs hidden layers to handle complex computations for challenging tasks. With training data, these neural networks can autonomously learn to process data through nonlinear operations that identify vital features essential for tasks like classification and regression [7,8]. The structure of networks also equips them to manage amounts of unstructured data, such as free text. Studies in the field of cardiology have indicated that the use of machine learning (ML) and Deep Learning (DL), especially when incorporating modalities, is more successful in forecasting cardiovascular or overall mortality rates than relying solely on individual, clinical or imaging modalities. For heart monitoring applications, delay is a crucial component since early identification of cardiovascular illnesses is vital to save lives. The work in [9,10] offers an instantaneous response by computing on the edge rather than in the cloud; however, battery life limitations, the most valuable resource for the edge of the network [11], restrict the duration of time the device can spend tracking cardiac rhythm. Many people suffer from their illnesses for decades without realizing it because of these issues [12]. In certain scenarios, deaths from cardiovascular disease would have been avoided if the condition had been identified more promptly [13]. Therefore, for those suffering from cardiovascular problems, persistent instantaneous-fashion ECG surveillance may be a lifesaver.

Artificial intelligence (AI) is essential to cardiac monitoring since it provides a number of benefits in terms of effectiveness, precision and prompt action [14]. Continuous streams of cardiac data, such as ECG readings, can be analyzed by AI algorithms to find minuscule irregularities that human observers might miss. Effective treatment and improved management of heart problems are made possible by early identification [15]. Healthcare workers may find it time-consuming to analyze large volumes of cardiac data; artificial intelligence streamlines this procedure. Healthcare professionals may concentrate on providing treatment, assessment and analysis to patients due to this automation, which also increases productivity. These AI-driven systems are capable of analyzing information about patients to generate personalized cardiac tracking models [16]. This improves results by allowing medical professionals to customize treatments and therapeutic strategies according to each patient's unique cardiac pattern. In artificial intelligence (AI), metaheuristic algorithms are frequently employed to tackle challenging optimization and exploration challenges. A crucial step in the creation of AI models is the adjustment of hyperparameters [17]. The hyperparameter space can be effectively searched using metaheuristic algorithms to identify the appropriate instances for AI-based models [18]. These algorithms can help in feature selection for datasets with numerous features. They aid in lowering dimensionality and improving effectiveness by assisting in the identification of the most pertinent group of features that affect a model's performance [19]. Optimization issues in the fields of image and signal processing are addressed by these methods. Among other applications, they can be applied to tasks like the extraction of features, signal denoising and image categorization.

1.1. Motivations of Current Research

The present research was conducted to address the following research questions related to ECG signal classification using AI:

R1: Is it possible to use AI models for the continuous analysis of ECG data to find small changes over time that would allow for proactive management and early diagnosis of cardiac abnormalities?

R2: In real-time scenarios, how might metaheuristic algorithms be optimized for the effective and precise classification of normal and anomalous ECG signals?

R3: Which feature representations work best for extracting pertinent information from ECG signals so that artificial intelligence (AI) algorithms can distinguish between normal and abnormal patterns?

1.2. Contributions of Current Research

The main contributions of this paper are as follows:
1. To develop an AI-driven solution for monitoring cardiac activities using ECG signals to classify them as normal or anomalous.
2. To employ red fox optimization, a bio-inspired metaheuristic technique, to choose the best characteristics of ECG signals in order to improve the classification accuracy of the model.
3. To implement i-AlexNet architecture for categorizing ECG signals and to demonstrate its distinct performance by comparing it with other works in the literature that focus on real-time cardiac monitoring.

1.3. Paper Organization

The remainder of this paper is organized as follows. Section 2 presents the related research conducted in recent times on the categorization of ECG signals for cardiac surveillance. Section 3 elaborates the proposed methodology for ECG signal classification using the i-AlexNet technique. Section 4 discusses the results obtained when applying the proposed technique to PTB as well as MIT_BIH databases. Section 5 concludes the present research.

2. Related Works

This section elaborates the application of artificial intelligence algorithms in cardiac monitoring using various devices as mentioned in Table 1. The authors in [20] used a structural framework and an approach based on machine learning to anticipate coronary artery disease. This work combines traditional machine learning methods with a collaborative categorization technique in order to foresee the experimental findings. This model, also known as a meta-classifier, predicts the results based on the largest number of choices [21]. Its inadequate precision and substantial complexity of computation are, nevertheless, issues. The specific kind of health condition was determined using biosensors in [22] that collect patient data via Internet protocol connections. The authors of paper [23] present the IoTDL HDD model, which combines IoT and Deep Learning technologies to diagnose diseases (CVDs) based on analyzing ECG signals [23]. On a server located in the cloud, data from the patients' connected humidity and heart rate monitors were analyzed using support vector machine learning techniques to identify unusual situations.

Internal analysis is only utilized to execute simple inspections on unprocessed information and mobilizing tasks for encapsulating the information gathered with conventional methods of communication in certain studies suggested in the research pertaining to ECG signal surveillance. However, a large body of research has been produced in the scientific community that uses artificial intelligence, even at the edge, for heart disease detection. Comparing this intelligence method to other conventional approaches based on artificial intelligence, the usage of Convolutional Neural Networks (CNNs) demonstrates potential in terms of reliability in detecting arrhythmias in ECG signals. In [24], hidden lexical examination approaches were employed to increase the network's predictive efficacy when compared to alternative approaches for interpreting the ECG waveform. The objective is to shift deduction to the edge of a lightweight gadget in order to minimize delay periods and power expenditure associated with mobile communications, as both training and deductive reasoning happen on the cloud end. The researchers of [25] introduced an ECG device called iKardo, which has the ability to automatically categorize ECG data as critical or non-critical. This addresses the issue of imbalanced datasets. IKardo is part of a healthcare system based on technology focusing on improving data accuracy by balancing the dataset using appropriate methods. This ensures the identification of ECG signals, achieving an impressive accuracy rate of 99.58%. Consequently, iKardo helps in accurate disease detection, making it a valuable tool for monitoring healthcare. The research team developed [26] a prototype machine that can provide real-time monitoring of devices. This innovation will help doctors access information to detect heart conditions from ECG images. The device showcased is suitable for patients with a resting heart rate ranging from 60 to 100 beats per minute. It serves as a protocol and conceptual tool for tracking heartbeats.

Table 1. Comparison of related works in the literature.

References	Techniques	Dataset Used	Performance
[11]	Deep Neural Networks	MIT-BIH database	Accuracy = 82.3% Precision = 81.6% Recall = 81.9%
[13]	Support Vector Machine	MIT-BIH normal sinus rhythm database	Accuracy = 84.9% Precision = 83.4% Recall = 84.5%
[14]	Logistic Regression	PTB database	Accuracy = 83.7% Precision = 82.8% Recall = 83.4%
[15]	Random Forests	MIT-BIH atrial fibrillation database	Accuracy = 86.6% Precision = 85.7% Recall = 86.1%
[17]	Sparse Autoencoders	European ST-T database	Accuracy = 92.3% Precision = 91.4% Recall = 91.8%
[18]	Bidirectional Long Short-Term Memory Networks	MIT-BIH normal sinus rhythm database	Accuracy = 93.6% Precision = 93.1% Recall = 92.8%
[20]	One-dimensional Convolutional Neural Networks	MIT-BIH atrial fibrillation database	Accuracy = 94.7% Precision = 93.5% Recall = 94.3%
[21]	Generative Adversarial Networks	European ST-T database	Accuracy = 95.7% Precision = 94.2% Recall = 95.2%

The Asymmetric Estimation and Parametric Derivative Distortion Elimination approach was developed by the authors of [27] to remove distortions in the ECG signal with the intent of distinguishing between arrhythmias. By employing Asymmetric Estimation to reduce high-powered disturbances, which was employed to decrease acoustic variability, the aspects of operation were handled. Using Parametric Derivative Distortion Elimination, the electrical connection disturbance was split up into various modulation settings, and distortion was eliminated using proportional polynomial extrapolation.

In [28] a study implemented a CNN BiLSTM method to classify ECG signals, for detecting artery disease (CAD). This approach combined CNN) and Bidirectional Long Short Term Memory (BiLSTM) layers, for ECG data analysis. A novel metric named Spatial Uncertainty Estimator (SUE) was introduced to assess the accuracy of the models' predictions. Cuckoo Search Optimization (CSO) and Logistic Regression (LR) were applied to identify features. In CSO LR CSO was used to select traits that would enhance the classification process and optimize LR coefficients. The LR model used in this research was evaluated for a set of categories. It was necessary to create a multiclass modelling categorization in order to make a precise determination. The feature identification method established by investigators in [29] was through the use of ECG, and the feature subset was chosen using kernel-based complicated coarse groups. Subsequently, optimization techniques satisfying several objectives were used to generate the classification of arrhythmia based on electrocardiogram (MC-ECG) for different varieties of labels. In order to obtain improved categorization, this optimization method is dependent on low-density restriction, modelling connections among ECG characteristics and arrhythmia illnesses. For the purpose of collecting the appropriate characteristic subsets, the authors in [30] introduced the Multifaceted Polynomial Bilateral Grey Wolf Optimization with Random Forests. The final requirement of the proposed method was the swarming location, which was used to distinguish the most compelling answer from solutions that were not dominated. Choosing erroneous indicators of fitness has a significant influence on categorization.

3. Proposed Methodology

The collected ECG signals were initially preprocessed in order to remove the distortions. Three different types of transform techniques, such as Fractional Discrete Cosine Transform, Radon Wavelet Transform and Fractional Wavelet Transform, were applied to extract the features. The optimal features from the previous step were selected using optimization techniques before sending them to the i-AlexNet architecture for performing the final classification. The workflow of the proposed system is presented in Figure 1.

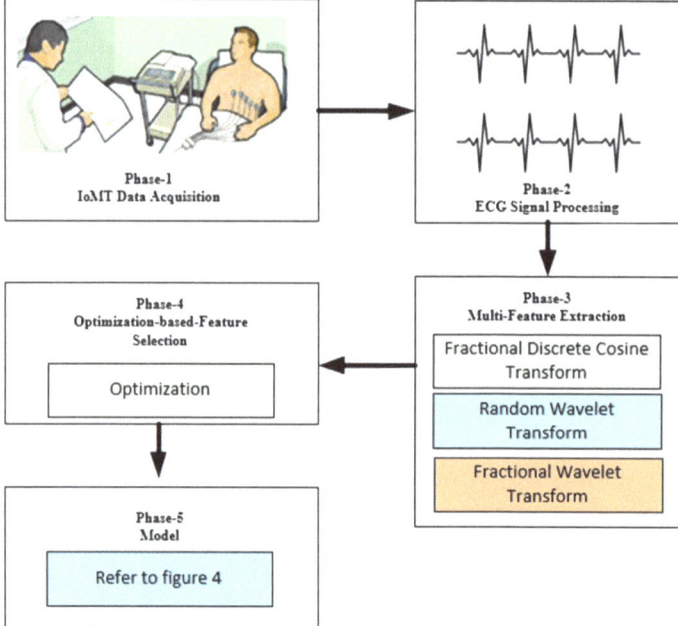

Figure 1. Proposed workflow.

3.1. ECG Signal Preprocessing

This is an essential phase to be performed while processing the ECG signals, as there is a high probability of the distortion of signals due to noises. The two important steps carried out in this work during ECG signal preprocessing were eliminating noise and segmenting beats. These signals are categorized into minimum and maximum rhythm entities as described in Equation (1):

$$c(k) = c_s(k) + \sum_{h-\infty}^{h_0} t_h(k) \tag{1}$$

In the above equation, $c_s(k)$ denotes the processed signal, s denotes the modelling parameters and $t_h(k)$ is the exhaustive signal. The consecutive exhaustive signal can be computed by iterating the representation in Equation (1) as given in Equation (2):

$$c_s(k) = c_{s+1}(k) + t_{h+1}(k) \tag{2}$$

3.1.1. Noise Elimination

The ECG signal, as shown in Figure 2, obtained from subjects might have been tainted by noise and other irregularities. Electricity cable disruption, the initial value slide, sensory movement, erroneous sensory proximity and skeletal muscle spasms are the sources of noise and aberrations. Incorrect data might have an impact on the characteristics that make heartbeats naturally unique. As a result, the ECG signal's adaptation is crucial to raising its quality for proper information representation. Noise is introduced into the ECG signal during recording and is dispersed across many harmonic ranges.

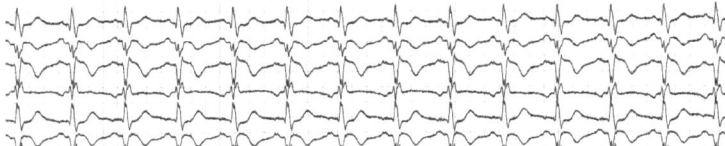

Figure 2. Sample raw signal.

Therefore, in order to create an ECG signal of excellent accuracy, as shown in Figure 3, filters covering several harmonic bands are typically utilized. As a result, a band pass filter that only needs a coefficient number of integers was applied to the signal. A filter with a low pass threshold and one with a high pass threshold were combined to create a band pass filtering device. The original ECG signal, which has less noise, is typically between 5 and 15 Hz in frequency. The representations for filters with low and high pass thresholds are represented in Equations (3) and (4):

$$f_{mD} = 2f_{(m-1)D} - f_{(m-2)D} + g_{mD} - 2g_{(m-6)D} + g_{(m-12)D} \tag{3}$$

$$f_{mD} = 32g_{(m-16)D} - (f_{(m-1)D} + g_{mD} - g_{(m-32)D}) \tag{4}$$

Denoised ECG

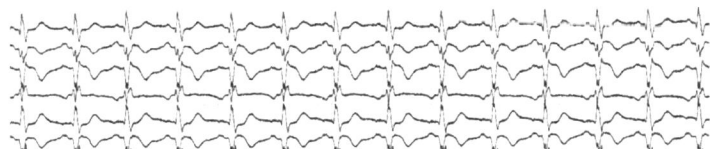

Figure 3. Denoising and segmentation results.

3.1.2. Segmentation of Beats

The identification of heartbeats from the denoised ECG signals was performed using the Hamiltonian-mean algorithm. This algorithm is proven to detect the QRS levels in the signals with high accuracy. The shift function and variance equation represented in Equations (5) and (6) were employed to determine the gradients of the QRS levels.

$$(x) = (1/8D)\left(-x^{-2} - 2x^{-1} + 2x^1 + x^2\right) \tag{5}$$

$$f_{mD} = (1/8D)[-g(mD-2D) - 2g(mD-D) + 2g(mD+D) + g(mD+2D)] \quad (6)$$

The rounding operation, which rounds the signal's value step-by-step, occurs following the slope estimation. The waveform data of R gradient is found by applying a window-shifting aggregator for a set of N samples as shown in Equation (7),

$$f_{mD} = \left(\frac{1}{M}\right)[g(mD - (M-1)D) + g(mD - (M-2)D) + \cdots + g(mD)] \quad (7)$$

Subsequently, the QRS structure of every individual heartbeat is identified using the dynamic screening approach. A time frame of size 600 ms surrounding the R-peak is defined for segmenting heartbeats when the R-peak is observed.

3.2. Multi-Feature Extraction

ECG characteristics were retrieved using temporal and harmonic set-based methodologies. Wavelet evaluation serves as an advantageous technique for the feature extraction process since ECG signals are inherently chaotic. Additionally, the ECG was subjected to wavelet transforms across multiple forms in order to extract pertinent features. In order to detect the time-based characteristics and extricate features, methods such as Fractional Discrete Cosine Transform, Radon Wavelet Transform and Fractional Wavelet Transform approaches were implemented.

3.2.1. Fractional Discrete Cosine Transform

Data in the temporal region can be transformed into the frequency domain using this technique. It investigates the duplication of data and decreases the number of parameters that are essential for describing evidence as an outcome. The mathematical representation of this transform is given in Equation (8):

$$FDC_T = ||\frac{1}{\sqrt{A}}\epsilon_x \cos\left(\frac{2\alpha(2\alpha+1)k}{4A}\right)| \quad (8)$$

3.2.2. Radon Wavelet Transform

The parameterization of signals and the assessment of its fundamentals form the basis of the Radon Transform. The Radon Transform's intrinsic qualities make it a helpful tool for capturing the spatial aspects of an input signal. The representation of Radon Wavelet Transform over the signal is as shown in Equation (9):

$$RWT(\beta, a) = \int_{-\infty}^{+\infty} v(\beta + ab, b) \, db \quad (9)$$

This transform, when applied to a function across two dimensions, can be represented as given in Equation (10):

$$H(h, \delta)[g(m,n)] = \int_{-\infty}^{+\infty} \int_{-\infty}^{+\infty} g(m,n) \, \gamma \, (h - m\cos\theta - n\sin\theta) \, dm \, dn \quad (10)$$

3.2.3. Fractional Wavelet Transform

This technique is the product of Fractional Fourier Transform and Wavelet Transform. Hence, it inherits the benefits of both transformations. Through the use of both these transforms, it ensures the potential to undertake analytical tasks with multiple resolutions and the mathematical modelling of signals in the fractional realm. This transform can be formulated mathematically as given in Equations (11) and (12):

$$Y_m^i(x,y) = \int_{-\infty}^{\infty} m(s) \, \mu_{i,x,y}^*(s) \, ds \quad (11)$$

$$\mu_{i,x,y}(s) = e^{-(\frac{y}{2})(h^2-r^2-(\frac{h-r}{l})^2)} \tag{12}$$

3.3. Optimization-Based Feature Selection

The red fox optimization technique was employed in this research to select the best characteristics to be supplied for the ECG signal categorization process. Red fox species are made up of both migratory individuals and those that depart on identifiable territory. The red fox is a skilled hunter of small game, both in and out of the home. As it moves across the area in search of food, the fox approaches its victim with stealth until it is close enough to launch a successful assault. The process by which the fox searches its domain and detects targets in the distance was modelled as an exhaustive search in this algorithm. A position as close to the target as possible before the assault was simulated as a regional search in the subsequent stage, which involved moving across the surroundings. The fitness of the foxes is the important parameter for initiating the exploration process. Based on this factor, the distance between each member in the group is computed as shown in Equation (13):

$$t((\bar{a}^x)^k, (\bar{a}^{best})^k) = \sqrt{||(\bar{a}^x)^k - (\bar{a}^{best})^k||} \tag{13}$$

The members in the group are migrated to the optimal locations using the representation given in Equation (14):

$$(\bar{a}^x)^k = (\bar{a}^x)^k + \beta sign((\bar{a}^{best})^k) - (\bar{a}^x)^k) \tag{14}$$

3.4. i-AlexNet Architecture

There is more than one hidden layer in a deep architecture. These hidden layers provide more effective analysis of features and augmentation. A large network, such as AlexNet, has many neurons, or between six hundred thousand and sixty million parameters. The activation function used in this network is Rectified Linear Unit, which outputs value 1 whenever the input is not less than zero. It is represented mathematically in Equation (15) as

$$b = \max(0, a) \tag{15}$$

For any input X with length l and breadth b, the convolution operation can be defined as shown in Equation (16):

$$H(l, b) = (X * k)(l, b) = \sum_m \sum_n X(l-m, b-n)k(m, n) \tag{16}$$

By convolution, the model can gain knowledge from the distinctive characteristics of input signals, and by sharing those variables, the degree of complexity is decreased. The characteristics that are extracted are diminished using the pooling layers. The feature map's layers for pooling take a collection of pixels in close proximity and produce parameters for inclusion. AlexNet uses max pooling to minimize the characteristic map. Using a 4 × 4 chunk from the characteristic map, max pooling creates a 2 × 2 chunk with the highest possible data. The fully connected layers in the model use SoftMax activation function and their values can be determined using Equation (17):

$$oftmax(a)_x = \frac{\exp(a_x)}{\sum_{y=1}^m \exp(a_y)} \; for \; x = 0, 1, 2, \ldots, m \tag{17}$$

A convolution layer, followed by a fully connected (fc) and ReLU layer, and a normalization layer and pooling layer constitute the layers of the i-AlexNet model. The architecture of the i-AlexNet model is presented in Figure 3. In order to make the AlexNet model consistent with the current investigation, the final three layers were eliminated. The original AlexNet model's remaining parameters were retained. There were 50 neurons in the newly added fully linked layer as shown in the Figure 4. The optimization algorithm implemented in this model to reduce the errors is represented as in (18):

$$\delta_{t+1} = \delta_t - \beta \nabla G(\delta_t) + \alpha(\delta_t - \delta_{t-1}) \tag{18}$$

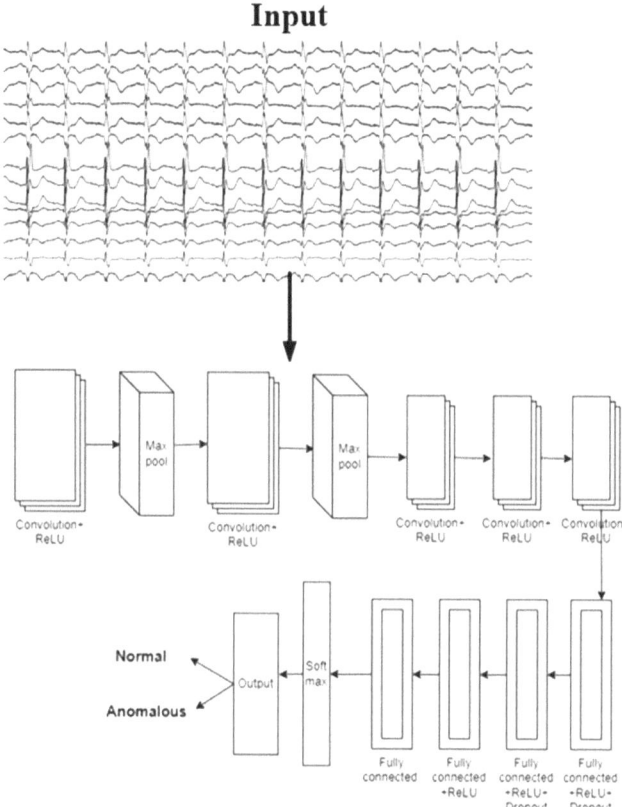

Figure 4. i-AlexNet architecture.

4. Results and Discussion

This section discusses the results of the application of the proposed approach to two different publicly accessible datasets, the PTB and MIT-BIH datasets. Further, the performance of the proposed model is also compared against other existing works.

4.1. Dataset Description
4.1.1. PTB Database

This database consists of samples taken from 290 individuals, and the total number of rows in this dataset is close to 550. The data in this database are a combination of both individuals with diseases and those without them. Records for 12 different types of arrhythmias are available in this database. The initial set of images for the ECG signals present is 4652, which is further augmented in order to create a larger dataset. This dataset can be accessed using the link below. The PTB XL dataset is not evenly distributed. Table 2 shows that the records are divided among the five classes of ECG findings. https://physionet.org/content/ptb-xl/1.0.3/ (accessed on 12 November 2023) [31].

Table 2. Distribution of records among diagnostic superclasses in the PTB-XL dataset.

Superclass	Description	Number of Records	Percentage of Total
NORM	Normal ECG	9514	43.57%
MI	Myocardial Infarction	5469	25.06%
STTC	ST/T Change	5235	23.97%
CD	Conduction Disturbance	4898	22.43%
HYP	Hypertrophy	2649	12.13%

The disparity is particularly evident in NORM with HYP, as HYP makes up around 12.13% of the dataset. This suggests that the dataset is not evenly distributed, showing a gap in record numbers across diagnostic categories. The dataset contains a range of ECG abnormalities grouped into categories, for simplicity. NORM (normal ECG) represents ECG readings without any abnormalities, used as the standard group. MI (Myocardial Infarction) indicates a heart attack where blood flow to a part of the heart is blocked, leading to heart muscle damage. STTC (ST/T Change) covers changes in the ST segment and T wave of the ECG, which can signal issues like ischemia, inflammation or other unspecified changes. CD (Conduction Disturbance) includes heart block types and disruptions in the heart's conduction system. HYP (Hypertrophy) shows the presence of Hypertrophy, where the heart muscle thickens due to factors like blood pressure or other heart conditions.

4.1.2. MIT-BIH Database

This dataset consists of data collected from fifty individuals for a duration of one hour. Data for seventeen different types of arrhythmias are available in this dataset. An aggregate of 1736 images for ECG signals is prepared and presented in the dataset. The available data are further augmented to create a total of seventeen thousand images for all the seventeen arrhythmia categories. This dataset can be downloaded using the link provided below: https://physionet.org/content/mitdb/1.0.0/ (accessed on 12 November 2023) [32].

4.2. Experimental Setup

This study used an NVIDIA Jetson Nano board. It is a compact, potent low-level board in the Jetson environment from NVIDIA. It enables simultaneous functioning of several neural networks for a range of uses, including language processing, recognition of items, categorization and visual grouping. It features libraries created for applications based on embedded systems, artificial intelligence, the Internet of Things, machine intelligence, visualizations and audio and video, together with an entire programming platform called Jetpack SDK. Applying the same CUDA cores to a Jetson Nano and a GeForce-capable GPU results in a very potent software development ecosystem. Furthermore, Jetson Nano features a hybrid architecture, meaning that the CPU can start the operating system and configure it to use the GPU's CUDA characteristics to accelerate difficult artificial intelligence tasks.

4.3. Performance Assessment

The dataset balancing was performed using RandomOverSampler from the imblearn library to handle class imbalance in the ECG dataset. RandomOverSampler was initialized with a fixed random state for reproducibility. The ECG data were reshaped into a 2D array format, as required by RandomOverSampler, which then generated additional samples for minority classes until all classes had equal representation. After resampling, the data were reshaped back to their original multi-dimensional form suitable for neural network input.

Class weights were calculated to further address class imbalance. The number of samples in each class was counted using np.bincount after resampling. Class weights were then computed as the inverse of these counts, assigning more importance to minority classes. These weights were converted into a PyTorch tensor for use in the loss function during model training. This approach ensures balanced class representation, enhancing the model's ability to learn and generalize across all classes while reducing bias towards the majority class. The following Algorithm 1, was used to rectify dataset imbalance.

Algorithm 1. To treat imbalance	
1	Reshape Data
2	n_samples, *input_shape = X.shape
3	X_reshaped = reshape(X, (n_samples, -1))
4	Initialize RandomOverSampler
5	ros = RandomOverSampler(random_state=random_state)
6	Resample Dataset
7	X_resampled = reshape(X_resampled, (len(X_resampled), *input_shape))
8	Compute Class Weights
9	class_counts = bincount(y_resampled)
10	class_weights = 1.0 / class_counts
11	class_weights_tensor = convert_to_tensor(class_weights, dtype=float32)

Figure 5 shows that the model produced a significant number of misclassifications, particularly as Healthy Controls, indicating that the model struggles to differentiate Myocardial Hypertrophy from normal ECGs. However, this result was generated without the module of weight imbalance and optimization. However, Figure 6 shows that the classification of diagnostic classes was produced by the module after weight imbalance and optimization were applied.

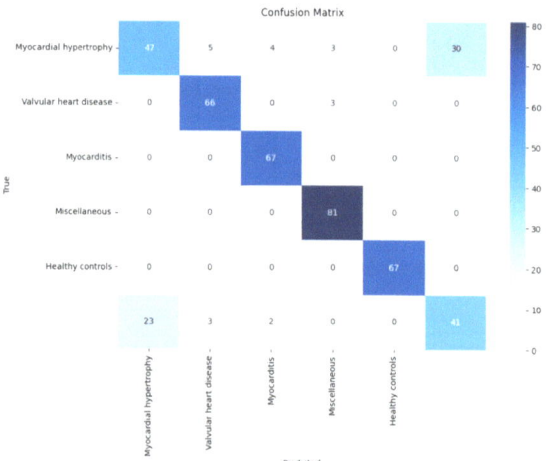

Figure 5. Confusion matrix for classification model performance.

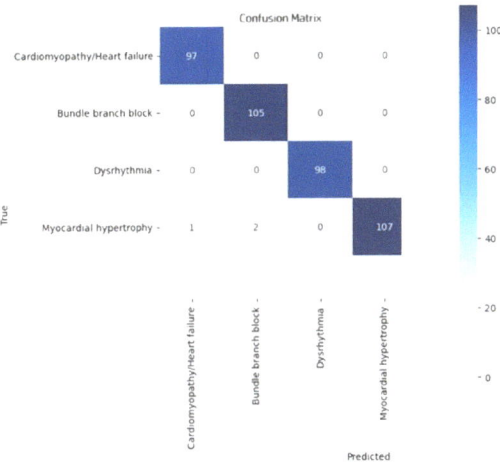

Figure 6. Confusion matrix for classification model performance.

The performance of the proposed i-AlexNet model was compared against the conventional algorithms to interpret its performance supremacy. The algorithms, such as Deep Neural Networks (DNNs), Fully Connected Neural Networks (FCNNs), Gated Recurrent Units (GRUs), VGG16, DenseNet and ResNet, were considered for evaluation. These algorithms were applied to the PTB and the MIT_BIH database and the obtained results are presented in Table 3 and Figures 6 and 7 The CNN model produced an accuracy of 89.8% for the PTB database and 91.3% for the MIT_BIH database. FCNN exhibited 90.8% accuracy, 89.8% precision, 89.5% recall and 90.4% F1 score for the PTB database. Also, the FCNN model produced 92.6% accuracy, 91.5% precision, 91.2% recall and 92.2% F1 score. The performance of the GRU and VGG16 models are closer to each other, with an accuracy of 91.7% and 92.7% for the PTB database and 93.2% and 94.7% for the MIT_BIH database, respectively. The DenseNet and ResNet models offer higher accuracy for both the ECG databases. However, the proposed i-AlexNet model produces efficient accuracy in classification, with 98.2% for the PTB database and 98.8% for the MIT_BIH database.

Table 3. Comparison of conventional algorithms.

Techniques	PTB Database				MIT_BIH Database			
	Accuracy (%)	Precision (%)	Recall (%)	F1 (%)	Accuracy (%)	Precision (%)	Recall (%)	F1 (%)
DNN	89.8	88.5	88.2	89.4	91.3	90.5	90.8	91.1
FCNN	90.8	89.8	89.5	90.4	92.6	91.5	91.2	92.2
GRU	91.7	90.2	90.4	91.3	93.2	92.4	92.6	93.1
VGG16	92.7	92.4	92.0	92.6	94.7	93.5	93.2	94.2
DenseNet	93.8	92.4	92.6	93.5	95.9	94.6	94.3	95.4
ResNet	95.3	94.2	94.6	95.1	96.3	95.2	94.7	95.8
Proposed	98.2	97.5	97.2	97.9	98.8	98.2	97.7	98.4

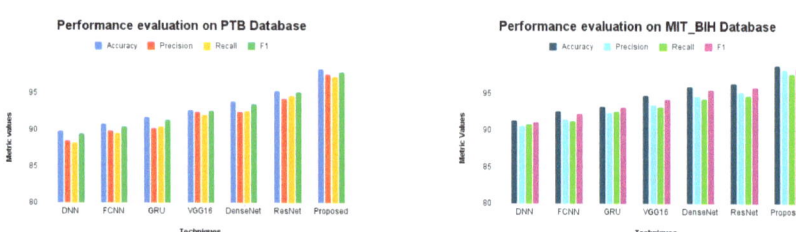

Figure 7. Performance evaluation of proposed system.

To see how well the model is learning, the training loss and validation loss are usually shown over the span of the training dataset's iterations (Figure 6). A drop in the validation loss suggests that the model is successfully extending to new data, and a decrease in the training loss shows that the model has learnt well from the training data. To improve extrapolation, normalization or changing the structure of the model may be required if the training loss keeps going down while the validation loss starts to rise. This could be an indication of overfitting. But this is not the case with the proposed approach, and it is depicted in Figure 8.

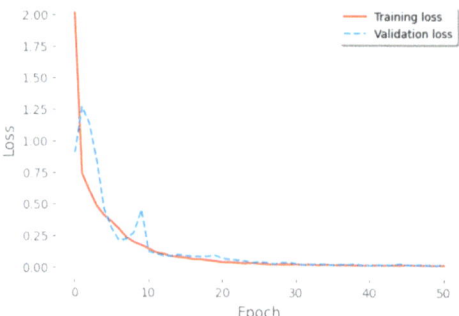

Figure 8. Training vs. validation loss.

The heartbeats were categorized into two groups as normal and anomalous, as presented in Figure 8. If the heartbeat is determined to be normal, the input is not sent to the cloud network. It is essential to ensure that the beats that are anomalous are classified with more precision. It is well known that the heart rate changes from its regular pattern during arrhythmias. Premature beats are characterized by rapid cardiac changes that arise when the chambers of the heart or ventricle burst prematurely or out of sync with the regular pulse. The anomalous beats' waveform differs from that of the typical beats.

Consequently, anomalous beats can be identified by the heart rate variability (HRV) and correlation of the beats. These have been utilized in conjunction with the first output block's result to determine if a beat is normal or anomalous. The output of the first convolutional is transmitted directly to the second classifier for additional analysis if the first output block flags a beat as anomalous. However, this evidence only serves to validate the classification of a beat as normal. The experimental results obtained during the classification of ECG signals are presented in Figure 9.

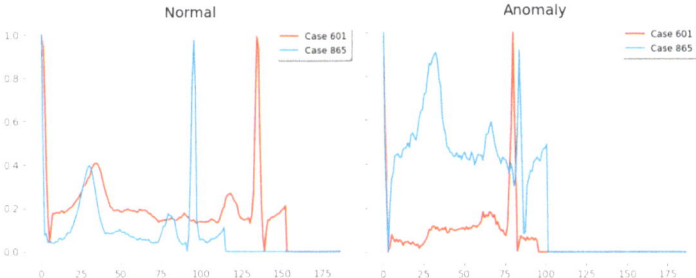

Figure 9. Sample normal and anomalous ECG data.

Furthermore, the outcomes of the proposed approach are also compared with the state-of-the-art methods in the literature, and the outcomes are shown in Table 4 and depicted in Figure 10. Our method, utilizing the AlexNet architecture, attained an accuracy rate of 98.8%, a precision of 98.2%, a recall of 97.7% and an F1 score of 98.4%. These outcomes suggest that our approach is highly competitive, with performance metrics aligning with those of cutting-edge methods. Originally crafted for image classification duties, the AlexNet structure displayed adaptability and effectiveness in managing ECG data. Its deep convolutional layers can adeptly capture patterns within the data, resulting in robust feature extraction and classification capabilities. This adaptability proves beneficial in ECG analysis scenarios where signal patterns are complex and vary significantly among patients. When compared to techniques like BiLSTM, FDDN and Deep Network, our method exhibits superior performance across all assessed metrics. While BiLSTM and FDDN achieved an F1 score of 88%, our approach attained 98.4%, showcasing an enhancement in performance. Similarly, although Deep Network scored a 97% on the F1 metric, our method surpassed it by a margin of 1.4%. Moreover, our methods' performance stands on par with that of the Modified ResNet18, CNN BiLSTM and Multi-Scale Fusion Neural Network approaches, all achieving good results. The slight differences in accuracy and completeness between these techniques and our suggested strategy showcase the effectiveness of the AlexNet design in maintaining a rounded performance across measurements. To sum up the proposed approach, utilizing the AlexNet design showcases a good degree of precision, accuracy, completeness and F1 score, establishing it as a trustworthy method for ECG signal categorization. The findings indicate that the AlexNet-driven technique can effectively rival and even outperform cutting-edge methods in instances, underlining its potential for broad application in ECG analysis and related domains.

Table 4. Comparison of existing vs. proposed techniques.

Techniques	Accuracy (%)	Precision (%)	Recall (%)	F1 (%)
BiLSTM -FDDN [23]	93	94	62	88
Modified ResNet18 [25]	99	1	99	1
Deep Network [26]	97	97	97	97
CNN-BiLSTM [28]	99	99	99	99
Multi-Scale Fusion Neural Network [30]	99	99	99	99
Proposed	98.8	98.2	97.7	98.4

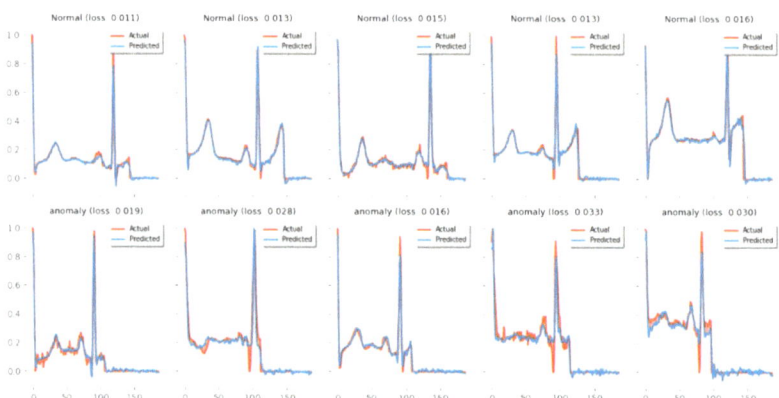

Figure 10. Experimental results of normal vs. anomalous classification.

We conducted experiments on the PTB and Mit_bih databases to confirm the strength and versatility of our suggested model. Each test included iterations with cross validation to ensure trustworthy outcomes. The data displayed in Table 3 and Figure 4 are an average of tests to consider variations and offer a level of confidence for the performance metrics reported. Our proposed i-AlexNet model consistently surpasses cutting-edge methods in all performance measures. The notable enhancements in accuracy, precision, recall and F1 score showcase the effectiveness of our approach. The comparative study underscores the advantages of our model, its capacity to utilize preprocessing techniques, and a robust neural network structure for superior performance. The incorporation of wavelet transform in preprocessing plays a role in boosting the model's capability to extract features from ECG signals thereby contributing to its high accuracy in classification. In summary, our suggested i-AlexNet model, with its preprocessing techniques and advanced feature extraction abilities, establishes a new standard for ECG classification. Through comparisons with existing methods, it highlights the progress achieved by our approach as shown in the Figure 11.

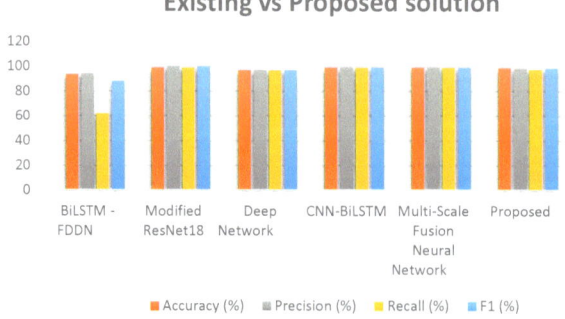

Figure 11. Performance comparison of existing vs. proposed methods [23,25,26,28,30].

The Healthcare Disease Diagnosis system powered by Deep Learning, known as IoTDL HDD, achieved an accuracy rate of 93.452% in classifying ECG signals, demonstrating its reliability as a tool for diagnosing cardiovascular conditions in real time. This system employs methods for its operation. One notable technique involves BiLSTM feature extraction utilizing Bidirectional Long Short-Term Memory networks to extract features from ECG signals. These networks excel at capturing dependencies in data, allowing the model to consider information from both future time steps. Moreover, the AFO algorithm optimizes the hyperparameters of the BiLSTM model by mimicking the natural propagation behavior of plants, efficiently enhancing performance and accurately extracting features from ECG signals. In addition, a Fuzzy Deep Neural Network classifier is utilized to assign labels to ECG signals. This classifier merges network learning with logic to effectively manage uncertainties and variations, in data ensuring classification with unclear input signals. By utilizing these methods, the IoTDL HDD model can precisely categorize ECG signals establishing itself as a tool for real time disease diagnosis. A study introduced an ECG device called iKardo that automatically sorts ECG beats as critical or non-critical. The tool utilizes machine learning and a Convolutional Neural Network (CNN) based on ResNet for accuracy. To handle datasets researchers applied SMOTE and BIRCH techniques for data balancing. Real time processing and sorting of ECG signals were conducted by integrating the system into an IoT based setup for monitoring purposes. IKardo achieved a 99.58% accuracy in distinguishing critical from critical ECG beats. Validation was carried out using metrics, like precision, recall and F1 score to evaluate classification outcomes. Incorporating power management resulted in decreased power consumption extending the devices lifespan. IKardo marks an advancement in healthcare tech by swiftly detecting critical heart conditions through ongoing monitoring. Combining machine learning with frameworks enhances health monitoring systems' capabilities, offering practical real-time healthcare solutions. iKardos's effectiveness in detecting heart issues and providing care is enhanced by employing sophisticated methods to balance data even when dealing with uneven datasets.

During surgeries, the evaluation of anesthesia heavily relies on ECG signals. However, understanding these signals can pose a challenge for medical professionals. In a study by the authors of [26], Convolutional Neural Networks were utilized to categorize types of ECG images to aid in anesthesia assessment. They created prototypes for IoT-based ECG measurements. They used neural networks to classify signals into various categories, such as QRS widening, sinus rhythm, ST depression and ST elevation. The accuracy and kappa statistics for the ResNet, AlexNet and SqueezeNet models were reported as (0.97, 0.96), (0.96, 0.95) and (0.75, 0.67), respectively. This research demonstrates the potential for real-time ECG measurement and classification while hinting at the possibility of expanding to include types of ECG signals, for practicality. The new CNN BiLSTM model performed well in accuracy (99.6%), sensitivity (99.8%) and specificity (98.2%) in sorting CAD from ECG signals. The SUE measure effectively differentiated between classified ECG segments, showing a connection between higher SUE values and correct classifications. Compared to models like CNN and DenseNet, the CNN BiLSTM model showed resilience and dependability in diverse noise environments [28]. The DMSFNet showed good performance on the dataset, achieving an F1 score of 82.8%, and on the PhysioNet/CinC_2017 dataset, with an F1 score of 84.1%. These findings surpassed models highlighting enhanced precision and reliability in categorizing types of arrhythmias [30].

5. Conclusions

In this current paper, continuous surveillance of patient's cardiac activities is achieved using AI and IoMT technologies. IoMT sensors are placed on the body of individuals to receive ECG signals in real time. These signals are preprocessed to remove noises and segment the heartbeats. The preprocessed signals are passed on to the feature extraction phase, in which three types of transforms are performed to extricate the pertinent characteristics. These extracted features are further optimally chosen using red fox optimization.

Finally, categorization of ECG signals is implemented using the Improved AlexNet model, which identifies normal and anomalous signals efficiently. The performance of the model is evaluated using various metrics and it is observed that the proposed model achieves an accuracy of 98.8%, a precision of 98.2%, a recall of 97.7% and an F1 score of 98.4%. One of the limitations with this system is that thorough validation is necessary before applying AI models developed in research settings to clinical settings. Healthcare practitioners' acceptance of AI-based ECG classification tools may be hampered by a lack of formal clinical validation. As an extension of the present research, strong security protocols and privacy controls can be implemented, as cyberattacks may target IoMT devices and AI systems, jeopardizing the integrity and anonymity of patient data.

Author Contributions: M.K.: Data curation, Formal analysis. Funding acquisition, investigation, Methodology, Project administration, Resources, Software, supervision, Validation, Visualization, Writing—original draft, Writing—review & editing. R.N.A.K.: Methodology, Project, administration, Resources, Software, Supervision, Validation. H.M.: Data curation, Formal analysis. A.M.A.R.: Funding acquisition, Supervision, Validation, Visualization, Writing—review & editing. All authors have read and agreed to the published version of the manuscript.

Funding: This work was supported by the Deanship of Scientific Research, Vice Presidency for Graduate Studies and Scientific Research, King Faisal University, Saudi Arabia Grant No. KFU241181.

Institutional Review Board Statement: Not applicable.

Informed Consent Statement: Not applicable.

Data Availability Statement: PTB database is available at https://www.physionet.org/content/ptbdb/1.0.0 (accessed on 14 November 2023).

Conflicts of Interest: The authors declare no conflict of interest.

References

1. Lin, J.; Fu, R.; Zhong, X.; Yu, P.; Tan, G.; Li, W.; Zhang, H.; Li, Y.; Zhou, L.; Ning, C. Wearable sensors and devices for real-time cardiovascular disease monitoring. *Cell Rep. Phys. Sci.* **2021**, *2*, 100541. [CrossRef]
2. Qureshi, M.A.; Qureshi, K.N.; Jeon, G.; Piccialli, F. Deep learning-based ambient assisted living for self-management of cardiovascular conditions. *Neural Comput. Appl.* **2022**, *34*, 10449–10467. [CrossRef]
3. Tuli, S.; Basumatary, N.; Gill, S.S.; Kahani, M.; Arya, R.C.; Wander, G.S.; Buyya, R. HealthFog: An ensemble deep learning based Smart Healthcare System for Automatic Diagnosis of Heart Diseases in inte-grated IoT and fog computing environments. *Future Gener. Comput. Syst.* **2020**, *104*, 187–200. [CrossRef]
4. Desai, S.; Patel, K.; Patel, A.; Jadav, N.K.; Tanwar, S. A Survey on AI-based Parkinson Disease Detection: Taxonomy, Case Study, and Research Challenges. *Scalable Comput. Pract. Exp.* **2024**, *25*, 1402–1423. [CrossRef]
5. Boch, A.; Ryan, S.; Kriebitz, A.; Amugongo, L.M.; Lütge, C. Beyond the Metal flesh: Understanding the intersection between bio- and ai ethics for robotics in healthcare. *Robotics* **2023**, *12*, 110. [CrossRef]
6. Theodore Armand, T.P.; Nfor, K.A.; Kim, J.I.; Kim, H.C. Applications of Artificial Intelligence, Machine Learning, and Deep Learning in Nutrition: A Systematic Review. *Nutrients* **2024**, *16*, 1073. [CrossRef] [PubMed]
7. Alomari, Y.; Andó, M.; Baptista, M.L. Advancing aircraft engine RUL predictions: An interpretable integrated approach of feature engineering and aggregated feature importance. *Sci. Rep.* **2023**, *13*, 13466. [CrossRef]
8. Muneer, S.; Farooq, U.; Athar, A.; Raza, M.A.; Ghazal, T.M.; Sakib, S. A Critical Review of Artificial Intelligence Based Approaches in Intrusion Detection: A Comprehensive Analysis. *J. Eng.* **2024**, *2024*, 3909173. [CrossRef]
9. Cheikhrouhou, O.; Mahmud, R.; Zouari, R.; Ibrahim, M.; Zaguia, A.; Gia, T.N. One-dimensional CNN approach for ECG arrhythmia analysis in fog-cloud environments. *IEEE Access* **2021**, *9*, 103513–103523. [CrossRef]
10. Sanamdikar, S.T.; Hamde, S.T.; Asutkar, V.G. Classification and analysis of cardiac arrhythmia based on incremental support vector regression on IOT platform. *Biomed. Signal Process. Control* **2021**, *64*, 102324. [CrossRef]
11. Kumar, A.; Kumar, S.; Dutt, V.; Dubey, A.K.; García-Díaz, V. IoT-based ECG monitoring for arrhythmia classification using Coyote Grey Wolf optimization-based deep learning CNN classifier. *Biomed. Signal Process. Control* **2022**, *76*, 103638. [CrossRef]
12. Belaid, S.; Hattay, J.; Mohamed, H.H.; Rezgui, R. Deep Cardiac Telemonitoring for Clinical Cloud Healthcare Applications. *Procedia Comput. Sci.* **2022**, *207*, 2843–2852. [CrossRef]
13. Shafi, J.; Obaidat, M.S.; Krishna, P.V.; Sadoun, B.; Pounambal, M.; Gitanjali, J. Prediction of heart abnormalities using deep learning model and wearabledevices in smart health homes. *Multimed. Tools Appl.* **2022**, *81*, 543–557. [CrossRef]
14. Rawal, V.; Prajapati, P.; Darji, A. Hardware implementation of 1D-CNN architecture for ECG arrhythmia classification. *Biomed. Signal Process. Control* **2023**, *85*, 104865. [CrossRef]

15. Cheng, L.H.; Bosch, P.B.; Hofman, R.F.; Brakenhoff, T.B.; Bruggemans, E.F.; van der Geest, R.J.; Holman, E.R. Revealing Unforeseen Diagnostic Image Features With Deep Learning by Detecting Cardiovascular Diseases From Apical 4-Chamber Ultrasounds. *J. Am. Heart Assoc.* **2022**, *11*, e024168. [CrossRef]
16. Dami, S.; Yahaghizadeh, M. Predicting cardiovascular events with deep learning approach in the context of the internet of things. *Neural Comput. Appl.* **2021**, *33*, 7979–7996. [CrossRef]
17. Ghosh, S.; Chattopadhyay, B.P.; Roy, R.M.; Mukherjee, J.; Mahadevappa, M. Non-invasive cuffless blood pressure and heart rate monitoring using impedance cardiography. *Intell. Med.* **2022**, *2*, 199–208. [CrossRef]
18. Pal, P.; Mahadevappa, M. Adaptive Multi-Dimensional dual attentive DCNN for detecting Cardiac Morbidities using Fused ECG-PPG Signals. *IEEE Trans. Artif. Intell.* **2022**, *4*, 1225–1235. [CrossRef]
19. Sadad, T.; Bukhari, S.A.C.; Munir, A.; Ghani, A.; El-Sherbeeny, A.M.; Rauf, H.T. Detection of Cardiovascular Disease Based on PPG Signals Using Machine Learning with Cloud Computing. *Comput. Intell. Neurosci.* **2022**, *2022*, 1672677. [CrossRef]
20. Patro, S.P.; Padhy, N.; Chiranjevi, D. Ambient assisted living predictive model for cardiovascular disease prediction using supervised learning. *Evol. Intell.* **2021**, *14*, 941–969. [CrossRef]
21. Nelson, I.; Annadurai, C.; Devi, K.N. An Efficient AlexNet Deep Learning Architecture for Automatic Diagnosis of Cardio-Vascular Diseases in Healthcare System. *Wirel. Pers. Commun.* **2022**, *126*, 493–509. [CrossRef]
22. Deka, B.; Kumar, S.; Datta, S. Dictionary Learning-Based Multichannel ECG Reconstruction Using Compressive Sensing. *IEEE Sens. J.* **2022**, *22*, 16359–16369. [CrossRef]
23. Khanna, A.; Selvaraj, P.; Gupta, D.; Sheikh, T.H.; Pareek, P.K.; Shankar, V. Internet of things and deep learning enabled healthcare disease diagnosis using biomedical electrocardiogram signals. *Expert Syst.* **2023**, *40*, e12864. [CrossRef]
24. Sun, L.; Wang, Y.; Qu, Z.; Xiong, N.N. BeatClass: A Sustainable ECG Classification System in IoT-Based eHealth. *IEEE Internet Things J.* **2021**, *9*, 7178–7195. [CrossRef]
25. Maji, P.; Mondal, H.K.; Roy, A.P.; Poddar, S.; Mohanty, S.P. iKardo: An Intelligent ECG Device for Automatic Critical Beat Identification for Smart Healthcare. *IEEE Trans. Consum. Electron.* **2021**, *67*, 235–243. [CrossRef]
26. Yeh, L.-R.; Chen, W.-C.; Chan, H.-Y.; Lu, N.-H.; Wang, C.-Y.; Twan, W.-H.; Du, W.-C.; Huang, Y.-H.; Hsu, S.-Y.; Chen, T.-B. Integrating ECG monitoring and classification via IoT and deep neural networks. *Biosensors* **2021**, *11*, 188. [CrossRef] [PubMed]
27. Ying, Z.; Zhang, G.; Pan, Z.; Chu, C.; Liu, X. FedECG: A Federated Semi-supervised Learning Framework for Electrocardiogram Abnormalities Prediction. *J. King Saud Univ. Comput. Inf. Sci.* **2022**, *35*, 101568. [CrossRef]
28. Seoni, S.; Molinari, F.; Acharya, U.R.; Lih, O.S.; Barua, P.D.; García, S.; Salvi, M. Application of spatial uncertainty predictor in CNN-BiLSTM model using coronary artery disease ECG signals. *Inf. Sci.* **2024**, *665*, 120383. [CrossRef]
29. Sivapalan, G.; Nundy, K.K.; James, A.; Cardiff, B.; John, D. Interpretable Rule Mining for Real-Time ECG Anomaly Detection in IoT Edge Sensors. *IEEE Internet Things J.* **2022**, *10*, 13095–13108. [CrossRef]
30. Wang, R.; Fan, J.; Li, Y.A. Deep Multi-Scale Fusion Neural Network for Multi-Class Arrhythmia Detection. *IEEE J. Biomed. Health Inform.* **2020**, *24*, 2461–2472. [CrossRef]
31. Goldberger, A.; Amaral, L.; Glass, L.; Hausdorff, J.; Ivanov, P.C.; Mark, R.; Mietus, J.E.; Moody, G.B.; Peng, C.K.; Stanley, H.E. PhysioBank, PhysioToolkit, and PhysioNet: Components of a new research resource for complex physiologic signals. *Circulation* **2000**, *101*, e215–e220. [CrossRef] [PubMed]
32. Moody, G.B.; Mark, R.G. The impact of the MIT-BIH Arrhythmia Database. *IEEE Eng. Med. Biol.* **2001**, *20*, 45–50. [CrossRef] [PubMed]

Disclaimer/Publisher's Note: The statements, opinions and data contained in all publications are solely those of the individual author(s) and contributor(s) and not of MDPI and/or the editor(s). MDPI and/or the editor(s) disclaim responsibility for any injury to people or property resulting from any ideas, methods, instructions or products referred to in the content.

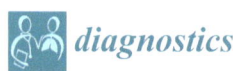

Article

Deep Neural Network Augments Performance of Junior Residents in Diagnosing COVID-19 Pneumonia on Chest Radiographs

Yangqin Feng [1], Jordan Sim Zheng Ting [2], Xinxing Xu [1,*], Chew Bee Kun [2], Edward Ong Tien En [2], Hendra Irawan Tan Wee Jun [2], Yonghan Ting [2], Xiaofeng Lei [1], Wen-Xiang Chen [2], Yan Wang [1], Shaohua Li [1], Yingnan Cui [1], Zizhou Wang [1], Liangli Zhen [1], Yong Liu [1], Rick Siow Mong Goh [1] and Cher Heng Tan [2,3]

[1] Institute of High Performance Computing (IHPC), Agency for Science, Technology and Research (A*STAR), 1 Fusionopolis Way, #16-16 Connexis, Singapore 138632, Singapore
[2] Department of Diagnostic Radiology, Tan Tock Seng Hospital, 11, Jalan Tan Tock Seng, Singapore 308433, Singapore
[3] Lee Kong Chian School of Medicine, 11, Mandalay Road, Singapore 308232, Singapore
* Correspondence: xuxinx@ihpc.a-star.edu.sg; Tel.: +65-9833-6289

Abstract: Chest X-rays (CXRs) are essential in the preliminary radiographic assessment of patients affected by COVID-19. Junior residents, as the first point-of-contact in the diagnostic process, are expected to interpret these CXRs accurately. We aimed to assess the effectiveness of a deep neural network in distinguishing COVID-19 from other types of pneumonia, and to determine its potential contribution to improving the diagnostic precision of less experienced residents. A total of 5051 CXRs were utilized to develop and assess an artificial intelligence (AI) model capable of performing three-class classification, namely non-pneumonia, non-COVID-19 pneumonia, and COVID-19 pneumonia. Additionally, an external dataset comprising 500 distinct CXRs was examined by three junior residents with differing levels of training. The CXRs were evaluated both with and without AI assistance. The AI model demonstrated impressive performance, with an Area under the ROC Curve (AUC) of 0.9518 on the internal test set and 0.8594 on the external test set, which improves the AUC score of the current state-of-the-art algorithms by 1.25% and 4.26%, respectively. When assisted by the AI model, the performance of the junior residents improved in a manner that was inversely proportional to their level of training. Among the three junior residents, two showed significant improvement with the assistance of AI. This research highlights the novel development of an AI model for three-class CXR classification and its potential to augment junior residents' diagnostic accuracy, with validation on external data to demonstrate real-world applicability. In practical use, the AI model effectively supported junior residents in interpreting CXRs, boosting their confidence in diagnosis. While the AI model improved junior residents' performance, a decline in performance was observed on the external test compared to the internal test set. This suggests a domain shift between the patient dataset and the external dataset, highlighting the need for future research on test-time training domain adaptation to address this issue.

Keywords: COVID-19; chest X-rays; deep neural networks; AI assistant for diagnosing

1. Introduction

The Severe Acute Respiratory Syndrome Coronavirus 2 (SARS-CoV-2) outbreak [1], initially detected in Wuhan, Hubei, China, has rapidly escalated into a worldwide pandemic [2]. The National Centre for Infectious Diseases (NCID) [3] has been at the forefront of Singapore's COVID-19 response. As of the time of writing, the Ministry of Health (MOH) has recorded over 2.2 million confirmed cases in Singapore [4].

Patients with COVID-19 pneumonia often exhibit similar symptoms to other viral diseases, such as Middle East Respiratory Syndrome [5], and their imaging findings are often

Citation: Feng, Y.; Sim Zheng Ting, J.; Xu, X.; Bee Kun, C.; Ong Tien En, E.; Irawan Tan Wee Jun, H.; Ting, Y.; Lei, X.; Chen, W.-X.; Wang, Y.; et al. Deep Neural Network Augments Performance of Junior Residents in Diagnosing COVID-19 Pneumonia on Chest Radiographs. *Diagnostics* **2023**, *13*, 1397. https://doi.org/10.3390/diagnostics13081397

Academic Editors: Sivaramakrishnan Rajaraman, Zhiyun Xue and Sameer Antani

Received: 2 March 2023
Revised: 5 April 2023
Accepted: 7 April 2023
Published: 12 April 2023

Copyright: © 2023 by the authors. Licensee MDPI, Basel, Switzerland. This article is an open access article distributed under the terms and conditions of the Creative Commons Attribution (CC BY) license (https://creativecommons.org/licenses/by/4.0/).

non-specific, presenting a diagnostic challenge [6–8]. Currently, the definitive method for diagnosing COVID-19 infection is the reverse transcriptase polymerase chain reaction (RT-PCR) [9]; however, limitations in diagnostic testing resources can hinder its accuracy [10–12]. In this context, chest imaging techniques [13], including computed tomography (CT) and chest radiography (CXR), are essential in the context of patient triaging and making treatment decisions [12,14]. Despite being less sensitive than CT, CXR is more widely adopted as it is faster, exposes patients to lower levels of radiation, and is potentially more cost-effective [7,15,16]. Therefore, junior residents, who are often the first point of contact, are expected to interpret CXRs of COVID-19 patients in many institutions.

In recent years, the application of deep learning models to clinical problems has shown significant potential in facilitating auto-diagnosis of diseases and providing real-time procedural support, particularly in the field of healthcare [17–19]. Several studies have explored the use of deep learning models for diagnosing COVID-19 through analysis of chest X-rays [20,21]. For instance, Jordan et al. collected a CXR dataset from NCID to train an AI model with the DenseNet as backbone to detect COVID-19 pneumonia. In response to the rapidly evolving global pandemic during COVID-19, they quickly deployed the trained model to NCID [22]. Abul et al. adopted a convolutional neural network (CNN) to extract feature representations from CXRs, and connected it with various classifiers, such as support vector machine (SVM), pattern recognition network (PRN), decision tree (DT), random forest (RF), and k-nearest neighbours (KNN), to perform COVID-19 detection [23]. Linda et al. introduced a novel COVID-Net for diagnosing COVID-19 from CXRs in publicly available datasets [24]. This approach incorporates an explainability method to not only provide clinicians with a deeper understanding of the critical factors associated with COVID-19 cases and improved screening, but also to enhance the transparency and accountability of COVID-Net by ensuring that its decisions are based on relevant information extracted from CXR images. However, the diagnostic performance of these models has yet to be validated in a clinical setting due to the limited size of CXR datasets used for training [24–26]. Moreover, it has been reported that lab-trained models may experience a significant decline in performance when deployed in clinical practice [27].

The motivation of this research is to harness AI's potential to improve the diagnostic process, optimize healthcare resources, and ultimately enhance patient care. Specifically, we develop a deep neural network to differentiate COVID-19 from other forms of pneumonia and explore the potential of AI techniques to enhance the diagnostic accuracy of junior residents, who often serve as the primary point-of-contact in the diagnostic process. In order to achieve the objectives of this study, an interdisciplinary approach has been adopted that combines clinical research, image diagnostics, and AI models. The primary aim of the study is to collect structured data, including CXRs and RT-PCR results, and use these data to develop a three-class classification AI model that can accurately distinguish between non-pneumonia, non-COVID-19 pneumonia, and COVID-19 pneumonia cases. Subsequently, the study seeks to assess the effectiveness of the AI model in enhancing the diagnostic precision of novice residents by implementing and evaluating its performance. Specifically, we collected a patient dataset and used it to train and validate the AI model. Then, the trained AI model has been deployed in the Tan Tock Seng Hospital (TTSH), where its effectiveness in improving junior residents' diagnostic accuracy has been evaluated. In addition, the study has investigated the performance of junior residents with different levels of training, both with and without the assistance of the deployed AI model.

2. Materials and Methods
2.1. Dataset

The dataset utilized in this work comprised a total of 5051 CXRs obtained from the NCID Screening Centre and Tan Tock Seng Hospital (TTSH) in Singapore. CXRs that were conducted between February 2020 and early April 2020 were included in the dataset. Two senior radiologists, each with over 15 years of experience, annotated the class label of the CXRs as pneumonia or non-pneumonia and used them as the reference standard.

All CXRs were reviewed independently by senior radiologists who were unaware of any clinical details.

Patients were classified into three groups based on their clinical presentation and diagnostic results. Patients were classified as positive for COVID-19 pneumonia if they tested positive on the PCR test and had a CXR positive for pneumonia. Patients were classified as having non-COVID-19 pneumonia if their CXR was positive for pneumonia, but they tested negative on the PCR test. The remaining patients were grouped to the non-pneumonia class.

The dataset contained a total of 607 COVID-19 pneumonia cases, 570 cases of non-COVID-19 pneumonia (including viral, bacterial, and fungal pneumonia), and 3874 non-pneumonia cases. To form the training, validation, and test sets, CXRs were chosen randomly from each category within the dataset. These three sets comprised 70%, 10%, and 20% of the total data, respectively. Table 1 provides a summary of the dataset split statistics.

Table 1. Statistics of training, validation, test, and external test sets.

	COVID-19 Pneumonia	Non-COVID-19 Pneumonia	Non-Pneumonia	Total
Training set	425	399	2712	3536
Validation set	61	57	387	505
Test set	121	114	775	1010
External test set	72	49	379	500

2.2. External Test Set

In order to assess the potential of AI assistance to improve the diagnostic accuracy of junior residents, a separate dataset consisting of 500 CXRs were used. This external test set was reviewed by three junior residents with varying levels of training, both with and without the assistance of the developed AI model.

The external dataset was also obtained from the same institution but was collected during a different time period. It included 72 cases of COVID-19 pneumonia, 49 cases of non-COVID-19 pneumonia, and 379 cases of non-pneumonia, as detailed in Table 1.

2.3. Neural Network Architecture and Training Strategy

The workflow of the AI model-aided diagnosis is presented in Figure 1. Initially, we developed an end-to-end CNN-based framework [28] to classify CXRs as non-pneumonia, non-COVID-19 pneumonia, or COVID-19 pneumonia. In the second stage, three junior residents, each with varying levels of training, were enlisted to review the external test set both with and without AI assistance. During the AI-assisted review, the junior residents were provided with the probability output and relevant heatmap for each case, generated by the trained model.

To extract the features of the input CXRs, we employed an EffcientNet-b7 [29] model as the backbone, replacing the output layer with one that includes three neurons with the softmax activation function to output the final predictions. The architecture of the EfficientNet-b7, comprising Block1 to Block7, Stem, and Final Layers, is illustrated in Figure 2. Given the imbalanced patient dataset, we minimized the weighted cross-entropy loss (WCEL) to optimize the AI model as follows:

$$\mathcal{L} = -\sum_{i=1}^{N}\sum_{j=1}^{C} w_j y_{ij} \log(p_{ij}), \tag{1}$$

where N is the number of samples in the dataset, C is the number of classes, w_j is the weight assigned to class j, y_{ij} is the true label for class j of sample i, and p_{ij} is the predicted probability of sample i belonging to class j obtained from the output of the model. In this work, the weight for each class is $w_j = \frac{N}{N_j}$ with N_j as the number of samples in class j.

We trained, validated, and tested our AI model on the internal dataset, choosing the model that displayed the top AUC score during validation to generate probability scores and heatmaps for use in our experiment.

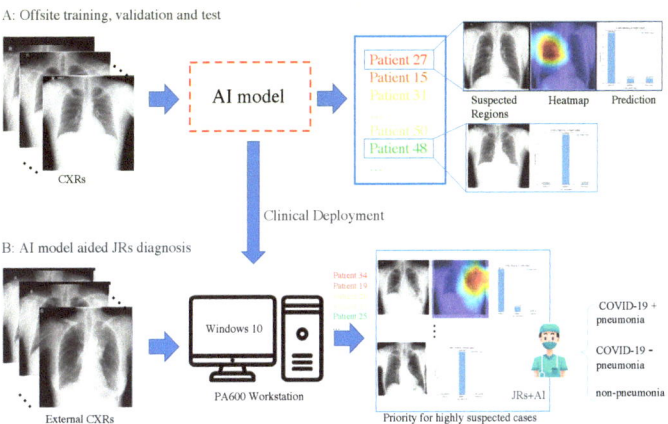

Figure 1. The workflow for training the AI model and conducting AI-aided diagnosis. Stage (**A**) involves training, validating, and testing the AI model for diagnosing CXRs. In Stage (**B**), the trained AI model is deployed in the hospital, and the junior residents (JRs) can upload CXRs to obtain the predictions and heatmaps generated by the AI model. By using AI results, the JRs can make more informed decisions.

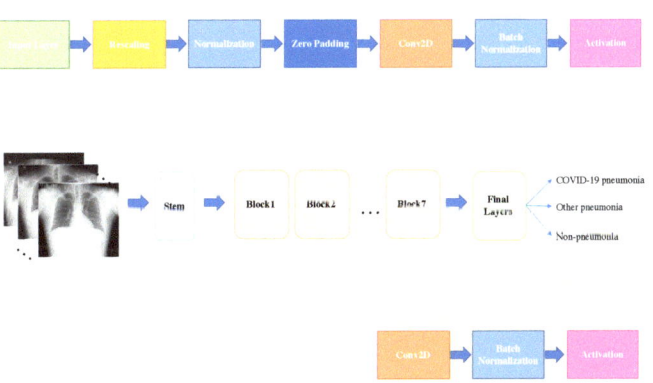

Figure 2. The architecture of EffcientNet-b7 for CXRs classification. The model takes CXRs as inputs and ultimately classifies them into three categories: non-pneumonia, non-COVID-19 pneumonia, and COVID-19 pneumonia.

2.4. AI Model Deployment & Diagnosis

In this study, the trained model was executed on a virtual machine running Ubuntu 18.04, which was hosted on a Windows 10 workstation equipped with two Nvidia 2080Ti GPUs, located within the Department of Diagnostic Radiology. In adherence to the hospital's security guidelines, formal authorization was secured from the Integrated Health Information Systems (IHiS) committee in Singapore, which is in charge of managing the IT risk and security for Tan Tock Seng Hospital.

To evaluate the impact of our AI model in enhancing the performance of junior residents, we recruited three junior residents with varying levels of training for the study. The residents independently reviewed the external dataset of 500 CXRs, initially without the aid of the AI model. After a deliberate 3-month hiatus, the same dataset of 500 CXRs was reviewed by all three junior residents, this time with the aid of AI in the form of probability outputs and relevant heatmaps.

3. Results
3.1. Verify on AI Model

The effectiveness of the developed AI model was verified by comparing it with five deep learning methods [6,30–33] designed for COVID-19 diagnosis using CT scans and CXRs. The performance of our method and the five peer methods for the test set and the external test set in terms of AUC scores (with the macro-averaging strategy) and 95% confidence interval (95% CI) are reported in Table 2, which show that our model outperforms the other five methods significantly, achieving an AUC score of 0.9520 (95% CI: 0.9479–0.9585) for the internal test set and 0.8588 (95% CI: 0.8570–0.8623) for the external test set. Specifically, it improves the AUC score of the peer methods by 1.25% and 4.26% for the test set and the external test set, respectively. This evidence suggests that the proposed AI model demonstrates efficacy in diagnosing pneumonia. All the tested methods demonstrated significant performance degradation on the external test, potentially due to a data distribution mismatch between the TTSH dataset (training, validation, and test set) and the external test set.

The AUC score of our AI model for each of the three classes (non-pneumonia, non-COVID-19 pneumonia, and COVID-19 pneumonia) is reported in Table 3. Our AI model achieved higher AUC scores, sensitivity, and specificity for each class on both the internal and external test sets, outperforming the second-best method (CV19-Net) by a large margin. Specifically, our AI model improves the AUC score of the second-best performing algorithms by 1.63% and 3.40% for the test set and the external test set on COVID-19 pneumonia, respectively. Moreover, our AI model improves the sensitivity and specificity of the peer methods by 1.39% and 7.24% for the external test set on COVID-19 pneumonia, respectively. The comparison of ROC curves is presented in Figure 3. Additionally, examples of heatmaps from Grad-CAM [34] and predictions generated by our model are shown in Figure 4. Our proposed model is capable of generating a set of three images for reference, pertaining to a given case of interest, such as JRs. The first image in the sequence corresponds to the original CXR, which is augmented with blue circles indicating the suspicious area showing signs of possible COVID-19 infection, computed by the AI model. The second image displays the heatmaps obtained from the model's predictions, which are overlaid onto the original CXRs. The regions highlighted by the heatmaps correspond to the anatomical areas that exert the greatest impact on the final model predictions. The final image in the set presents the predicted probabilities for each class, thereby providing an integrated summary of the model's diagnostic accuracy.

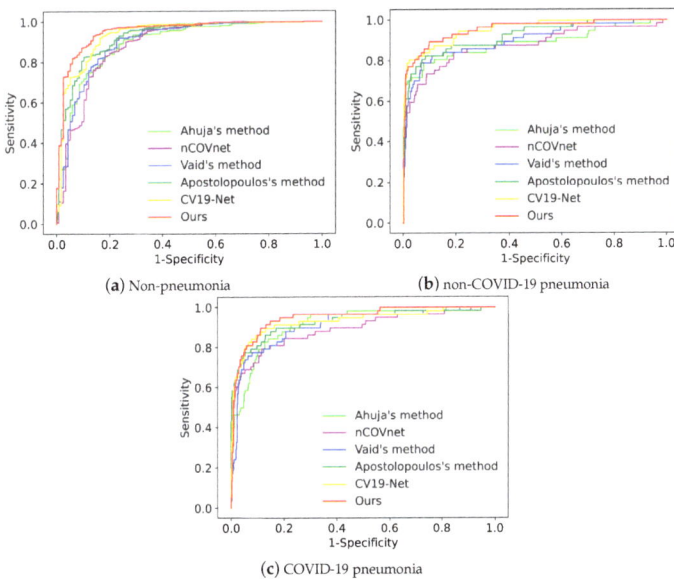

Figure 3. The ROC curve of the peer methods (i.e., Ahuja's method [30], nCOVnet [31], Apostolopoulos's method [33], and CV19-Net [6]) and ours on the three classes.

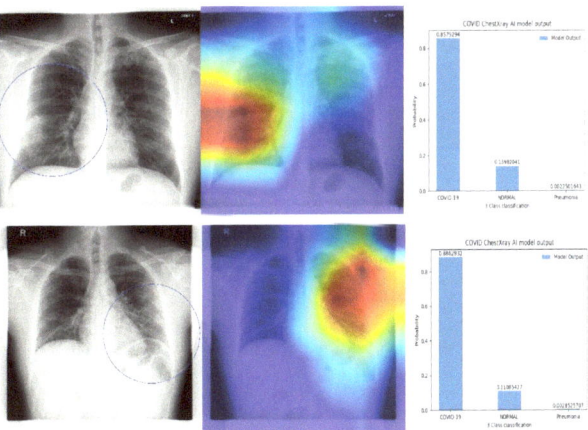

Figure 4. Examples of heatmaps and predictions generated by the AI model. The left-most image displays grayscale chest radiographs with superimposed blue circles indicating the suspicious area showing signs of possible COVID-19 infection based on the AI model's heatmaps. The middle image shows the heatmaps overlaid on the original CXRs, with the highlights indicating the anatomical regions that contribute most to the final model predictions. The right-most image displays the predicted probabilities for each class.

Table 2. Performance comparison of the proposed model with that of peer methods for the test set and the external test set in terms of AUC scores and 95% confidence interval (95% CI).

	Test Set		External Test Set	
	AUC	95% CI	AUC	95% CI
Ahuja's [30]	0.8982	0.8968–0.8993	0.7680	0.7651–0.7704
nCOVnet [31]	0.8876	0.8854–0.8897	0.6837	0.6012–0.6859
Vaid's [32]	0.9021	0.8996–0.9038	0.7402	0.7379–0.7425
Apostolopoulos's [33]	0.9279	0.9229–0.9294	0.8162	0.8145–0.8185
CV19-Net [6]	0.9395	0.9361–0.9407	0.7987	0.7952–0.8032
Ours	0.9520 *	0.9479–0.9585	0.8588 *	0.8570–0.8623

* Denotes statistically significant ($p > 0.05$). AUC = the area under the receiver operating characteristic.

Table 3. Performance comparison for each class on the test set and the external test set in terms of AUC scores, Sensitivity, and Specificity.

		Test Set			External Test Set		
		AUC	Sensitivity	Specificity	AUC	Sensitivity	Specificity
Ahuja's [30]	COVID-19 pneumonia	0.9185	0.8966	0.7768	0.7309	0.7361	0.5491
	Non-COVID-19 pneumonia	0.8886	0.8421	0.8136	0.7762	0.7755	0.6408
	Non-pneumonia	0.8964	0.8429	0.8000	0.7740	0.7784	0.6116
nCOVnet [31]	COVID-19 pneumonia	0.8897	0.8793	0.7312	0.6437	0.7083	0.5117
	Non-COVID-19 pneumonia	0.8817	0.8639	0.7739	0.7251	0.7347	0.5322
	Non-pneumonia	0.8882	0.8596	0.7864	0.6860	0.7230	0.5124
Vaid's [32]	COVID-19 pneumonia	0.9088	0.8448	0.8064	0.7154	0.7500	0.6005
	Non-COVID-19 pneumonia	0.9024	0.8421	0.8500	0.7387	0.6735	0.5854
	Non-pneumonia	0.9010	0.8613	0.8087	0.7451	0.7704	0.5785
Apostolopoulos's [33]	COVID-19 pneumonia	0.9284	0.8793	0.8497	0.7856	0.7917	0.6519
	Non-COVID-19 pneumonia	0.9234	0.8772	0.8182	0.7938	0.7347	0.7251
	Non-pneumonia	0.9285	0.8586	0.8174	0.8250	0.7863	0.7438
CV19-Net [6]	COVID-19 pneumonia	0.9327	0.8966	0.8360	0.7787	0.8194	0.5958
	Non-COVID-19 pneumonia	0.9565	0.8947	0.8091	0.7882	0.7959	0.5987
	Non-pneumonia	0.9380	0.9241	0.8261	0.8038	0.8470	0.6033
Ours	COVID-19 pneumonia	0.9490	0.9310	0.8519	0.8196	0.8333	0.7243
	Non-COVID-19 pneumonia	0.9541	0.9123	0.8500	0.8348	0.8776	0.7073
	Non-pneumonia	0.9522	0.9338	0.8261	0.8694	0.8918	0.6446

3.2. AI-Aided Diagnosis

In order to investigate the extent to which the proposed AI model improves the performance of junior residents (JRs), we conducted a comparison of the performances of the JRs with and without AI assistance, as presented in Table 4. The JRs who participated in this study possessed varying levels of expertise. Specifically, JR1, JR2, and JR3 had approximately 6 months, 1 year, and more than 2 years of experience in interpreting CXRs, respectively. The results indicate that the performance of the junior residents improved in proportion to their level of training. Even without AI assistance, the JR with the most experience (JR3) achieved an AUC score of 0.8657 (95% CI: 0.8633–0.8676), while the JR with the least experience (JR1) attained an AUC score of 0.7813 (95% CI: 0.7785–0.7827). Following AI augmentation, we observed improvements for both JR1 and JR2, achieving AUC scores of 0.8482 (95% CI: 0.8452–0.8511) and 0.8511 (95% CI: 0.8493–0.8526), respectively. Additionally, Table 4 presents Cohen's kappa score for each JR, with the scores of JR1 (0.5574) and JR2 (0.4651) being smaller than that of JR3 (0.7400), indicating that the AI model had a greater impact on JR1 and JR2 compared to JR3. The detailed performance of all JRs before and after AI assistance is presented in Table 5. From Table 5 we can find that: with the AI model's assistance, the JR1's sensitivity has been improved from 0.3889 to 0.6250 on COVID-19 pneumonia diagnosis, the specificity has been improved from 0.7317 to 0.9002 on non-COVID-19 pneumonia, the AUC score has been improved from 0.8121 to 0.8417 and the specificity has been improved from 0.9091 to 0.9339 on non-pneumonia. JR2's sensitivity has been improved from 0.5000 to 0.5833 on COVID-19 pneumonia diagnosis, the specificity has been improved from 0.8226 to 0.8514 on non-COVID-19 pneumonia, and the specificity has been improved from 0.9008 to 0.9835 on non-pneumonia. Notably, even JR3 with higher training level, the AI model was found to improve sensitivity, from 0.8681 to 0.8902, demonstrating the broad applicability and effectiveness of the model.

Table 4. Performance comparison of JRs and JRs+AI for the external test set in terms of AUC score, 95% confidence interval (95% CI), and Cohen's kappa score.

Expertise Level	JR1 (~6 Months)		JR2 (~1 Year)		JR3 (>2 Year)	
	w/o AI	+AI	w/o AI	+AI	w/o AI	+AI
AUC	0.7813	0.8482 *	0.8214	0.8511 *	0.8657	0.8609
95% CI	0.7785–0.7827	0.8452–0.8511	0.8197–0.8232	0.8493–0.8526	0.8633–0.8676	0.8585–0.8624
Cohen's kappa score [1]	0.5574		0.4651		0.7400	

* Denotes statistically significant ($p > 0.05$). [1] 0.41–0.60 moderate agreement, 0.61–0.80 substantial agreement.

Table 5. Performance comparison for each class on the test set and the external test set in terms of AUC scores, Sensitivity, and Specificity.

		JRs			JRs+AI		
		AUC	Sensitivity	Specificity	AUC	Sensitivity	Specificity
JR1 ~ 6 months	COVID-19 pneumonia	0.6524	0.3889	0.9159	0.7424	0.6250	0.8598
	Non-COVID-19 pneumonia	0.7026	0.6735	0.7317	0.6848	0.4694	0.9002
	Non-pneumonia	0.8121	0.7150	0.9091	0.8878	0.8417	0.9339
JR2 ~ 1 year	COVID-19 pneumonia	0.7079	0.5000	0.9159	0.7239	0.5833	0.8645
	Non-COVID-19 pneumonia	0.6868	0.5510	0.8226	0.6604	0.4694	0.8514
	Non- pneumonia	0.8581	0.8153	0.9008	0.8981	0.8127	0.9835
JR3 > 2 years	COVID-19 pneumonia	0.7681	0.6250	0.9112	0.7542	0.5972	0.9112
	Non-COVID-19 pneumonia	0.7518	0.6122	0.8914	0.7693	0.5918	0.9468
	Non- pneumonia	0.8968	0.8681	0.9256	0.8902	0.9208	0.8595

4. Discussion

Several recent studies have highlighted the potential of chest CT in diagnosing COVID-19 pneumonia, particularly in its early stages [35,36]. However, in healthcare systems with limited resources, CT may not always be available, and CXR is the more commonly used imaging method in clinical practice. Additionally, concerns have been raised by international workgroups regarding the untested specificity of CT in cases where the pretest probability of COVID-19 infection is low, and CXR is preferred to reduce the risk of nosocomial transmission [37–39]. Recent reports have demonstrated that CXR findings correlate well with clinical severity and can be used to predict severe pneumonia [24]. Therefore, the development of AI models that aid in diagnosing COVID-19 pneumonia using CXRs remains an area of active research and is of significant importance.

Junior residents are often the first healthcare professionals to interpret CXRs for suspected COVID-19 patients in clinical practice. However, interpreting CXRs can be challenging, especially when the radiological report may impact patient disposition. This study presents an AI model capable of performing three-class classification for non-pneumonia, non-COVID-19 pneumonia, and COVID-19 pneumonia. The proposed model demonstrates superiority in AUC score, sensitivity, and specificity compared to five peer methods. Although all methods experience performance degradation when tested on the external test set, our model performs better, achieving an AUC score of 0.8594 (95% CI: 0.8594–0.8602), and outperforming the second-best method by a large margin [33].

This study provides compelling evidence for the potential of a trained AI model to enhance the diagnostic performance of junior residents in the field of chest radiography by providing probability outputs and heatmaps. Although previous studies have investigated the augmentation of radiologists' performance using AI in distinguishing COVID-19 from other types of pneumonia on chest CTs [40], this study specifically focuses on the performance of junior residents, which may have significant implications for both diagnostic imaging and education. The participating JRs possessed varying levels of expertise, with JR1, JR2, and JR3 having approximately 6 months, 1 year, and more than 2 years of experience in interpreting CXRs, respectively. The findings suggest that the performance of the junior residents improved in proportion to their level of training. Furthermore, in addition to the quantitative improvements observed, all three junior residents reported increased confidence when using AI assistance, suggesting that AI may have positive qualitative outcomes as well.

In this study, the adoption of EfficientNet as the backbone for diagnosing COVID-19 pneumonia, and non-COVID-19 pneumonia from CXRs was proposed. Although the model achieved promising performance for the test set and improved decision-making for junior residents, several limitations were noted. Specifically, a significant decrease in performance was observed on the external test set, which is not unique to our method but common in medical image analysis due to domain shift problems [41–43]. The training process did not account for differences in data distributions between the TTSH dataset and the external test set, leading to a drop in performance. Medical datasets are often drawn from different domains, even within the same institution, which can pose challenges for deep learning models that assume similar data distributions between training and test sets [43]. Deep learning typically assumes that both the distributions of the training and test sets are similar [44]. If the distributions of both datasets are dissimilar, the performance may drop dramatically. In future work, domain adaption techniques will be explored to align the distributions of different datasets for automated disease diagnoses from CXRs. Furthermore, a purposeful 3-month hiatus was implemented, during which three JRs were tasked with interpreting the same dataset of 500 CXRs with and without AI assistance. Over this three-month period, the diagnostic abilities of the JRs may have improved, potentially influencing the accuracy enhancement achieved when using AI as an assistant.

In summary, our proposed method exhibited a high degree of accuracy in performing a three-class classification of non-pneumonia, non-COVID-19 pneumonia, and COVID-19 pneumonia. Furthermore, the method was observed to improve the diagnostic performance of junior residents in identifying COVID-19 pneumonia on CXRs, a potentially valuable asset in triage and education during the ongoing pandemic.

5. Conclusions

This study proposes an AI model that utilizes EfficientNet-b7 [29] as the backbone to differentiate non-pneumonia, non-COVID-19 pneumonia, and COVID-19 pneumonia from CXRs. The training dataset was collected from Tan Tock Seng Hospital and was annotated by experienced senior radiologists. This study showcases the innovative creation of an AI model for three-category CXR classification, emphasizing its ability to enhance the diagnostic precision of less experienced residents. Validated with external data, the model demonstrates practical relevance in real-world scenarios. Upon deployment, the AI model demonstrated its ability to assist junior residents in CXR interpretation and increase their confidence in diagnostic accuracy. Although the proposed AI model improved the performance of junior residents, a performance drop was observed on the external test in comparison to the results on the test set. It indicated that there has been a domain shift between the collected patient dataset (including the training, validation, and test set) and the external dataset. Domain shift is a common issue in practical applications of AI, especially in clinical practice. The clinical practice presents much more heterogeneous acquisition conditions [17] which may lead to the performance of the trained model on external test datasets (or a dataset it encounters when deployed) degrading.

To address the domain gap issue between the training dataset and the external test dataset, we plan to investigate and develop a test-time training domain adaptation model in future work. This model will aim to align the tested CXR in real time with the training data, which is expected to enhance the model's performance after deployment. By aligning the test CXR with the training dataset, the test-time training domain adaptation model is expected to be more effective and mitigate performance degradation to a large extent. Moreover, it is expected to be more robust to the changing acquisition conditions during CXR screening.

Author Contributions: Conceptualization, X.X.; methodology, Y.F. and J.S.Z.T.; software, W.-X.C.; validation, Y.W., C.B.K., E.O.T.E. and H.I.T.W.J.; formal analysis, Z.W. and L.Z.; investigation, Y.C.; resources, Y.T.; data curation, X.L.; writing—original draft preparation, Y.F.; writing—review and editing, J.S.Z.T.; visualization, S.L.; supervision, C.H.T.; project administration, R.S.M.G.; funding acquisition, Y.L. and R.S.M.G. All authors have reviewed and approved the published version of the manuscript.

Funding: This research was supported by A*STAR through its AME Programmatic Funding Scheme Under Project grant number A20H4b0141.

Institutional Review Board Statement: This research obtained approval from the relevant organizations' ethics committees (Approval code: 2017/00683-AMD0005) and adhered to the Health Insurance Portability and Accountability Act regulations. Owing to the study's retrospective design and low associated risks, permission to waive consent was granted.

Informed Consent Statement: Not applicable.

Data Availability Statement: The data are not publicly available due to privacy restrictions.

Conflicts of Interest: All authors declared no conflict of interest.

References

1. Lai, C.C.; Shih, T.P.; Ko, W.C.; Tang, H.J.; Hsueh, P.R. Severe acute respiratory syndrome coronavirus 2 (SARS-CoV-2) and coronavirus disease-2019 (COVID-19): The epidemic and the challenges. *Int. J. Antimicrob. Agents* **2020**, *55*, 105924. [CrossRef] [PubMed]
2. Zu, Z.Y.; Jiang, M.D.; Xu, P.P.; Chen, W.; Ni, Q.Q.; Lu, G.M.; Zhang, L.J. Coronavirus disease 2019 (COVID-19): A perspective from China. *Radiology* **2020**, *296*, E15–E25. [CrossRef] [PubMed]
3. Facilities and Services, National Centre for Infectious Diseases (NCID). Available online: https://www.ncid.sg/Facilities-Services/Pages/default.aspx (accessed on 21 October 2022).
4. UPDATES ON COVID-19 (CORONAVIRUS DISEASE 2019) LOCAL SITUATION, Ministry of Health. Available online: https://www.moh.gov.sg/COVID-19/statistics (accessed on 26 February 2023).
5. Kooraki, S.; Hosseiny, M.; Myers, L.; Gholamrezanezhad, A. Coronavirus (COVID 19) outbreak: What the department of radiology should know. *J. Am. Coll. Radiol.* **2020**, *17*, 447–451. [CrossRef]
6. Zhang, R.; Tie, X.; Qi, Z.; Bevins, N.B.; Zhang, C.; Griner, D.; Song, T.K.; Nadig, J.D.; Schiebler, M.L.; Garrett, J.W.; et al. Diagnosis of COVID-19 Pneumonia Using Chest Radiography: Value of Artificial Intelligence. *Radiology* **2020**, *24*, 202944.
7. Pereira, R.M.; Bertolini, D.; Teixeira, L.O.; Silla, C.N., Jr.; Costa, Y.M. COVID-19 identification in chest X-ray images on flat and hierarchical classification scenarios. *Comput. Methods Programs Biomed.* **2020**, *8*, 105532. [CrossRef]
8. Rahimzadeh, M.; Attar, A. A modified deep convolutional neural network for detecting COVID-19 and pneumonia from chest X-ray images based on the concatenation of Xception and ResNet50V2. *Inform. Med. Unlocked* **2020**, *26*, 100360. [CrossRef]
9. Khan, I.U.; Aslam, N.; Anwar, T.; Alsaif, H.S.; Chrouf, S.M.B.; Alzahrani, N.A.; Alamoudi, F.A.; Kamaleldin, M.M.A.; Awary, K.B. Using a deep learning model to explore the impact of clinical data on COVID-19 diagnosis using chest X-ray. *Sensors* **2022**, *22*, 669. [CrossRef] [PubMed]
10. Ai, T.; Yang, Z.; Hou, H.; Zhan, C.; Chen, C.; Lv, W.; Tao, Q.; Sun, Z.; Xia, L. Correlation of chest CT and RT-PCR testing in coronavirus disease 2019 (COVID-19) in China: A report of 1014 cases. *Radiology* **2020**, *26*, 200642. [CrossRef]
11. Stephanie, S.; Shum, T.; Clevel, H.; Challa, S.R.; Herring, A.; Jacobson, F.L.; Hatabu, H.; Byrne, S.C.; Shashi, K.; Araki, T.; et al. Determinants of Chest X-Ray Sensitivity for COVID-19: A Multi-Institutional Study in the United States. *Radiol. Cardiothorac. Imaging* **2020**, *2*, e200337. [CrossRef]

12. Rubin, G.D.; Ryerson, C.J.; Haramati, L.B.; Sverzellati, N.; Kanne, J.P.; Raoof, S.; Schluger, N.W.; Volpi, A.; Yim, J.J.; Martin, I.B.; et al. The role of chest imaging in patient management during the COVID-19 pandemic: A multinational consensus statement from the Fleischner Society. *Radiology* **2020**, *296*, 172–180. [CrossRef]
13. Hayden, G.E.; Wrenn, K.W. Chest radiograph vs. computed tomography scan in the evaluation for pneumonia. *J. Emerg. Med.* **2009**, *36*, 266–270. [CrossRef]
14. Li, Y.; Xia, L. Coronavirus disease 2019 (COVID-19): Role of chest CT in diagnosis and management. *Am. J. Roentgenol.* **2020**, *214*, 1280–1286. [CrossRef] [PubMed]
15. Gaur, L.; Bhatia, U.; Jhanjhi, N.Z.; Muhammad, G.; Masud, M. Medical image-based detection of COVID-19 using deep convolution neural networks. *Multimed. Syst.* **2021**, *28*, 1–10. [CrossRef]
16. Wong, H.Y.; Lam, H.Y.; Fong, A.H.; Leung, S.T.; Chin, T.W.; Lo, C.S.; Lui, M.M.; Lee, J.C.; Chiu, K.W.; Chung, T.; et al. Frequency and distribution of chest radiographic findings in COVID-19 positive patients. *Radiology* **2020**, *27*, 201160. [CrossRef] [PubMed]
17. Feng, Y.; Wang, Z.; Xu, X.; Wang, Y.; Fu, H.; Li, S.; Zhen, L.; Lei, X.; Cui, Y.; Ting, J.S.; et al. Contrastive domain adaptation with consistency match for automated pneumonia diagnosis. *Med. Image Anal.* **2023**, *83*, 102664. [CrossRef]
18. Wang, Y.; Feng, Y.; Zhang, L.; Zhou, J.T.; Liu, Y.; Goh, R.S.; Zhen, L. Adversarial multimodal fusion with attention mechanism for skin lesion classification using clinical and dermoscopic images. *Med. Image Anal.* **2022**, *81*, 102535. [CrossRef] [PubMed]
19. Feng, Y.; Xu, X.; Wang, Y.; Lei, X.; Teo, S.K.; Sim, J.Z.; Ting, Y.; Zhen, L.; Zhou, J.T.; Liu, Y.; et al. Deep supervised domain adaptation for pneumonia diagnosis from chest x-ray images. *IEEE J. Biomed. Health Inform.* **2021**, *26*, 1080–1090. [CrossRef]
20. El-Rashidy, N.; Abdelrazik, S.; Abuhmed, T.; Amer, E.; Ali, F.; Hu, J.W.; El-Sappagh, S. Comprehensive survey of using machine learning in the COVID-19 pandemic. *Diagnostics* **2021**, *11*, 1155. [CrossRef]
21. Hertel, R.; Benlamri, R. Deep learning techniques for COVID-19 diagnosis and prognosis based on radiological imaging. *ACM Comput. Surv.* **2023**, *55*, 1–39. [CrossRef]
22. Sim, J.Z.; Ting, Y.H.; Tang, Y.; Feng, Y.; Lei, X.; Wang, X.; Chen, W.X.; Huang, Z.; Wong, S.T.; Lu, Z.; et al. Diagnostic performance of a deep learning model deployed at a national COVID-19 screening facility for detection of pneumonia on frontal chest radiographs. *Healthcare* **2022**, *10*, 175. [CrossRef]
23. Azad, A.K.; Ahmed, I.; Ahmed, M.U. In Search of an Efficient and Reliable Deep Learning Model for Identification of COVID-19 Infection from Chest X-ray Images. *Diagnostics* **2023**, *13*, 574. [CrossRef]
24. Wang, L.; Lin, Z.Q.; Wong, A. Covid-net: A tailored deep convolutional neural network design for detection of COVID-19 cases from chest X-ray images. *Sci. Rep.* **2020**, *10*, 19549. [CrossRef] [PubMed]
25. Narin, A.; Kaya, C.; Pamuk, Z. Automatic detection of coronavirus disease (COVID-19) using x-ray images and deep convolutional neural networks. *Pattern Anal. Appl.* **2021**, *24*, 1207–1220. [CrossRef]
26. Zhang, J.; Xie, Y.; Li, Y.; Shen, C.; Xia, Y. Covid-19 screening on chest x-ray images using deep learning based anomaly detection. *arXiv* **2020**, arXiv:2003.12338.
27. Kitamura, G.; Deible, C. Retraining an open-source pneumothorax detecting machine learning algorithm for improved performance to medical images. *Clin. Imaging* **2020**, *61*, 15–19. [CrossRef] [PubMed]
28. Goodfellow, I.; Bengio, Y.; Courville, A. *Deep Learning*; MIT Press: Cambridge, UK, 2016; Volume 1, No. 2.
29. Tan, M.; Le Q. Efficientnet: Rethinking model scaling for convolutional neural networks. In Proceedings of the International Conference on Machine Learning, Long Beach, CA, USA, 9–15 June 2019; pp. 6105–6114.
30. Ahuja, S.; Panigrahi, B.K.; Dey, N.; Rajinikanth, V.; Gandhi, T.K. Deep transfer learning-based automated detection of COVID-19 from lung CT scan slices. *Appl. Intell.* **2021**, *51*, 571–585. [CrossRef]
31. Panwar, H.; Gupta, P.K.; Siddiqui, M.K.; Morales-Menendez, R.; Singh, V. Application of deep learning for fast detection of COVID-19 in X-Rays using nCOVnet. *Chaos Solitons Fractals* **2020**, *138*, 109944. [CrossRef]
32. Vaid, S.; Kalantar, R.; Bhandari, M. Deep learning COVID-19 detection bias: Accuracy through artificial intelligence. *Int. Orthop.* **2020**, *44*, 1539–1542. [CrossRef]
33. Apostolopoulos, I.D.; Mpesiana, T.A. COVID-19: Automatic detection from X-ray images utilizing transfer learning with convolutional neural networks. *Phys. Eng. Sci. Med.* **2020**, *43*, 635–640. [CrossRef]
34. Selvaraju, R.R.; Cogswell, M.; Das, A.; Vedantam, R.; Parikh, D.; Batra, D. Grad-cam: Visual explanations from deep networks via gradient-based localization. In Proceedings of the IEEE International Conference on Computer Vision, Venice, Italy, 22–29 October 2017; pp. 618–626.
35. Kang, H.; Xia, L.; Yan, F.; Wan, Z.; Shi, F.; Yuan, H.; Jiang, H.; Wu, D.; Sui, H.; Zhang, C.; et al. Diagnosis of coronavirus disease 2019 (COVID-19) with structured latent multi-view representation learning. *IEEE Trans. Med. Imaging* **2020**, *39*, 2606–2614. [CrossRef]
36. Han, R.; Huang, L.; Jiang, H.; Dong, J.; Peng, H.; Zhang, D. Early clinical and CT manifestations of coronavirus disease 2019 (COVID-19) pneumonia. *AJR Am. J. Roentgenol.* **2020**, *215*, 338–343. [CrossRef] [PubMed]
37. Revel, M.P.; Parkar, A.P.; Prosch, H.; Silva, M.; Sverzellati, N.; Gleeson, F.; Brady, A.; European Society of Radiology (ESR) and the European Society of Thoracic Imaging (ESTI). COVID-19 patients and the Radiology department—Advice from the European Society of Radiology (ESR) and the European Society of Thoracic Imaging (ESTI). *Eur. Radiol.* **2020**, *30*, 4903–4909. [CrossRef] [PubMed]

38. Nair, A.; Rodrigues, J.C.; Hare, S.; Edey, A.; Devaraj, A.; Jacob, J.; Johnstone, A.; McStay, R.; Denton, E.; Robinson, G. A British Society of Thoracic Imaging statement: Considerations in designing local imaging diagnostic algorithms for the COVID-19 pandemic. *Clin. Radiol.* **2020**, *75*, 329–334. [CrossRef] [PubMed]
39. Skulstad, H.; Cosyns, B.; Popescu, B.A.; Galderisi, M.; Salvo, G.D.; Donal, E.; Petersen, S.; Gimelli, A.; Haugaa, K.H.; Muraru, D.; et al. COVID-19 pandemic and cardiac imaging: EACVI recommendations on precautions, indications, prioritization, and protection for patients and healthcare personnel. *Eur. Heart J.-Cardiovasc. Imaging* **2020**, *21*, 592–598. [CrossRef]
40. Bai, H.X.; Wang, R.; Xiong, Z.; Hsieh, B.; Chang, K.; Halsey, K.; Tran, T.M.L.; Choi, J.W.; Wang, D.-C.; Shi, L.-B.; et al. AI augmentation of radiologist performance in distinguishing COVID-19 from pneumonia of other etiology on chest CT. *Radiology* **2020**, *296*, 201491. [CrossRef]
41. Sun, B.; Feng, J.; Saenko, K. Return of frustratingly easy domain adaptation. In Proceedings of the AAAI Conference on Artificial Intelligence, Phoenix, AZ, USA, 12–17 February 2016; Volume 30, No. 1.
42. Kamnitsas, K.; Baumgartner, C.; Ledig, C.; Newcombe, V.; Simpson, J.; Kane, A.; Menon, D.; Nori, A.; Criminisi, A.; Rueckert, D.; et al. Unsupervised domain adaptation in brain lesion segmentation with adversarial networks. In Proceedings of the 25th International Conference on Information Processing in Medical Imaging, IPMI 2017, Boone, NC, USA, 25–30 June 2017; Springer International Publishing: Cham, Switzerland, 2017; pp. 597–609.
43. Varsavsky, T.; Orbes-Arteaga, M.; Sudre, C.H.; Graham, M.S.; Nachev, P.; Cardoso, M.J. Test-time unsupervised domain adaptation. In Proceedings of the 23rd International Conference on Medical Image Computing and Computer Assisted Intervention–MICCAI 2020, Lima, Peru, 4–8 October 2020; Springer International Publishing: Cham, Switzerland, 2020; pp. 428–436.
44. Wang, X.; Liang, G.; Zhang, Y.; Blanton, H.; Bessinger, Z.; Jacobs, N. Inconsistent performance of deep learning models on mammogram classification. *J. Am. Coll. Radiol.* **2020**, *17*, 796–803. [CrossRef]

Disclaimer/Publisher's Note: The statements, opinions and data contained in all publications are solely those of the individual author(s) and contributor(s) and not of MDPI and/or the editor(s). MDPI and/or the editor(s) disclaim responsibility for any injury to people or property resulting from any ideas, methods, instructions or products referred to in the content.

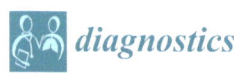

Article

Developing a Deep-Learning-Based Coronary Artery Disease Detection Technique Using Computer Tomography Images

Abdul Rahaman Wahab Sait [1,*] and Ashit Kumar Dutta [2]

[1] Department of Documents and Archive, Center of Documents and Administrative Communication, King Faisal University, P.O. Box 400, Hofuf 31982, Al-Ahsa, Saudi Arabia
[2] Department of Computer Science and Information Systems, College of Applied Sciences, AlMaarefa University, Riyadh 13713, Saudi Arabia
* Correspondence: asait@kfu.edu.sa

Abstract: Coronary artery disease (CAD) is one of the major causes of fatalities across the globe. The recent developments in convolutional neural networks (CNN) allow researchers to detect CAD from computed tomography (CT) images. The CAD detection model assists physicians in identifying cardiac disease at earlier stages. The recent CAD detection models demand a high computational cost and a more significant number of images. Therefore, this study intends to develop a CNN-based CAD detection model. The researchers apply an image enhancement technique to improve the CT image quality. The authors employed You look only once (YOLO) V7 for extracting the features. Aquila optimization is used for optimizing the hyperparameters of the UNet++ model to predict CAD. The proposed feature extraction technique and hyperparameter tuning approach reduces the computational costs and improves the performance of the UNet++ model. Two datasets are utilized for evaluating the performance of the proposed CAD detection model. The experimental outcomes suggest that the proposed method achieves an accuracy, recall, precision, F1-score, Matthews correlation coefficient, and Kappa of 99.4, 98.5, 98.65, 98.6, 95.35, and 95 and 99.5, 98.95, 98.95, 98.95, 96.35, and 96.25 for datasets 1 and 2, respectively. In addition, the proposed model outperforms the recent techniques by obtaining the area under the receiver operating characteristic and precision-recall curve of 0.97 and 0.95, and 0.96 and 0.94 for datasets 1 and 2, respectively. Moreover, the proposed model obtained a better confidence interval and standard deviation of [98.64–98.72] and 0.0014, and [97.41–97.49] and 0.0019 for datasets 1 and 2, respectively. The study's findings suggest that the proposed model can support physicians in identifying CAD with limited resources.

Keywords: coronary artery disease; UNet++; cardiac arrests; convolutional neural networks; hyperparameter tuning

Citation: Wahab Sait, A.R.; Dutta, A.K. Developing a Deep-Learning-Based Coronary Artery Disease Detection Technique Using Computer Tomography Images. *Diagnostics* 2023, 13, 1312. https://doi.org/10.3390/diagnostics13071312

Academic Editors: Sivaramakrishnan Rajaraman, Zhiyun Xue and Sameer Antani

Received: 28 February 2023
Revised: 26 March 2023
Accepted: 30 March 2023
Published: 31 March 2023

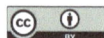

Copyright: © 2023 by the authors. Licensee MDPI, Basel, Switzerland. This article is an open access article distributed under the terms and conditions of the Creative Commons Attribution (CC BY) license (https://creativecommons.org/licenses/by/4.0/).

1. Introduction

Across the globe, cardiovascular diseases (CVD) are the leading cause of mortality, which accounts for an estimated 17.9 million deaths annually [1]. The most prevalent form of CVD is coronary artery disease (CAD), which frequently results in cardiac arrest. Coronary artery blockage leads to heart failure [2–7]. The heart relies on blood flow from the coronary arteries [8]. In developing countries, heart disease diagnosis and treatment are difficult due to the limited number of medical resources and professionals [9]. In order to avoid further damage to the patient, there is a demand for practical diagnostic tools and techniques. Both economically developed and underdeveloped nations are experiencing significant surges in the number of deaths from CVD [10]. Early CAD identification can save lives and lower healthcare costs [11–16]. Developing a reliable and non-invasive approach for early CAD identification is desirable. During the past few years, practitioners have significantly increased their utilization of computer technology to make decisions [17].

Physicians utilize conventional invasive methods to diagnose heart disease based on a patient's medical history, physical tests, and symptoms [18]. Angiography is one of the most precise approaches for analyzing heart issues using conventional methods. However, it has a few limitations, such as a high cost, multiple side effects, and the requirement for extensive technological expertise [19]. Due to human error, conventional approaches frequently result in inaccurate diagnoses and additional delays. The coronary artery assessment through computed tomography (CT) is called coronary CT angiography (CCTA). A high-speed CT scan is performed on the cardiovascular system by administering a contrast agent through the intravenous route to the patient [20,21]. CCTA is used to identify atherosclerotic disease and evaluate abnormalities in the heart or blood vessels [22].

Machine learning (ML) is rapidly emerging as a game-changing tool for improving patient diagnoses in the healthcare sector [17]. It is an analytical method for huge and challenging programming tasks, including information transformation from medical records, pandemic forecasting, and genetic data analysis. Several studies suggest multiple approaches for identifying cardiac issues using machine learning [23–26]. The ML approach consists of several processes, including image preprocessing, feature extraction, training and parameter tuning, evaluating the model, and subsequently making predictions using the model. The classifier's performance is based on the feature selection process. Several metrics have been described in the recent literature [27] for the evaluation of the ML-based model. These metrics include accuracy, sensitivity, specificity, and F1-score. Healthcare practitioners are primarily concerned about the ML-based model's reliability and performance [28]. In addition, simplicity, interpretability, and computational complexity are essential criteria for implementing the CAD detection model in healthcare centers [29].

Deep learning (DL) is a relatively new ML technique with great promise for various classification problems [30]. DL offers a practical approach to building an end-to-end model using the raw medical image to predict a crucial disease [31]. In particular, the CNN model outperforms other methods in several image categorization problems. CNN identifies the key features and classifies images [32]. However, image annotation is one of the critical phases in medical image classification. High dataset dimensionality is a crucial issue for ML approaches [33]. The algorithm's performance can be improved by weighting features, which reduce redundant data and prevent overfitting [33–37].

Alothman A. F. et al. [4] developed a CAD detection model using the DL technique. They employed the CNN model for classifying the CCTA images. In [7], the authors contributed to developing an automated classifier for patients with congestive heart failure. This classifier differentiates between individuals with a low risk and those with a high risk of complications. In [9], the authors presented a deep neural network technique for categorizing electrocardiogram data. The authors of [10] developed a clinical decision support system to evaluate heart failure. The researchers examined the efficacy of several ML classifiers, including neural networks, support vector machines, fuzzy rule systems, and random forest.

The existing CAD detection models demand high computational costs and training time for producing a reasonable outcome. It requires valuable features to identify an image's key pattern. The recent models face difficulties in overcoming underfitting and overfitting issues. In addition, an effective feature extraction technique and hyperparameter-tuned CNN model can address the shortcomings of the existing CAD detection models. Therefore, this study intends to develop a CAD detection model using a CNN technique. The contributions of the study are:

1. An image enhancement technique to improve the quality of the CT images.
2. An intelligent feature extraction approach for extracting key features.
3. A hyperparameter-tuned CNN technique for identifying CAD.

The remaining part of the paper is organized as follows: Section 2 presents the methodology of the proposed study. It highlights the research phases, dataset characteristics, and hyperparameter-tuning process. Section 3 outlines the experimental results on CCTA datasets. Section 4 discusses the study's contribution and limitations. Finally, Section 5 concludes the study with its future directions.

2. Materials and Methods

The proposed CAD detection model uses the CNN technique for identifying CAD from the CT images. Figure 1 highlights the proposed CAD detection model. It contains image enhancement, feature extraction, and hyperparameter-tuned UNet++ models for predicting CAD using CCTA images.

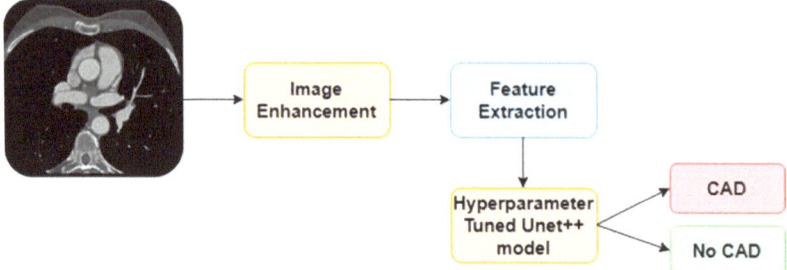

Figure 1. Proposed CAD detection model.

2.1. Dataset Characteristics

A total of two datasets are employed to train the models. Dataset 1 is publicly available in the repository [5]. The CCTA images of 500 patients are stored in the dataset. The images are classified into normal (50%) and abnormal (50%). The image is represented in 18 multiple views of a straightened coronary artery. The images are divided into training, validation, and test images. The authors have included 2364 images to balance the dataset.

The 3D CCTA images of 1000 patients are deposited in dataset 2. The images were captured using a Siemens 128-slice dual-source scanner. The size of the images is $512 \times 512 \times (206\text{--}275)$ voxels. The images were collected from the Guangdong Provincial People's hospital between April 2012 and December 2018. The average ages of females and males were 59.98 and 57.68 years, respectively. The dataset repository [6] is publicly available for the researchers. In addition, it offers an image segmentation method for extracting images of coronary arteries from raw 3D images. Figure 2a,b are the raw images of datasets 1 and 2, respectively. Table 1 presents the characteristics of the dataset.

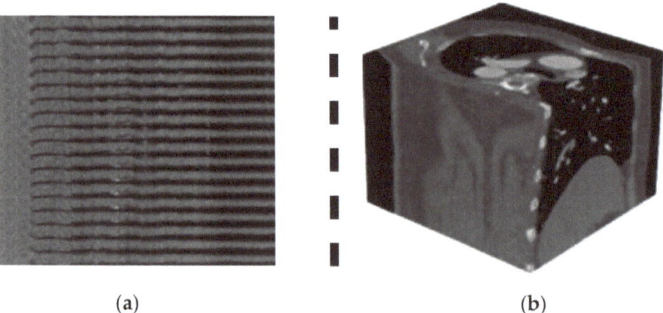

Figure 2. (a) Dataset 1. (b) Dataset 2.

Table 1. Dataset characteristics.

Dataset	Number of Images	Number of Patients	CAD	No CAD	Classifications
Dataset 1	2364	500	1182	1182	2
Dataset 2	1000	1000	503	497	2

2.2. Proposed Methodology

Figure 3 highlights the research phases of the study. Phase 1 outlines the image preprocessing and feature extraction processes. Phase 2 describes the processes for classifying the CCTA images into CAD and No CAD. In this phase, the Aquila optimization (AO) algorithm [21] is employed for tuning the hyperparameters of the UNet++ model. Lastly, phase 3 presents the performance evaluation of the proposed model.

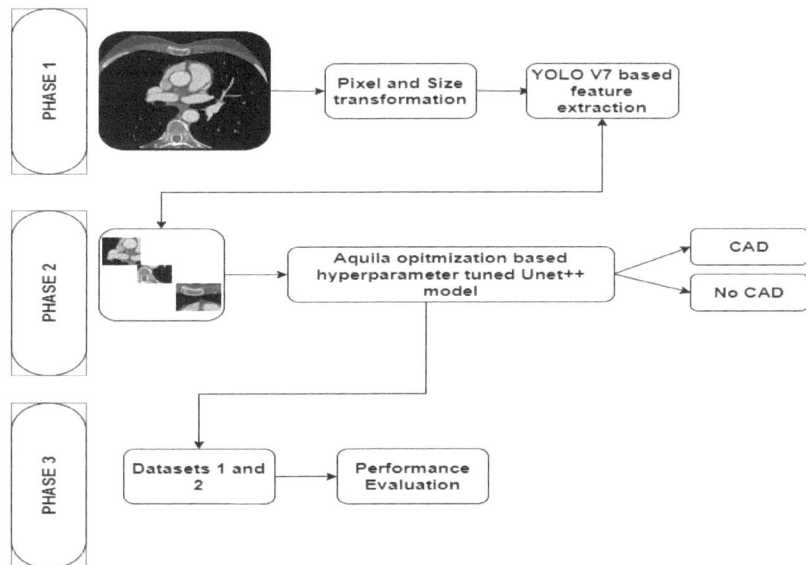

Figure 3. Research methodology.

2.2.1. Feature Extraction

In phase 1, the researchers follow the methods of [18] to enhance the image quality. A fuzzy function processes the standard CCTA image in the raster format. A discrete space is used to represent the height and width of an image. A mapping function maps the fuzzy image and the discrete space. The spatial information of the fuzzy image is located using a neighborhood function. The researchers modified the membership function of [18] to increase the pixel value. The membership function includes a rescaling function to enable the YOLO V7 model to rescale the images during feature extraction. Equation (1) shows the fuzzification process.

$$\text{Fuzzy}(\text{CCTA Image}) = Int_{H,w}(CCTA\ image) + Mem_{H,w}(CCTA\ Image) \quad (1)$$

where $Int_{H,w}$ and $Mem_{H,w}$ are intensity and membership functions, and H and W are the height and width of the CCTA image. The defuzzification function applies the maxima for generating the enhanced CCTA image. Using the enhanced image, the researchers transform the images into different sizes and supply them to the subsequent phases.

The images in dataset 2 are represented in 3D form, whereas the images of dataset 1 are expressed as the standard straightened arteries. To generate the straightened arteries from the 3D CCTA images, the researchers apply the centerline extraction [19] using the YOLO V7 model [20]. The YOLO V7 model identifies the centerlines using the anchor point between the coronary ostia and cardiac chambers. The arterial characteristics are generated using the central lines and area around the coronary vessels. In the subsequent steps, YOLO V7 extracts the features, which are forwarded to the CAD detection model.

2.2.2. Fine-Tuned CNN Model

In phase 2, the author applies the AO algorithm and the UNet++ model to generate the outcome. CCTA image features are convolutionally processed using a linear filter and merged with a bias term. Then, the resulting feature map is passed through a non-linear activation function. Hence, each neuron gains input from an N × N area of a subset of feature maps of the prior or input layer. This neuron's receptive fields comprise the combined regions of its receptive fields. As the same filter in the convolutional layer is used to probe all tolerable receptive fields of prior feature maps, the weights of neurons in the same feature map are always the same.

During the training phase, the system acquires the shared weights, which may also be filters or kernels. The activation function is a mathematical equation for determining the outcome of a neural network [20]. The process is linked to each neuron of the network. The active neuron is used to support the model to make a prediction. The activation function determines the outcome of a neuron. The pooling layer triggers the non-linear function. This layer is assigned to reduce the number of values in the feature maps by identifying the important values of the previous convolutional layer. The dropout technique includes an additional hyperparameter and dropout rate, influencing the chance of removing or keeping layer outputs.

With UNet++, decoders from different U-Nets are densely coupled at the exact resolution [21]. As a result of structural improvements, UNet++ offers the following benefits. First, UNet++ embeds U-Nets of various depths in its design. The encoding and decoding processes of these U-Nets are interconnected, and the encoders are partially shared. All the individual UNets are trained in parallel with a standard image representation assistance by training UNet++ under deep supervision. This architecture enhances the total segmentation performance, and model pruning is made possible during the inference phase. In addition, the encoder and decoder of the UNet++ model allow the feature maps to be fused at a similar rate. The aggregation layer can determine how to merge feature maps transported via skip connections with decoder feature maps using UNet++'s new skip connections. The following section discusses the number of layers and the outcome of the training phase. In order to tune the hyperparameters of the UNet++ model, the researchers employ the specific features of the AO algorithm. Let P be the set of hyperparameters and consider a population of candidate solutions with the upper bound (U) and lower bound (L). In each iteration, an optimal solution is attained. Equations (2) and (3) present the candidate and random solutions for P.

$$P = \begin{bmatrix} P_{1,1} & \cdots & P_{1,j} & P_{1,Dim-1} & P_{1,Dim} \\ P_{2,1} & \cdots & P_{2,j} & \cdots & P_{2,Dim} \\ \vdots & \vdots & \vdots & \vdots & \vdots \\ P_{N,1} & \cdots & P_{N,j} & P_{N,Dim-1} & P_{2,Dim} \end{bmatrix} \quad (2)$$

where P represents the hyperparameters, N is the total number of parameters, and Dim is the dataset size.

$$P_{i,j} = rand * (U_j - L_j) + L_j \quad i = 1, 2, \ldots N; \ j = 1, 2, \ldots, Dim \quad (3)$$

where rand is the function to generate an anchor point for searching the parameter, i and j are the total number of parameters of the UNet++ model and the dataset's size. The researchers derive narrowed exploration and exploitation features of the AO algorithm for finding the suitable hyperparameters of the UNet++ model. The AO agent considers the locations of hyperparameters as a prey area from a high soar and narrowly explores it using Equations (4) and (5).

$$M_1(t+1) = M_{1best}(t) \times Levy(s) + M_{1R}(t) + (Y - M_1) \tag{4}$$

where $M_1(t+1)$, M_{1best}, and M_{1R} are the generative outcome at each iteration(t), s is the space, Y is the random location of the search space, and Levy(s) is a flight distribution function presented in Equation (5).

$$Levy(s) = \frac{c * n * \sigma}{|m|^{\frac{1}{\beta}}} \tag{5}$$

where c, n, m, σ, and β are the constants for finding the hyperparameters.

Furthermore, narrow exploitation searches the hyperparameter using stochastic movements. Equation (6) shows the mathematical expression for the narrow exploitation.

$$M_2(t+1) = Q * M_{2best}(t) - (G_1 * M_2(t) * rand) \\ -(G_2 * Levy(s) * rand) + G_1 \tag{6}$$

where $M_2(t+1)$ is the generative solution at iteration (t), Q represents the quality function, and G_1 and G_2 are movements of the AO agent. The researchers modified the quality function according to the UNet++ model's performance.

2.2.3. Performance Evaluation

Finally, the third phase evaluates the proposed method using the evaluation metrics, including accuracy, precision, recall, F1-score, Matthews correlation coefficient (MCC), and Kappa. The datasets are divided into a train set (70%) and a test set (30%). The number of parameters, learning rate, and testing time are computed for each model. The researchers compute the area under the receiver operating characteristic (AU-ROC) and the precision-recall (PR) curve for each CAD detection model. In addition, the confidence interval (CI) and the standard deviation (SD) are calculated to find the outcome's uncertainty levels.

3. Results

To evaluate the performance of the proposed model, the researchers implemented the model in Windows 10 professional with an i7 processor, NVIDIA GeForce RTX 3060 Ti, and 8 GB RAM. Python 3.9, Keras, and Tensorflow libraries are used for constructing the proposed model. Yolo V7 [20] and UNet++ [21] are employed for developing the proposed model. In addition, the Alothman A.F. et al. model [4], Papandrianos N et al. model [7], Moon, J.H. et al. model [8], and Banerjee, R. et al. model [9] are used for performance comparison. The researcher trains the UNet++ model using datasets 1 and 2 under the AO environment. During the process, the proposed model scores a superior outcome at the 36th epoch and around the 34th epoch for datasets 1 and 2, respectively. The dropout ratios of 0.3 and 0.4 are used for datasets 1 and 2. These are used to address overfitting and underfitting issues. Finally, six layers, including two dropout layers, three fully connected layers, and a softmax layer, are integrated with the UNet++ model.

Table 2 presents the performance analysis of the proposed model on dataset 1. It indicates that the proposed model achieves an average accuracy and F1-measure of 98.85 and 98.37 during the training phase. In contrast, in the testing phase, it obtains a superior accuracy and F1-measure of 99.40 and 98.60.

Table 2. Performance analysis for dataset 1.

Methods/Measures	Accuracy	Precision	Recall	F1-Measure	MCC	Kappa
Training						
CAD	98.60	98.10	98.60	98.35	95.30	95.60
No CAD	99.10	98.40	98.40	98.40	95.40	94.90
Average	98.85	98.25	98.50	98.37	95.35	95.25
Testing						
CAD	99.20	98.60	98.60	98.65	95.60	95.20
No CAD	99.60	98.40	98.70	98.55	95.10	94.80
Average	99.40	98.50	98.65	98.60	95.35	95.00

Table 3 reflects the proposed model performance on dataset 2. It is evident that the image enhancement and feature extraction processes support the proposed model to detect normal and abnormal CCTA images with optimal accuracy and F1-measure.

Table 3. Performance analysis for dataset 2.

Methods/Measures	Accuracy	Precision	Recall	F1-Measure	MCC	Kappa
Training						
CAD	98.70	98.80	98.70	98.75	96.40	96.30
No CAD	99.10	99.20	99.40	99.30	96.30	96.10
Average	98.90	99.00	99.05	99.02	96.35	96.20
Testing						
CAD	99.40	98.80	98.60	98.70	96.40	96.30
No CAD	99.60	99.10	99.30	99.20	96.30	96.20
Average	99.50	98.95	98.95	98.95	96.35	96.25

Table 4 outlines the comparative analysis outcome of CAD using dataset 1. The proposed model outperforms the existing models by achieving accuracy, precision, recall, F1-measure, MCC, and Kappa of 99.40, 98.50, 98.65, 98.60, 95.35, and 95.00, respectively.

Table 4. Comparative analysis of CAD detection models using dataset 1.

Models/Measures	Accuracy	Precision	Recall	F1-Measure	MCC	Kappa
Alothman A.F. et al. [4] model	98.60	98.20	97.80	98.00	94.10	94.20
Papandrianos, N. et al. [7] model	98.90	97.80	98.10	97.95	94.80	94.60
Moon, J.H. et al. [8] model	98.50	97.60	98.20	97.90	95.10	93.80
Banerjee, R. et al. [9] model	98.20	97.80	98.30	98.05	94.30	93.70
Proposed model	99.40	98.50	98.65	98.60	95.35	95.00

Likewise, Table 5 displays the outcome of CAD detection models using dataset 2. The proposed model's dropout and fully connected layers supported the UNet++ model to overcome the existing challenges of the CNN models in classifying the images. Thus, the performance of the proposed model is better compared to the baseline models. Figures 4 and 5 highlight the performance of the CAD detection models on datasets 1 and 2, respectively.

Table 5. Comparative analysis of CAD detection models using dataset 2.

Models/Measures	Accuracy	Precision	Recall	F1-Measure	MCC	Kappa
Alothman A.F. et al. [4] model	98.60	98.20	98.10	98.15	95.30	95.10
Papandrianos, N. et al. [7] model	98.30	98.60	97.40	98.00	95.40	94.90
Moon, J.H. et al. [8] model	98.50	97.90	97.60	97.75	95.70	94.70
Banerjee, R. et al. [9] model	98.70	98.20	98.40	98.30	94.80	95.20
Proposed model	99.50	98.95	98.95	98.95	96.35	96.25

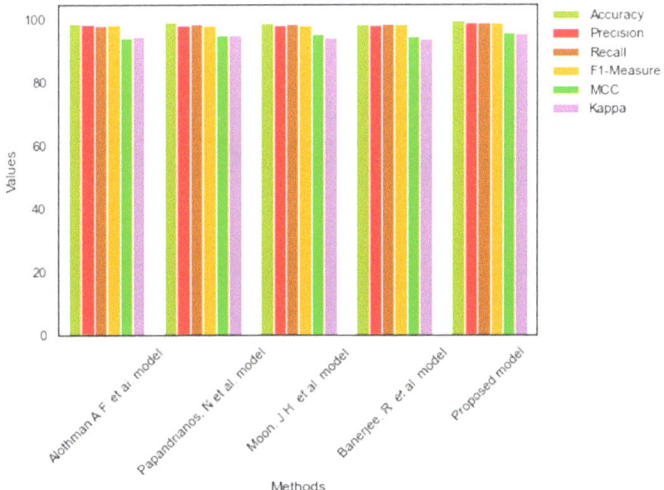

Figure 4. Comparative analysis of dataset 1 [4,7–9].

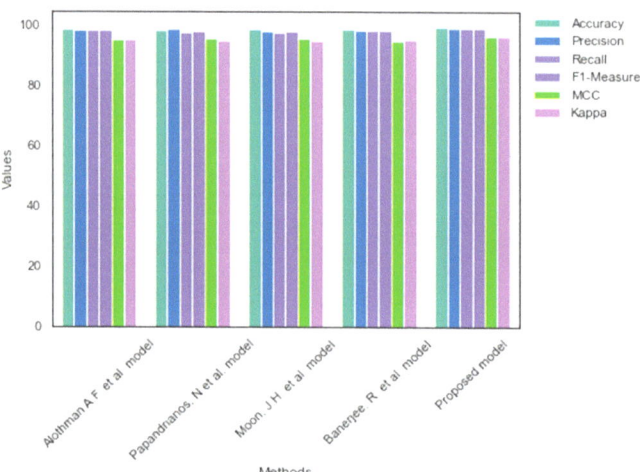

Figure 5. Comparative analysis of dataset 2 [4,7–9].

Figure 6 shows the AU-ROC and PR curves of the models using dataset 1. The proposed model learns the environment efficiently and handles the images effectively. In contrast, the current models face challenges in managing images of dataset 1. The proposed model obtained the AU-ROC and PR curve values of 0.97 and 0.95, which were higher than the baseline models of dataset 1.

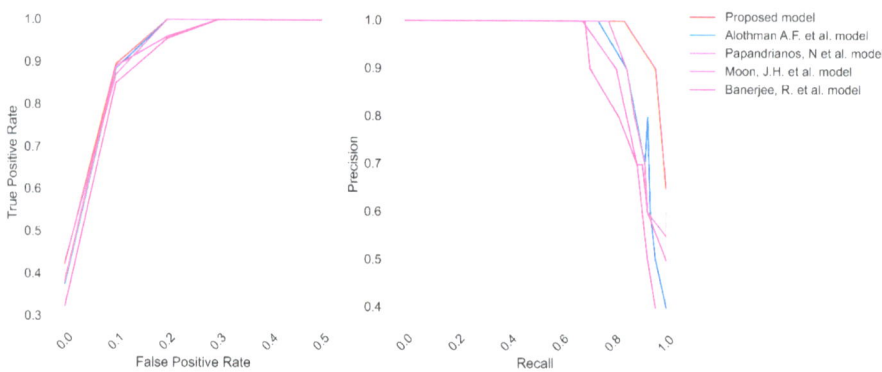

Figure 6. AU-ROC and PR curve of CAD for dataset 1 [4,7–9].

Similarly, Figure 7 represents the AU-ROC and PR curve for dataset 2. Dataset 2 contains a smaller number of images compared to dataset 1. The recent models failed to generate a better AU-ROC and PR curve. In contrast, the proposed model generates the AU-ROC and PR curve values of 0.96 and 0.94, respectively.

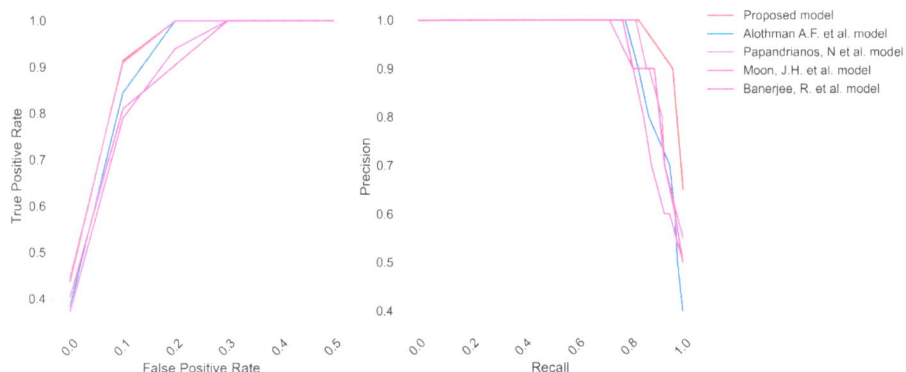

Figure 7. AU-ROC and PR curve of CAD for dataset 2 [4,7–9].

Table 6 highlights the computation cost of each model. The proposed model predicted the existence of CAD with fewer parameters in a shorter learning rate (1×10^{-4}). In contrast, the Alothman A.F. et al. [4] model, Papandrianos N. et al. [7] model, Moon, J.H. et al. [8] model, and Banerjee R. et al. [9] model consumed a learning rate of 1×10^{-4}, 1×10^{-3}, 1×10^{-3}, and 1×10^{-3}, respectively.

Table 6. Computational requirements for the CAD detection model.

Methods/Dataset	Dataset 1			Dataset 2		
	No. of Parameters	Learning Rate	Learning Time (seconds)	No. of Parameters	Learning Rate	Learning Time (seconds)
Alothman A.F. et al. [4] model	4.3 M	1×10^{-4}	1.92	5.2 M	1×10^{-3}	1.98
Papandrianos, N. et al. [7] model	11.2 M	1×10^{-3}	2.1	6.3 M	1×10^{-3}	2.45
Moon, J.H. et al. [8] model	7.4 M	1×10^{-3}	2.36	11.2 M	1×10^{-4}	2.27
Banerjee, R. et al. [9] model	14.6 M	1×10^{-3}	2.3	6.1 M	1×10^{-5}	2.3
Proposed model	3.6 M	1×10^{-4}	1.4	3.7 M	1×10^{-4}	1.5

Table 7 reveals the CI and SD of the outcomes generated by the CAD detection models. The higher CI and SD values indicate that the proposed method's results are highly reliable.

Table 7. Uncertainty levels of the CAD detection model outcomes.

Methods/Dataset	Dataset 1		Dataset 2	
	CI	SD	CI	SD
Alothman A.F. et al. [4] model	[98.55–98.61]	0.0017	[96.62–96.71]	0.0021
Papandrianos, N. et al. [7] model	[97.41–97.48]	0.0021	[95.37–95.41]	0.0042
Moon, J.H. et al. [8] model	[97.32–97.42]	0.0016	[95.82–95.91]	0.0029
Banerjee, R. et al. [9] model	[97.91–98.02]	0.0019	[95.96–96.02]	0.0031
Proposed model	[98.64–98.72]	0.0014	[97.41–97.49]	0.0019

4. Discussion

Recently, there has been a demand for a lightweight CAD detection model for diagnosing patients at earlier stages. The CAD detection model helps the individual to recover from the illness. CCTA is one of the primary tools in detecting CAD. It offers a non-invasive evaluation of atherosclerotic plaque on the artery walls. The current CAD detection models require substantial computational resources and time. The researchers proposed a CAD detection model for classifying the CCTA images and identifying the existence of CAD.

Therefore, the researchers built a model using YOLO V7 and UNet++ models. The effectiveness of the model is evaluated using two datasets. Initially, the images are enhanced through a quality improvement process. Generally, the images are in grayscale with low quality. The proposed image enhancement increases the pixel size and removes the irrelevant objects from the primary images. Subsequently, YOLO V7 is applied to extract the CCTA images' features. It is widely applied in object detection techniques. The researchers used this technique to identify the key features. Finally, the AO algorithm is used to tune the hyperparameters of the UNet++ model. The findings highlight that transfer learning can replace large datasets in potential AI-powered medical imaging to automate repetitive activities and prioritize unhealthy patients. The proposed method obtained an average accuracy of 99.40 and 99.50 for datasets 1 and 2, respectively. The outcome shows that the model correctly classifies CAD and No CAD from the CCTA images. The proposed feature extraction provided the critical features to the UNet++ model in making the decision. Precision, recall, and F1-measure values of 98.50, 98.65, and 98.60 for dataset 1 represent the effectiveness of the proposed model's classification. The proposed model identified the relevant features of the straightened coronary arteries of dataset 1. In addition, the proposed model achieved superior precision, recall, and F1-measure values for dataset 2. The presented data preprocessing and feature extraction methods supplied the crucial features of straightened arteries to the UNet++ model. MCC and Kappa values of 96.35 and 96.25 highlight the binary classification ability of the suggested CAD detection model. Figures 6 and 7 outline the AU-ROC and PR curve of the CAD detection models. It indicates the effectiveness of the proposed CAD detection model's capability to handle true positive and false positive objects.

However, the CNN model can produce a poor outcome due to the generalization ability. Thus, annotating or labeling the images is necessary to improve the performance of the YOLO V7 model. Transfer learning prevents overfitting and allows the generalization of tasks for other domains. It supports the UNet++ model to adjust the final weights concerning the features. The advantages of transfer learning using image embeddings with a feature extraction technique generate the highest average AUROC of 0.97 and 0.96 for datasets 1 and 2, respectively. The time necessary to train the proposed model was a few minutes, eliminating the requirement for a significant amount of computing resources and extensive training timeframes. The researcher achieves the study's goal with limited resources by employing the CNN model. CAD detection models have demonstrated strong visual analysis, comprehension, and classification performance. The proposed model gradually reduces the input size, extracting features in parallel using convolutional layers. Images can be embedded to represent the input in a lower-dimensional environment properly. The fuzzy function offers an opportunity to improve the quality of images in the datasets. Improving the grayscale images enables the YOLO V7 model to identify valuable features.

Furthermore, narrowed exploration and exploitation of the AO algorithm have identified the optimal set of hyperparameters for the UNet++ model. Although the UNet++ model contains an array of Unet models, it does not sufficiently address the overfitting issues. However, the hyperparameter optimization integrated a set of dropouts and fully connected layers with the UNet++ model. Thus, the proposed model achieves the study's objective by developing a CAD detection model. The findings reveal that the proposed CAD detection model can help healthcare centers to identify CAD using limited computing resources. The CI and SD outcomes show that the results are reliable. The following outcomes of the comparative analysis reveal the proposed model's significance in detecting CAD.

Alothman A.F. et al. [4] suggested a feature extraction strategy and a CNN model to identify CAD in the shortest amount of time while maintaining the highest level of accuracy. The effectiveness of the suggested model is examined using two datasets. The experimental results for the benchmark datasets reveal that the model achieved a better outcome with limited resources. However, the proposed model outperforms the model by producing a superior outcome. Papandrianos et al. [7] developed a model for detecting CAD using single-photon emission CT images. They applied an RGB-based CNN model for CAD detection. The model achieved an AUC score of 0.936. However, the proposed model obtained an AUC score of 0.97 and 0.96 on datasets 1 and 2. In addition, it produces a better outcome on grayscale CCTA images.

Likewise, Moon J.H. et al. [8] proposed a DL model to detect CAD from 452 proper coronary artery angiography movie clips. In line with [8], the proposed model employs the YOLO V7 technique, which can be used for video clips. Moreover, the proposed model outperforms the Moon J.H. et al. model with limited resources. Table 6 outlines the computational complexities of the CAD detection models. It is evident that the proposed CAD detection model generated results with a few sets of parameters and a lower learning rate. Banerjee et al. [9] found a CNN long short-term memory approach for detecting CAD from the electrocardiogram images. Tables 4 and 5 show that the Bannerjee et al. model produces low accuracy and F1-measure. The proposed model achieved a better outcome than the recent image classification [11–18]. The feature extraction technique supplied the practical features to support the proposed model and generate better insights from the CCTA images.

The proposed CAD detection generates an effective outcome on imbalanced datasets. However, there is a demand for future studies to overcome a few limitations of the proposed model. The multiple layers of the CNN model may require an additional training period. The UNet++ architecture requires an extensive search due to the varying depths. In an imbalanced dataset, the skip connection process may impose a restrictive fusion scheme to simultaneously force sub-networks to aggregate the feature maps.

5. Conclusions

The authors proposed a CAD detection model using the computed tomography images in this study. They intended to improve the performance of the CAD detection model using the effective feature extraction approach. The recent models require high computational costs to generate the outcome. Therefore, the authors proposed a three-phase method for detecting CAD from the images. In the first phase, an image enhancement technique using a fuzzy function improves an image's quality. In addition, the authors applied the YOLO V7 technique to extract critical features. They improved the pixel value of the images to increase the YOLO V7 performance in extracting features from the grayscale images. The second phase used the AO algorithm for optimizing the hyperparameters of the UNet++ model with CCTA image datasets. The dropout layers are integrated with the model to address the overfitting issues. Finally, the third phase evaluated the performance of the proposed model. The state-of-the-art CAD detection models are compared with the proposed model. The comparative analysis revealed that the proposed model outperformed the recent CAD detection models. In addition, the computational cost required for the proposed model was lower than the others. The findings highlighted that the proposed model could support the healthcare center in developing countries to identify CAD in the initial stages. Moreover, the proposed model can be implemented with limited computational resources. However, future studies are required to minimize the training time and improve the performance of the CAD models with unbalanced data.

Author Contributions: Conceptualization, A.R.W.S.; Methodology, A.R.W.S.; Software, A.R.W.S.; Validation, A.R.W.S.; Formal analysis, A.R.W.S. and A.K.D.; Investigation, A.K.D.; Resources, A.R.W.S. and A.K.D.; Writing—original draft, A.R.W.S. and A.K.D.; Writing—review & editing, A.R.W.S. All authors have read and agreed to the published version of the manuscript.

Funding: This work was supported by the Deanship of Scientific Research, Vice Presidency for Graduate Studies and Scientific Research, King Faisal University, Saudi Arabia (Grant No. 3002).

Institutional Review Board Statement: Not applicable.

Informed Consent Statement: Not applicable.

Data Availability Statement: The datasets can be found in the following repositories: https://data.mendeley.com/datasets/fk6rys63h9/1 (accessed on 27 February 2023) and https://github.com/XiaoweiXu/ImageCAS-A-Large-Scale-Dataset-and-Benchmark-for-Coronary-Artery-Segmentation-based-on-CT (accessed on 27 February 2023).

Conflicts of Interest: The authors declare no conflict of interest.

References

1. WHO. Available online: https://www.who.int/health-topics/cardiovascular-diseases#tab=tab_1 (accessed on 15 December 2022).
2. Lin, A.; Kolossváry, M.; Motwani, M.; Išgum, I.; Maurovich-Horvat, P.; Slomka, P.J.; Dey, D. Artificial intelligence in cardiovascular imaging for risk stratification in coronary artery disease. *Radiol. Cardiothorac. Imaging* **2021**, *3*, e200512. [CrossRef] [PubMed]
3. Han, D.; Liu, J.; Sun, Z.; Cui, Y.; He, Y.; Yang, Z. Deep learning analysis in coronary computed tomographic angiography imaging for the assessment of patients with coronary artery stenosis. *Comput. Methods Programs Biomed.* **2020**, *196*, 105651. [CrossRef] [PubMed]
4. AlOthman, A.F.; Sait, A.R.W.; Alhussain, T.A. Detecting Coronary Artery Disease from Computed Tomography Images Using a Deep Learning Technique. *Diagnostics* **2022**, *12*, 2073. [CrossRef] [PubMed]
5. Demirer, M.; Gupta, V.; Bigelow, M.; Erdal, B.; Prevedello, L.; White, R. Image dataset for a CNN algorithm development to detect coronary atherosclerosis in coronary CT angiography. *Mendeley Data* **2019**. [CrossRef]
6. Zeng, A.; Wu, C.; Huang, M.; Zhuang, J.; Bi, S.; Pan, D.; Ullah, N.; Khan, K.N.; Wang, T.; Shi, Y.; et al. ImageCAS: A Large-Scale Dataset and Benchmark for Coronary Artery Segmentation based on Computed Tomography Angiography Images. *arXiv* **2022**, arXiv:2211.01607.
7. Papandrianos, N.; Papageorgiou, E. Automatic Diagnosis of Coronary Artery Disease in SPECT Myocardial Perfusion Imaging Employing Deep Learning. *Appl. Sci.* **2021**, *11*, 6362. [CrossRef]
8. Moon, J.H.; Cha, W.C.; Chung, M.J.; Lee, K.S.; Cho, B.H.; Choi, J.H. Automatic stenosis recognition from coronary angiography using convolutional neural networks. *Comput. Methods Programs Biomed.* **2021**, *198*, 105819. [CrossRef]
9. Banerjee, R.; Ghose, A.; Mandana, K.M. A hybrid CNN-LSTM architecture for detection of coronary artery disease from ECG. In Proceedings of the International Joint Conference on Neural Networks (IJCNN), Glasgow, UK, 19–24 July 2020; pp. 1–8.
10. Liu, C.Y.; Tang, C.X.; Zhang, X.L.; Chen, S.; Xie, Y.; Zhang, X.Y.; Qiao, H.Y.; Zhou, C.S.; Xu, P.P.; Lu, M.J.; et al. Deep learning powered coronary CT angiography for detecting obstructive coronary artery disease: The effect of reader experience, calcification and image quality. *Eur. J. Radiol.* **2021**, *142*, 109835. [CrossRef]
11. Yi, Y.; Xu, C.; Xu, M.; Yan, J.; Li, Y.Y.; Wang, J.; Yang, S.J.; Guo, Y.B.; Wang, Y.; Li, Y.M.; et al. Diagnostic improvements of deep learning–based image reconstruction for assessing calcification-related obstructive coronary artery disease. *Front. Cardiovasc. Med.* **2021**, *8*, 758793. [CrossRef]
12. Hampe, N.; Wolterink, J.M.; Van Velzen, S.G.; Leiner, T.; Išgum, I. Machine learning for assessment of coronary artery disease in cardiac CT: A survey. *Front. Cardiovasc. Med.* **2019**, *6*, 172. [CrossRef]
13. Baskaran, L.; Ying, X.; Xu, Z.; Al'Aref, S.J.; Lee, B.C.; Lee, S.E.; Danad, I.; Park, H.B.; Bathina, R.; Baggiano, A.; et al. Machine learning insight into the role of imaging and clinical variables for the prediction of obstructive coronary artery disease and revascularization: An exploratory analysis of the CONSERVE study. *PLoS ONE* **2020**, *15*, e0233791. [CrossRef] [PubMed]
14. Chen, M.; Wang, X.; Hao, G.; Cheng, X.; Ma, C.; Guo, N.; Hu, S.; Tao, Q.; Yao, F.; Hu, C. Diagnostic performance of deep learning-based vascular extraction and stenosis detection technique for coronary artery disease. *Br. J. Radiol.* **2020**, *93*, 20191028. [CrossRef] [PubMed]
15. Li, Y.; Wu, Y.; He, J.; Jiang, W.; Wang, J.; Peng, Y.; Jia, Y.; Xiong, T.; Jia, K.; Yi, Z.; et al. Automatic coronary artery segmentation and diagnosis of stenosis by deep learning based on computed tomographic coronary angiography. *Eur. Radiol.* **2022**, *32*, 6037–6045. [CrossRef]
16. Yang, W.; Chen, C.; Yang, Y.; Chen, L.; Yang, C.; Gong, L.; Wang, J.; Shi, F.; Wu, D.; Yan, F. Diagnostic performance of deep learning-based vessel extraction and stenosis detection on coronary computed tomography angiography for coronary artery disease: A multi-reader multi-case study. *La Radiol. Med.* **2023**, *3*, 307–315. [CrossRef]

17. Nous, F.M.; Budde, R.P.; Lubbers, M.M.; Yamasaki, Y.; Kardys, I.; Bruning, T.A.; Akkerhuis, J.M.; Kofflard, M.J.; Kietselaer, B.; Galema, T.W.; et al. Impact of machine-learning CT-derived fractional flow reserve for the diagnosis and management of coronary artery disease in the randomized CRESCENT trials. *Eur. Radiol.* **2020**, *30*, 3692–3701. [CrossRef]
18. Hurtik, P.; Molek, V.; Hula, J. Data preprocessing technique for neural networks based on image represented by a fuzzy function. *IEEE Trans. Fuzzy Syst.* **2019**, *28*, 1195–1204. [CrossRef]
19. Candemir, S.; White, R.D.; Demirer, M.; Gupta, V.; Bigelow, M.T.; Prevedello, L.M.; Erdal, B.S. Automated coronary artery atherosclerosis detection and weakly supervised localization on coronary CT angiography with a deep 3-dimensional convolutional neural network. *Comput. Med. Imaging Graph.* **2020**, *83*, 101721. [CrossRef]
20. Wang, C.Y.; Bochkovskiy, A.; Liao, H.Y.M. YOLOv7: Trainable bag-of-freebies sets new state-of-the-art for real-time object detectors. *arXiv* **2022**, arXiv:2207.02696.
21. Zhou, Z.; Siddiquee, M.M.R.; Tajbakhsh, N.; Liang, J. UNet++: Redesigning skip connections to exploit multiscale features in image segmentation. *IEEE Trans. Med. Imaging* **2019**, *39*, 1856–1867. [CrossRef]
22. Abualigah, L.; Yousri, D.; Abd Elaziz, M.; Ewees, A.A.; Al-Qaness, M.A.; Gandomi, A.H. Aquila optimizer: A novel meta-heuristic optimization algorithm. *Comput. Ind. Eng.* **2021**, *157*, 107250. [CrossRef]
23. Overmars, L.M.; van Es, B.; Groepenhoff, F.; De Groot, M.C.; Pasterkamp, G.; den Ruijter, H.M.; van Solinge, W.W.; Hoefer, I.E.; Haitjema, S. Preventing unnecessary imaging in patients suspect of coronary artery disease through machine learning of electronic health records. *Eur. Heart J.-Digit. Health* **2022**, *3*, 11–19. [CrossRef] [PubMed]
24. Tian, F.; Gao, Y.; Fang, Z.; Gu, J. Automatic coronary artery segmentation algorithm based on deep learning and digital image processing. *Appl. Intell.* **2021**, *51*, 8881–8895. [CrossRef]
25. Kawasaki, T.; Kidoh, M.; Kido, T.; Sueta, D.; Fujimoto, S.; Kumamaru, K.K.; Uetani, T.; Tanabe, Y.; Ueda, T.; Sakabe, D.; et al. Evaluation of significant coronary artery disease based on CT fractional flow reserve and plaque characteristics using random forest analysis in machine learning. *Acad. Radiol.* **2020**, *27*, 1700–1708. [CrossRef] [PubMed]
26. Lei, Y.; Guo, B.; Fu, Y.; Wang, T.; Liu, T.; Curran, W.; Zhang, L.; Yang, X. Automated coronary artery segmentation in coronary computed tomography angiography (CCTA) using deep learning neural networks. In Proceedings of the Medical Imaging 2020: Imaging Informatics for Healthcare, Research, and Applications, Houston, TX, USA, 16–17 February 2020; Volume 11318, pp. 279–284.
27. van Hamersvelt, R.W.; Zreik, M.; Voskuil, M.; Viergever, M.A.; Išgum, I.; Leiner, T. Deep learning analysis of left ventricular myocardium in CT angiographic intermediate-degree coronary stenosis improves the diagnostic accuracy for identification of functionally significant stenosis. *Eur. Radiol.* **2019**, *29*, 2350–2359. [CrossRef]
28. Chu, M.; Wu, P.; Li, G.; Yang, W.; Gutiérrez-Chico, J.L.; Tu, S. Advances in Diagnosis, Therapy, and Prognosis of Coronary Artery Disease Powered by Deep Learning Algorithms. *JACC Asia* **2023**, *3*, 1–14. [CrossRef]
29. Al'Aref, S.J.; Anchouche, K.; Singh, G.; Slomka, P.J.; Kolli, K.K.; Kumar, A.; Pandey, M.; Maliakal, G.; Van Rosendael, A.R.; Beecy, A.N.; et al. Clinical applications of machine learning in cardiovascular disease and its relevance to cardiac imaging. *Eur. Heart J.* **2019**, *40*, 1975–1986. [CrossRef]
30. Denzinger, F.; Wels, M.; Breininger, K.; Taubmann, O.; Mühlberg, A.; Allmendinger, T.; Gülsün, M.A.; Schöbinger, M.; André, F.; Buss, S.J.; et al. How scan parameter choice affects deep learning-based coronary artery disease assessment from computed tomography. *Sci. Rep.* **2023**, *13*, 2563. [CrossRef]
31. Jiang, Y.; Yang, Z.G.; Wang, J.; Shi, R.; Han, P.L.; Qian, W.L.; Yan, W.F.; Li, Y. Unsupervised machine learning based on clinical factors for the detection of coronary artery atherosclerosis in type 2 diabetes mellitus. *Cardiovasc. Diabetol.* **2022**, *21*, 259. [CrossRef]
32. Lu, H.; Yao, Y.; Wang, L.; Yan, J.; Tu, S.; Xie, Y.; He, W. Research Progress of Machine Learning and Deep Learning in Intelligent Diagnosis of the Coronary Atherosclerotic Heart Disease. *Comput. Math. Methods Med.* **2022**, *2022*, 3016532. [CrossRef]
33. Kolossváry, M.; De Cecco, C.N.; Feuchtner, G.; Maurovich-Horvat, P. Advanced atherosclerosis imaging by CT: Radiomics, machine learning and deep learning. *J. Cardiovasc. Comput. Tomogr.* **2019**, *13*, 274–280. [CrossRef]
34. Muscogiuri, G.; Chiesa, M.; Trotta, M.; Gatti, M.; Palmisano, V.; Dell'Aversana, S.; Baessato, F.; Cavaliere, A.; Cicala, G.; Lottreno, A.; et al. Performance of a deep learning algorithm for the evaluation of CAD-RADS classification with CCTA. *Atherosclerosis* **2020**, *294*, 25–32. [CrossRef] [PubMed]
35. Dong, C.; Xu, S.; Li, Z. A novel end-to-end deep learning solution for coronary artery segmentation from CCTA. *Med. Phys.* **2022**, *49*, 6945–6959. [CrossRef] [PubMed]
36. Mathur, P.; Srivastava, S.; Xu, X.; Mehta, J.L. Artificial intelligence, machine learning, and cardiovascular disease. *Clin. Med. Insights: Cardiol.* **2020**, *14*, 1179546820927404. [CrossRef] [PubMed]
37. Paul, J.F.; Rohnean, A.; Giroussens, H.; Pressat-Laffouilhere, T.; Wong, T. Evaluation of a deep learning model on coronary CT angiography for automatic stenosis detection. *Diagn. Interv. Imaging* **2022**, *103*, 316–323. [CrossRef] [PubMed]

Disclaimer/Publisher's Note: The statements, opinions and data contained in all publications are solely those of the individual author(s) and contributor(s) and not of MDPI and/or the editor(s). MDPI and/or the editor(s) disclaim responsibility for any injury to people or property resulting from any ideas, methods, instructions or products referred to in the content.

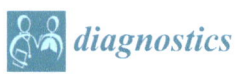

Article

Performance and Agreement When Annotating Chest X-ray Text Reports—A Preliminary Step in the Development of a Deep Learning-Based Prioritization and Detection System

Dana Li [1,2,*], Lea Marie Pehrson [1,3], Rasmus Bonnevie [4], Marco Fraccaro [4], Jakob Thrane [4], Lea Tøttrup [4], Carsten Ammitzbøl Lauridsen [1,5], Sedrah Butt Balaganeshan [6], Jelena Jankovic [1], Tobias Thostrup Andersen [1], Alyas Mayar [7], Kristoffer Lindskov Hansen [1,2], Jonathan Frederik Carlsen [1,2], Sune Darkner [3] and Michael Bachmann Nielsen [1,2]

[1] Department of Diagnostic Radiology, Copenhagen University Hospital, Rigshospitalet, 2100 Copenhagen, Denmark
[2] Department of Clinical Medicine, University of Copenhagen, 2100 Copenhagen, Denmark
[3] Department of Computer Science, University of Copenhagen, 2100 Copenhagen, Denmark
[4] Unumed Aps, 1055 Copenhagen, Denmark
[5] Radiography Education, University College Copenhagen, 2200 Copenhagen, Denmark
[6] Novo Nordisk Foundation Center for Protein Research, Faculty of Health and Medical Sciences, University of Copenhagen, 2100 Copenhagen, Denmark
[7] Department of Health Sciences, Panum Institute, University of Copenhagen, 2100 Copenhagen, Denmark
* Correspondence: dana.li@regionh.dk

Abstract: A chest X-ray report is a communicative tool and can be used as data for developing artificial intelligence-based decision support systems. For both, consistent understanding and labeling is important. Our aim was to investigate how readers would comprehend and annotate 200 chest X-ray reports. Reports written between 1 January 2015 and 11 March 2022 were selected based on search words. Annotators included three board-certified radiologists, two trained radiologists (physicians), two radiographers (radiological technicians), a non-radiological physician, and a medical student. Consensus labels by two or more of the experienced radiologists were considered "gold standard". Matthew's correlation coefficient (MCC) was calculated to assess annotation performance, and descriptive statistics were used to assess agreement between individual annotators and labels. The intermediate radiologist had the best correlation to "gold standard" (MCC 0.77). This was followed by the novice radiologist and medical student (MCC 0.71 for both), the novice radiographer (MCC 0.65), non-radiological physician (MCC 0.64), and experienced radiographer (MCC 0.57). Our findings showed that for developing an artificial intelligence-based support system, if trained radiologists are not available, annotations from non-radiological annotators with basic and general knowledge may be more aligned with radiologists compared to annotations from sub-specialized medical staff, if their sub-specialization is outside of diagnostic radiology.

Keywords: chest X-ray; deep learning; artificial intelligence; agreement; performance; text annotation; data; radiologists; development

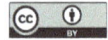

1. Introduction

Chest X-rays (CXRs) are the most commonly performed diagnostic image modality [1]. Recent technological advancements have made it possible to create systems that support and increase radiologists' efficiency and accuracy when analyzing CXR images [2]. Thus, interest in developing artificial intelligence-based systems for detection and prioritization of CXR findings has increased, including how to efficiently gather training data [3].

For training, validating, and testing a deep learning algorithm, labeled data are required [4]. Previous ontological schemes have been developed to have consistent labeling. Labeling schemes can vary, from hierarchical labeling systems with 180+ unique labels [5]

to few selected labels [6,7]. Label creation for deep learning development may be unique to each project, since they are dependent on factors such as imaging modality, body part, algorithm type, etc. [4]. In a previous study we developed a labeling scheme for annotation of findings in CXRs to obtain consistent labeling [8]. Our labeling scheme was tested for inter- and intra-observer agreement when used to annotate CXR images [8], and iterations have been ongoing to potentially increase consistent use of labels for annotation of CXR image and text reports.

Optimally, CXR training data should consist of manually labeled findings on the radiographic images, marked with e.g., bounding boxes for location, and radiologists are often needed to perform such a task to ensure the most accurate labeling [9]. Gathering data for training an algorithm may therefore be time-consuming and expensive. Several systems for automatic extraction of labels from CXR text reports have therefore been developed, including natural language processing models based on either feature engineering [6,10] or deep learning technology [11]. Labels that are extracted this way can then be linked to the corresponding CXR image to provide large, labeled image datasets using minimal time and cost [5].

To fully automate the labeling process, researchers have attempted to develop unsupervised machine learning engineering to extract labels [12]. However, these methods still seem inferior compared to solutions with components of supervision [13,14]. Therefore, just as with images, text labeling algorithms still need manually labeled data for training.

Labeling of text for training a deep learning algorithm needs to be consistent [15]. However, unlike images, labeling and annotation of text may not require specialized radiologists, since radiological reports are used for communication with other specialty fields in health care and therefore should be understood by a much more diverse group of people than just radiologists [16]. Only a few studies have been done on reading comprehension and understanding findings in radiological text reports, when readers are health care workers with differentiated levels of radiological experience [17]. Understanding how variability in radiological knowledge impacts reading comprehension of a radiological text report, could not only be beneficial in the development of a deep learning algorithm but could also give insight to pitfalls of a radiological text report as a communicative tool between medical staff [18].

In this study we aimed to investigate how differentiated levels of radiological task experience impact reading comprehension and labeling performance on CXR text reports. We also field-tested the text report labeling scheme by measuring label-specific agreement between predicted and actual labels as to decrease any potential bias to reading comprehension created by the labeling process itself.

2. Materials and Methods

Ethical approval was obtained on 11 May 2022 by the Regional Council for Region Hovedstaden (R-22017450). Approval for data retrieval and storage was obtained on 19 May 2022 by the Knowledge Center on Data Protection Compliance (P-2022-231).

2.1. Diagnostic Labeling Scheme for Text Annotations

The initial structure and development of the labeling scheme have previously been highlighted [8]. In summary, the labels were generated to match existing CXR ontologies such as Fleischner criteria and definitions [19] and other machine learning labeling schemes [5–7]. Labels were ordered hierarchically, where a high-level class such as "decreased translucency" was divided to lower-level classes that increased in specificity. The labeling scheme was previously tested for inter- and intra-observer agreement in CXR image annotation [8]. Iterations were since made to increase the agreement; (1) labels were made to be as descriptive as possible and (2) interpretive labels were added under the category "Differential diagnosis", because of increased detailed information that was present in chest X-ray text reports compared to chest X-ray images (Figure 1).

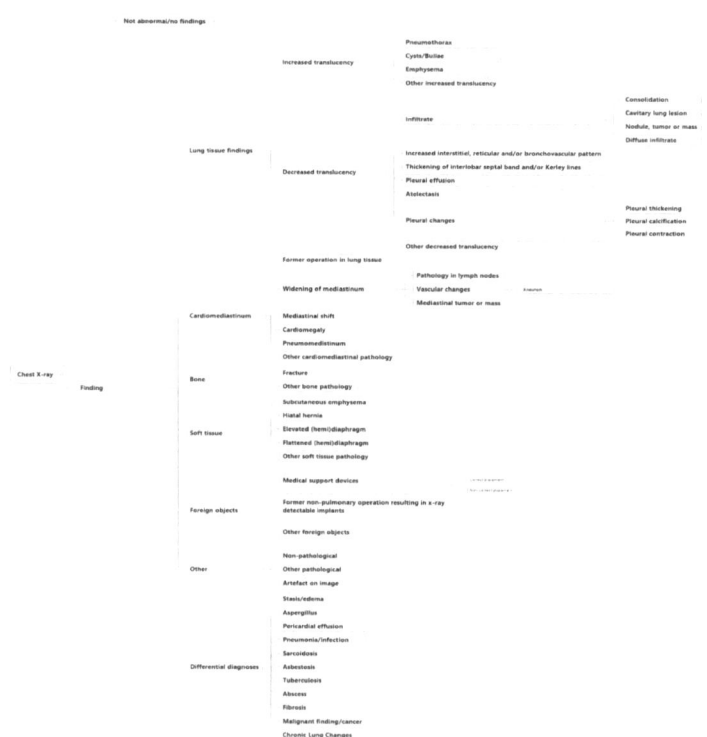

Figure 1. Labeling hierarchy for chest X-ray text report annotation.

2.2. Dataset

A selection of a total of 200 de-anonymized CXR reports from 1 January 2015 to 11 March 2022 were collected at the Department of Diagnostic Radiology at Rigshospitalet through the PACS system (AGFA Impax Client 6, Mortsel, Belgium). The CXR reports were retrieved through two methods:

Firstly, through a computerized search algorithm, CXR reports were selected using search words found in the text. A minimum of six CXR reports were required to be present for each of the following search words; pneumothorax, cysts/bullae, emphysema, infiltrate, consolidation, diffuse infiltrate, pleural effusion, atelectasis, lung surgery, chronic lung changes, pneumonia infection, tuberculosis, abscess, and stasis/edema. This method resulted in 84 reports.

Secondly, for the remaining 116 reports, a computerized search algorithm was used to find and distribute an equal number of cases, between the following criteria (29 cases each):

(1) Truly randomly selected.
(2) Randomly selected cases containing any abnormal findings.
(3) Randomly selected cases, within the top 10% of all cases that had the greatest number of associated labels per case relative to the length of the report.
(4) Randomly selected cases, within the bottom 10% of cases that had the least number of labels associated per case relative to the length of the report.

2.3. Participants and Annotation Process

A total of three board-certified radiologists were included as annotators to determine labels for the cases in the text annotation set to form the "gold standard" labels (actual labels). All three radiologists had specialized training ranging from 14 to 30+ years each. Six annotators with varying degrees of radiological experience were included to annotate the 200 text reports with labels from the labeling scheme (Figure 1). Annotators included a(n): intermediate radiologist (physician with radiological experience, 6 years), novice radiologist (physician with radiological experience, 2 years), experienced radiographer (radiological technician, with radiographer experience of 15 years), novice radiographer (radiological technician with radiographer experience of 3 years), non-radiological physician (7 years of other specialized, clinical experience, post-graduation), and a senior medical student (planning to graduate from university within 6 months).

The annotation process began on 25 August 2022, and ended on 25 October 2022. All 200 text reports were imported to a proprietary annotation software developed by Unumed Aps (Copenhagen, Denmark). Annotators were instructed to find and label each piece of text describing both positive and negative findings (Figure 2). Annotators were blinded to the X-ray images and other annotators' annotations.

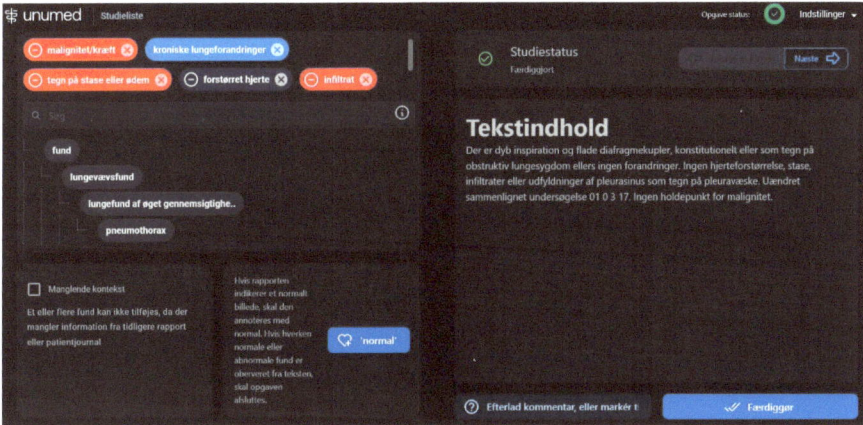

Figure 2. Annotation software for text report annotations. The full-text report is displayed on the right side and labels in the labeling hierarchy are displayed on the left. On the top left, selected labels are showcased; red labels for negative findings and blue labels for positive findings.

2.4. Presentation of Data and Statistical Analysis

"Gold standard" labels were defined as consensus on a label in a text report between two or more of the three board-certified radiologists. "Majority" vote labels were defined by consensus on a label between four or more of the six annotators and "majority excl. intermediate radiologist" were defined as consensus vote on a label between three or more of the remaining annotators after removing the intermediate radiologist as an annotator. Frequency counts reflected the total cumulative counts of a label's use in all text reports in the annotation set. Time spent on annotation was done by calculating the average time spent on a text report from opening the report to annotation completion.

Matthew's correlation coefficient (MCC) [20] was used to compare annotator performance to "gold standard" labeling and to compare annotators' performance to each other. The MCC was based on values selected for a 2 × 2 confusion matrix (Table 1) where true positive (TP) described the number of labels that matched "gold standard" labels for all positive and negative findings separately. True negative (TN) described the number of labels that were not used by annotators which also matched labels that were not used by both "gold standard" for all positive and negative findings separately. False positives (FP) described the number of labels that annotators used, but "gold standard" did not use, and false negative (FN) described all labels that "gold standard" used but annotators did not use.

Table 1. An example of 2 × 2 confusion matrix for the calculations of Matthew's Correlation Coefficient. TP, true positive; FP, false positive; FN, false negative; TN, true negative.

		Gold Standard	
		Labels used	Labels NOT used
Annotator(s)	Labels used	TP	FP
	Labels NOT used	FN	TN

MCC was then defined by following equation [20]:

$$MCC = \frac{(TP * TN) - (FP * FN)}{\sqrt{(TP + FP)(TP + FN)(TN + FP)(TN + FN)}}$$

To achieve this, MCC was calculated using Python 3.8.10 (https://www.python.org/) with the Pandas [21] and Numpy [22] libraries for each label and then micro-averaged [23] to give an overall coefficient for all positive and negative labels. MCC ranges between -1 and 1, where 1 represents perfect positive correlation, 0 represents correlation not better than random, and -1 represents total disagreement between labels of the "gold standard" set (actual) and the set of labels chosen by the annotator (predicted) [20].

One weakness of MCC and other standard agreement statistics is that they fail to take partial agreement into account in structured and taxonomic annotation tasks like ours. In addition, they do not clearly identify tendencies towards over- or under-annotation by any single annotator. To this end, we performed a separate analysis for any pair of annotators. An annotator here means either an individual human annotator or a constructed annotator such as "gold standard" or any of the "majority"-categories. For each annotator pair, we ran a maximum weight matching algorithm on a graph constructed from their individual annotations, trying to pair the labels from the two annotators as best as possible. We used the implementation available in the Python library networkx (version 2.8.8) [24].

We employed a weighting that enforced the following criteria in descending order:
(1) Match with the exact same label, or
(2) Match with an ancestral or descendent node (e.g., for "vascular changes" it could be either "aneurism" or "widening of mediastinum" etc. (Figure 1))

The hierarchical order in which the labels are placed, categorizes labels into similar groups and findings of similar characterization become more distinguishable from each other with each branch division. This is done to reduce the number of unusable labels caused by inter-reader variability [25] as disagreement on a label in a branched division could have common ascending nodes. Annotators do not manually mark a piece of text to a label, so to maximize data, we post-processed by discarding matched pairs of labels that did not belong to the same branch, since we operated on the assumption that the same piece of text/finding should not lead to annotation with labels that did not belong within the same category. The statistical algorithm would pair up any remaining annotations at random after all matches with positive weight had been made. If the annotators made an unequal number of annotations, such that it was impossible to pair all annotations, or if matched labels did not belong within the same branch or were not in a direct line of descending/ascending order we denoted the remaining annotations as unmatched.

Descriptive statistics were thus calculated to investigate specific agreements by comparing counts of "matched" and "unmatched" labels between annotators and "gold standard". In addition to presenting matched and unmatched labels as representation for individual annotator agreements, the number of matched and unmatched counts was also presented for each label.

3. Results

A total of 63 positive labels and 62 negative labels were possible to use for annotation (Figure 1). A pareto chart showed that 25 labels covered 80% of all labeled positive findings, and four labels covered 80% of all negative findings. The top 5 most used labels for positive findings were: "infiltrate", "pleural effusion", "cardiomegaly", "atelectasis", and "stasis/edema". The top 5 most used labels for negative findings were: "pleural effusion", "infiltrate", "stasis/edema", "cardiomegaly", and "pneumothorax" (Figure 3a,b).

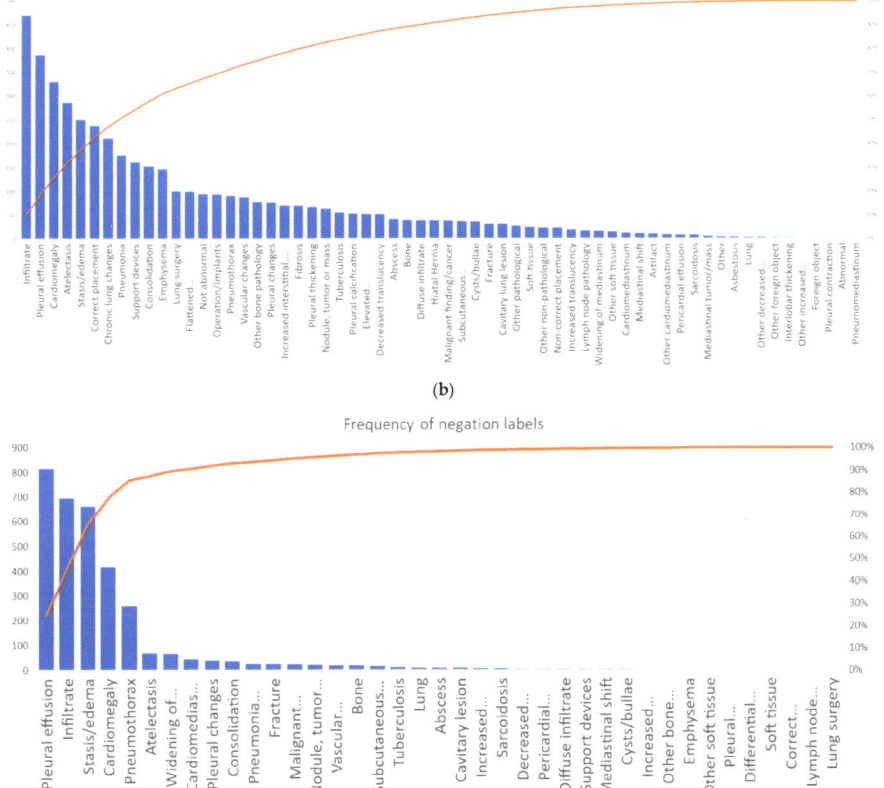

Figure 3. Pareto chart of all annotators accumulated use of labels for (**a**) positive findings and (**b**) negative findings.

For labels that represented positive findings, the novice radiographer had more annotations for "bone" (16 cases vs. 0–8 cases) and "decreased translucency" (29 cases vs.

0–10 cases) compared to other annotators. The novice radiologist had more annotations for "other non-pathological" compared to other annotators (18 cases vs. 0–2 cases), and the senior medical student had more annotations on "diffuse infiltrate" compared to other annotators (22 cases vs. 0–5 cases) (Table A1 in Appendix A).

For negative findings, the experienced radiographer had more annotations on "consolidation" (23 cases vs. 0–4 cases) and "pleural changes" (20 cases vs. 0–6 cases) compared to the other annotators. The non-radiological physician had more annotations on "cardiomediastinum" than other annotators (21 cases vs. 0–7 cases) (Table A2 in Appendix A).

The average time spent on annotating a text report was: 98.1 s for the intermediate radiologist, 76.2 s for the novice radiologist, 232.1 s for the experienced radiographer, 135 s for the novice radiographer, 99.4 s for the non-radiological physician, 145.8 s for the senior medical student, and each "gold standard" annotator took on average 135.2 s per text report.

3.1. Annotator Performance and Agreement

Table 2a,b showed the MCC values for each annotator for positive and negative findings, respectively. The intermediate radiologist had the best MCC compared to other annotators, both for labels representing positive findings and negative findings (MCC 0.77 and MCC 0.92). The senior medical student had comparable MCC values to the novice radiologist for both negative and positive findings (Table 2a,b).

Table 2. Matthew's correlation coefficients (MCC) for annotators' performance in annotating chest X-ray text reports compared to gold standard annotation set for (**a**) positive findings and (**b**) negative findings.

	Radiologist, Intermediate	Radiologist, Novice	Radiographer, Experienced	Radiographer, Novice	Physician, Non-Radiologist	Senior Medical Student
MCC	0.77	0.71	0.57	0.65	0.64	0.71

(a)

	Radiologist, Intermediate	Radiologist, Novice	Radiographer, Experienced	Radiographer, Novice	Physician, Non-Radiologist	Senior Medical Student
MCC	0.92	0.88	0.64	0.88	0.77	0.88

(b)

For both positive and negative findings, the senior medical student achieved better MCC than the non-radiological physician (0.71 vs. 0.64 for positive findings and 0.88 vs. 0.77 for negative findings). This tendency was also present for the radiographers. The novice radiographer achieved better MCC for both positive and negative findings compared to the experienced radiographer (0.65 vs. 0.57 for positive findings and 0.88 vs. 0.64 for negative findings).

All annotators achieved higher MCC for negative findings compared to their own MCC for positive findings (Table 2a,b).

The number of labels that were a match (Table 3) and unmatched (Table A3) between different pairs of annotators was used as representation for degree of agreement between different annotators.

Table 3 showed the number of matched labels between each annotator for both positive and negative findings. The intermediate radiologist, novice radiologists and senior medical student had the most label matches with each other. The novice radiographer had more matches with the "gold standard" (710 labels matched) compared with the experienced radiographer's matches with "gold standard" (589 labels matched). The senior medical student had more matches with "gold standard" (741 labels matched) compared with the non-radiological physician's matches with "gold standard" (665 labels matched).

Table 3. Number of matched labels of both positive and negative findings for each annotator, majority of annotators, and gold standard.

	Radiologist, Intermediate	Radiologist, Novice	Radiographer, Experienced	Radiographer, Novice	Physician, Non-Radiologist	Senior Medical Student	Majority	Majority excl. Intermed. Radiologist	Gold Standard
Radiologist, intermediate		849	679	785	753	832	794	810	766
Radiologist, novice	849		654	763	744	811	779	815	740
Radiographer, experienced	679	654		642	597	669	664	680	589
Radiographer, novice	785	763	642		710	791	753	801	710
Physician, non-radiologist	753	744	597	710		741	714	746	665
Senior medical student	832	811	669	791	741		783	823	741
Majority	794	779	664	753	714	783		824	702
Majority excl. Intermed. Radiologist	810	815	680	801	746	823	824		723
Gold Standard	766	740	589	710	665	741	702	723	

Fewest matched (worst) — 50% fractile — Most matched (best)

Table A3 in the Appendix A showed the number of unmatched labels that were left after subtracting the number of matched labels to each annotator's total label use. The intermediate radiologist had the least number of unmatched labels left compared with the "gold standard" (201), however, the other annotators closely followed (203–234). The "majority" vote achieved the lowest number of unmatched labels against "gold standard" annotations compared with any individual annotator (122). "Gold standard" generally used fewer labels per text report compared with any annotator. (e.g., 32 unmatched labels leftover for "gold standard" when matched to the intermediate radiologist vs. 201 unmatched labels leftover for the intermediate radiologist when matched to "gold standard").

The "majority excl. the intermediate radiologist" voting (723) had more labels that matched with "gold standard" compared with the "majority" voting which included the intermediate radiologist (702) (Table 3). Even though the number of unmatched labels increased (162) when excluding the intermediate radiologist majority vote compared with majority voting including the intermediate radiologist (122), there were still fewer unmatched labels than any individual annotator (Table A3).

3.2. Label Specific Agreement

Tables 4 and 5 showed the cumulative cases of matches on a specific label for labels in the "lung tissue findings" category and "cardiomediastinum" category, respectively. "Atelectasis", "infiltrate", and "pleural effusion" were lung tissue related labels with the most matches (219, 687, and 743, respectively) (Table 4), while "cardiomegaly" (472) was the label with the most matches in the "cardiomediastinum" category (Table 5), and "medical device, correct placement" (115), and "stasis/edema" (576) were the labels with the most matches in the rest of the labeling scheme (Table A4).

Table 4. Number of matched cases (accumulated) on specific labels in the labeling scheme related to "lung tissue findings". * Rows and columns not belonging to the parent node "lung tissue findings" and that did not have any label disagreements have been pruned and thus number of rows does not match number of columns.

		Gold Standard *									
Annotators *		Atelectasis	Consolidation	Cysts/Bullae	Increased Interstitial	Infiltrate	Decreased Translucency	Nodule, Tumor or Mass	Pleural Calcification	Pleural Changes	Pleural Effusion	Pleural Thickening
	Atelectasis	219										
	Cavitary lesion					8						
	Consolidation		22	21		53	3					
	Cysts/bullae											
	Diffuse infiltrate					30						
	Increased interstitial...				20							
	Infiltrate		4			687	1	10				
	Lung	1		1		1					2	
	Decreased translucency	1	3		1	5	5	2		1	9	1
	Nodule, tumor or mass					8		28				
	Pleural calcification								32			
	Pleural changes								10	10		13
	Pleural effusion										743	
	Pleural thickening											30

0 labels matched — 100+ labels matched

For the label "infiltrate", the annotators had a greater spread across different labels compared to "gold standard". When "gold standard" used the label "infiltrate", annotators matched with six labels other than "infiltrate". Four of these labels were more specific i.e., descendants of "infiltrate" and two were less specific i.e., ancestors of "infiltrate" (Figure 1 and Table 4). For comparison, "gold standard" matched only with two descendent labels and one ancestral label (Table 4).

The opposite tendency was seen in the labels "decreased translucency", "pleural changes", and "atelectasis"—"gold standard" had greater spread and used more specific labels compared to annotators (Table 4).

Table 5. Number of matched cases (accumulated) on specific labels in the labeling scheme related to "cardiomediastinal findings". * Rows and columns not belonging to the parent node "cardiomediastinal findings" and that did not have any label disagreements have been pruned and thus number of rows does not match number of columns.

		Gold Standard *					
		Cardiomediastinum	Cardiomegaly	Widening of Mediastinum	Lymph Node Pathology	Other Cardiomediastinum	Vascular Changes
Annotators *	Cardiomediastinum	1	16	8	1	1	
	Cardiomegaly	3	472				
	Widening of Mediastinum	1		36	1		
	Lymph node pathology				9		
	Mediastinal tumor			1			
	Other cardiomediastinum					4	
	Vascular changes			2			32

0 labels matched — 100+ labels matched

When annotators used "cardiomediastinum" it was most often matched with more specific, descendent nodes such as "cardiomegaly", "widening of mediastinum", and "lymph node pathology" by "gold standard" (Table 5). Annotators were also less specific when "gold standard" used "lymph node pathology" since annotators only matched with using ancestral nodes besides the label itself (Table 5).

For the rest of the labeling scheme "gold standard" also used more specific labels compared to annotators (Table A4).

For unmatched labels, annotators had more different types of unmatched labels compared to "gold standard" (60 different types of labels vs. 41). Annotators had labeled 760 findings that were unmatched with "gold standard" labels, while "gold standard" only had 131 findings that did not find a match within the annotators' labels.

4. Discussion

There were three main findings in our study: (1) for radiologists, annotation performance of CXR text reports increased when radiological experience increased, (2) annotators had better performance on annotating negative findings compared to positive findings, and (3) annotators with less radiological experience tended to use a greater amount of less specific labels compared to experienced radiologists.

4.1. Performance of Annotators

Generally, all annotators showed high correlation [20] to "gold standard" annotations of CXR text reports (Table 2a,b). This finding was comparable to a previous study which showed a similar level of agreement between radiologists and non-radiological physicians and medical students when reading and comprehending radiology reports [26]. However, disagreements in reading and reporting radiological findings exist even between readers of the same specialty [27]. Previous studies suggested that the free-form structure of a radiological text report permitted the use of sentences that were ambiguous and inconsistent [28]. The variability in using these phrases could contribute to the annotation variability observed between the annotators. The intermediate radiologist's specialized experience may enable them to be better aligned with the "gold standard" annotators in interpreting whether an ambiguously worded sentence suggested that a finding was relevant and/or important enough to be annotated [26,29].

Our study also showed that the senior medical student and the novice radiographer performed better in annotation than the non-radiological physician and the experienced radiographer, respectively (Table 2a,b). Previous studies have demonstrated the difference between adaptive and routine expertise [30]. Experienced medical staff are encouraged to increase their specialization over time, thus, narrowing, but deepening their field of knowledge and therefore do not often engage in unknown situations [31,32], contrary to younger medical staff in active training. The novice radiographer and the medical student may have been more receptive to the change in their usual tasks, making them quicker to adapt to the annotation process itself [33,34]. The inherent routine expertise the experienced radiographer and the non-radiological physician have, may affect their behavior to value efficiency higher than thoroughness [35,36], and to only annotate findings that they would usually find relevant and disregard other findings [26,37]. A previous study aligned with our findings and showed that radiologists in training had slightly better performance compared to sub-specialist radiologists when reading and understanding reports outside their sub-specialty [38]. Another study showed that clinicians extract information from a radiological report based on their clinical bias [39,40] which may also contribute to the result of lesser correlation with "gold standard" annotations by the non-radiological physician compared to e.g., the senior medical student.

We found that labeling negative findings or labeling normal cases from abnormal cases may result in more consistent data for training a decision support system. Our findings were congruent with previous findings where it was demonstrated that negative findings were described more unambiguously in text reports, and that this may contribute to less difficulty in reading and comprehending negative findings compared to positive findings [27]. Negations may be a useful resource in the development of artificial intelligence-based algorithms for radiological decision support systems and studies [10,41,42] have shown that they are just as crucial to identify in a text, as positive findings [43].

4.2. Majority Vote Labeling

The results of our research indicated that there could be a reduction in false positive labels when using majority labeling compared to the labels used by an individual annotator (Table A3). Recent efforts have been made to outsource labeling to more annotators of lesser specialized experience as a way to reduce the time and cost of data gathering compared to sourcing and reimbursing field experts in the same tasks [44]. Several methods have been proposed to clean data labeled by multiple, less experienced annotators to obtain high-quality datasets efficiently, including using majority-vote labeling [45–47]. More inexperienced annotators may tend to overinterpret and overuse labels due to lack of training [48] or fear of missing findings [49]. Our study suggested that using majority labeling instead of using labels by individual annotators may eliminate some of the noisy and dispensable labels created by inexperienced annotators. Even when we eliminated the most experienced annotator from the majority voting (intermediate radiologist), there was still a reduction in false positive labels compared to any individual annotator (Table A3).

4.3. The Labeling Scheme

"Atelectasis", "infiltrate", "pleural effusion", "cardiomegaly", "correctly placed medical device", and "stasis/edema" were the labels that were most frequently agreed upon from our labeling scheme (Tables 4, 5 and A4 in Appendix A). While some labeling taxonomies are highly detailed with more labels than our labeling scheme [5], our labels were comparable to previously used annotation taxonomies which used text mining methods to extract labels [6,50]. An increased number of labels may introduce noise in data gathering [51], which there is a particularly high risk of when interpreting CXR and thoracic findings [52]. Fewer and broader labels may therefore be more desirable since this may enable higher agreement on a label from different readers.

Although "infiltrate" was one of the most agreed-upon labels, the differential diagnosis "pneumonia/infection" was not, despite it being one of the most common referral reasons for a CXR [53]. The "pneumonia/infection" diagnosis is usually based on a combination of clinical and paraclinical findings [54]. Radiologists are aware of this and may oftentimes not be conclusive in their reports, thus, introducing larger uncertainty to words associated with "pneumonia" compared to "infiltrate" [52]. Comparable with previous results from labeling CXR images [8], our study suggested that labels which are descriptive may be preferred to interpretive diagnostic labels. When annotating CXR reports, uncertainty of the radiologist in making diagnostic conclusions may introduce increased annotation bias in text reports.

4.4. Bias, Limitations and Future Studies

Due to time constraints, only a limited number of CXR text reports were included in our study. Previous studies have mentioned the limitations of using Cohen's kappa when it comes to imbalanced datasets, specifically, when the distribution of true positives and true negatives is highly skewed [55]. The limitations have been shown to be most prevalent when readers show negative or no correlation [56]. In anticipation of a label imbalance in our dataset and a risk of none to negative correlation between an annotator and "gold standard", we used Matthew's correlation coefficient over Cohen's kappa. However, as shown by Chicco et al. [56] MCC and Cohen's kappa are closely related, especially when readers show positive correlation. In our study, all readers had positive correlation coefficients with "gold standard" and the interpretation of results would therefore likely not have changed if we had used Cohen's kappa instead of MCC.

A limitation of the number of annotators included in our study was due to a combination of time constraints and participant availability. We recognize that as with the "gold standard" labels, ideally each level of annotator-experience should consist of multiple annotators' consensus vote. However, we found it relevant that our study reflected the real-world obstacles of data-gathering for deep learning development projects since recruitment of human annotators is already a well-known problem. We presented "majority" voting categories as solutions to, not only the limited number of annotators in our study, but also as a solution when there is a lack of annotators in deep learning development projects in general.

Annotations by the board-certified experienced radiologists may not reflect true labels, since factors such as the annotation software and subjective opinions may influence a radiologist's annotations. We attempted to reduce these elements of reader bias through consensus between the experienced radiologists by majority voting [57]. Furthermore, since annotators did not manually link each specific text piece to a label, we could not guarantee that annotators labeled the exact same findings with the same labels. We used an algorithm for matching labels in this study, since that algorithm would also be used for developing the final artificial intelligence-based support system.

Our study did not investigate whether an artificial intelligence-based algorithm would perform better when trained on annotations from less experienced medical staff compared to experienced radiologists. The assumption behind our study was that radiologists could provide annotations of the highest quality to train an algorithm, and that annotators with higher correlation to those annotations would produce high quality data [9]. Further studies are needed to investigate the differences in algorithm performance based on training data annotated by experienced radiologists compared to other medical staff. We did not investigate whether our annotators' text report labels corresponded to the CXR image, since this was not within the scope of our study but could be a topic of interest for future studies.

5. Conclusions

Trained radiologists were most aligned with experienced radiologists in understanding a chest X-ray report. For the purpose of labeling text reports for the development of an artificial intelligence-based decision support system, performance increased with radiological experience for trained radiologists. However, as annotators, medical staff with general and basic knowledge may be preferred to experienced medical staff, if the experienced medical staff have sub-specialized routine experience in other domains than diagnosing thoracic radiological findings.

Author Contributions: Conceptualization, D.L., J.F.C., K.L.H., R.B., M.F., J.T., L.T., S.D. and M.B.N.; methodology, D.L., J.F.C., M.F., J.T., R.B. and M.B.N.; software, R.B., J.T., L.T. and M.F.; formal analysis, D.L. and R.B.; investigation, D.L., L.M.P, C.A.L., J.J., T.T.A., S.B.B., A.M. and R.B.; resources, S.D. and M.B.N.; data curation, J.T., R.B. and M.F.; writing—original draft preparation, D.L.; writing—review and editing, D.L., L.M.P., C.A.L., J.J., T.T.A., S.B.B., A.M., J.T., R.B., M.F., K.L.H., J.F.C., S.D. and M.B.N.; visualization, D.L., J.T. and R.B.; supervision, K.L.H., J.F.C., S.D. and M.B.N.; project administration, D.L.; funding acquisition, S.D. and M.B.N. All authors have read and agreed to the published version of the manuscript.

Funding: This research was funded by Innovation Fund Denmark (IFD) with grant no. 0176-00013B for the AI4Xray project.

Institutional Review Board Statement: The study was conducted in accordance with the Declaration of Helsinki and approved by the Regional Council for Region Hovedstaden (R-22017450, 11 May 2022) and Knowledge Center on Data Protection Compliance (P-2022-231, 19 May 2022).

Informed Consent Statement: Informed consent was obtained from all readers/annotators involved in the study. Informed consent from patients was waived by the Regional Council for Region Hovedstaden.

Data Availability Statement: Not applicable.

Acknowledgments: We acknowledge and are grateful for any support given by the Section of Biostatistics at the Department of Public Health at Copenhagen University.

Conflicts of Interest: The authors declare no conflict of interest.

Appendix A

Table A1. Frequency counts of labels used by each annotator for positive findings.

		Annotators								
Labels		Radiologist, Inter-Mediate	Radiologist, Novice	Radiographer, Experienced	Radiographer, Novice	Physician, Non-Radiologist	Senior Medical Student	Senior Radiologist 3	Senior Radiologist 2	Senior Radiologist 1	All
	Abnormal	0	0	1	0	0	0	0	0	0	1
	Abscess	6	5	5	3	5	5	5	6	1	41
	Asbestosis	0	1	1	0	1	0	0	0	1	4
	Atelectasis	33	31	31	32	33	33	35	35	23	286
	Bone	0	6	0	16	5	3	8	1	0	39
	Cardiomediastinum	0	0	0	1	9	0	1	1	0	12
	Cardiomegaly	39	37	38	38	34	36	36	39	33	330
	Cavitary lesion	2	2	8	6	3	4	2	0	4	31
	Chronic lung changes	33	33	17	28	17	29	21	26	7	211
	Consolidation	25	29	33	5	12	25	12	7	5	153
	Correct placement	32	42	11	29	34	7	27	24	32	238
	Cysts/bullae	4	2	7	4	4	3	4	4	4	36
	Decreased translucency	3	0	0	29	10	3	4	3	0	52
	Diffuse infiltrate	3	5	0	0	22	3	0	5	0	38
	Elevated (hemi)diaphragm	7	7	7	6	6	6	6	6	2	53
	Emphysema	16	15	18	24	19	18	10	10	17	147
	Enlarged mediastinum	2	2	2	2	0	2	2	2	2	16
	Fibrosis	12	10	11	8	10	7	7	4	2	71
	Flattened (hemi)diaphragm	8	13	14	13	12	13	15	10	2	100

Table A1. Cont.

	Annotators								
	Radiologist, Inter-Mediate	Radiologist, Novice	Radiographer, Experienced	Radiographer, Novice	Physician, Non-Radiologist	Senior Medical Student	Senior Radiologist 3	Senior Radiologist 2	Senior Radiologist 1	All
Foreign object	0	0	0	1	0	0	0	0	0	1
Fracture	7	1	4	0	1	4	3	4	7	31
Hiatal hernia	5	5	4	3	3	5	4	5	4	38
Increased interstitial....	6	10	5	1	5	16	3	11	14	71
Increased translucency	1	0	1	2	13	1	0	1	0	19
Infiltrate	52	45	53	64	39	62	60	31	64	470
Interlobar septal thickening	0	1	1	0	0	0	0	0	0	2
Lung	0	0	0	0	1	2	0	0	0	3
Lung surgery	5	12	7	17	15	19	5	14	7	101
Lymph node pathology	2	3	2	2	0	2	2	3	1	17
Malignant/cancer	3	3	4	5	7	7	2	7	0	38
Mediastinal shift	2	3	1	0	0	1	1	2	1	11
Mediastinal tumor	0	1	2	0	0	1	0	0	1	5
Nodule, tumor or mass	6	8	3	4	10	6	8	3	16	64
Not abnormal	9	23	13	2	16	10	12	6	4	95
Non-correct placement	2	2	3	4	1	1	3	6	1	23
Operation/implants	23	10	8	1	6	3	17	10	16	94
Artifact	0	7	2	0	0	0	0	1	0	10
Other bone pathology	11	9	7	5	12	11	5	12	6	78

Table A1. Cont.

	Annotators									
	Radiologist, Inter-Mediate	Radiologist, Novice	Radiographer, Experienced	Radiographer, Novice	Physician, Non-Radiologist	Senior Medical Student	Senior Radiologist 3	Senior Radiologist 2	Senior Radiologist 1	All
Other cardiomediastinum	1	1	0	0	1	3	1	1	1	9
Other	1	0	0	0	0	0	0	3	0	4
Other foreign object	0	0	0	1	0	0	1	0	0	2
Other decreased translucency	1	0	0	0	1	0	0	1	0	3
Other increased translucency	0	0	0	0	1	0	0	0	0	1
Other non-pathological	1	18	2	0	0	0	0	2	0	23
Other pathological	8	1	11	0	2	3	1	1	0	27
Other soft tissue	0	0	1	1	3	5	1	1	3	15
Pericardial effusion	1	0	0	1	1	1	3	1	0	8
Pleural calcification	8	8	1	2	8	7	5	8	7	54
Pleural changes	11	6	13	13	11	8	7	4	4	77
Pleural contraction	0	0	1	0	0	0	0	0	0	1
Pleural effusion	41	43	42	38	41	47	49	44	42	387
Pleural thickening	10	10	0	5	8	6	7	10	12	68
Pneumomediastinum	0	0	1	0	0	0	0	0	0	1
Pneumonia	32	32	19	18	29	14	0	30	2	176
Pneumothorax	10	10	10	10	13	10	10	10	8	91
Sarcoidosis	1	1	1	1	1	1	0	1	1	8
Soft tissue	0	1	0	8	11	0	4	0	0	24
Stasis/edema	30	31	23	23	32	26	29	29	27	250

Table A1. Cont.

	Annotators							
	Radiologist, Inter-Mediate	Radiologist, Novice	Radiographer, Experienced	Radiographer, Novice	Physician, Non-Radiologist	Senior Medical Student	Senior Radiologist 3	Senior Radiologist 2	Senior Radiologist 1	All
Subcutaneous emphysema	6	6	4	0	5	5	2	5	3	37
Support devices	10	0	34	40	12	12	11	17	3	162
Tuberculosis	8	8	3	6	8	8	6	6	8	56
Vascular changes	15	0	15	11	0	0	16	11	0	88

Table A2. Frequency counts of labels used by each annotator for negative findings.

		Annotators								
		Radiologist, Inter-Mediate	Radiologist, Novice	Radiographer, Experienced	Radiographer, Novice	Physician, Non-Radiologist	Senior Medical Student	Senior Radiologist 3	Senior Radiologist 2	Senior Radiologist 1	All
Labels	Abscess	1	1	1	1	1	1	1	1	0	8
	Atelectasis	9	8	8	10	6	8	5	8	7	69
	Bone	3	3	0	3	1	2	4	2	0	18
	Cardiomediastinum	0	7	1	0	21	5	5	5	0	44
	Cardiomegaly	52	45	50	53	31	48	43	42	55	417
	Cavitary lesion	0	0	3	2	0	1	1	0	1	8
	Consolidation	2	1	23	1	0	4	1	1	2	35
	Correct placement	0	0	1	0	0	0	0	0	0	1
	Cysts/bullae	0	0	3	0	0	0	0	0	0	3
	Differential diagnosis	0	0	1	0	3	0	0	1	0	1
	Decreased translucency	0	0	0	0	1	0	0	1	0	5
	Diffuse infiltrate	0	0	2	0	1	0	0	1	0	4
	Emphysema	0	0	0	1	0	0	1	0	0	2

Table A2. Cont.

	Annotators								
	Radiologist, Inter-Mediate	Radiologist, Novice	Radiographer, Experienced	Radiographer, Novice	Physician, Non-Radiologist	Senior Medical Student	Senior Radiologist 3	Senior Radiologist 2	Senior Radiologist 1	All
Enlarged mediastinum	18	9	2	8	0	6	11	11	1	66
Fracture	3	4	3	1	3	3	3	3	3	26
Increased interstitial	1	0	1	1	0	1	1	1	1	7
Increased translucency	0	0	0	1	1	0	0	0	0	2
Infiltrate	86	73	60	84	65	88	81	77	82	696
Lung	2	1	0	0	0	5	0	0	0	8
Lung surgery	0	0	0	0	0	0	0	1	0	1
Lymph node pathology	0	0	0	0	0	0	1	0	0	1
Malignant/cancer	3	3	5	3	4	2	2	2	0	24
Mediastinal shift	1	1	1	0	0	0	0	0	0	3
Nodule, tumor or mass	1	9	1	1	2	2	1	1	4	22
Other bone pathology	0	0	0	1	1	0	0	0	0	2
Other soft tissue	0	0	0	1	0	0	0	0	0	1
Pericardial effusion	0	0	2	1	0	0	2	0	0	5
Pleural changes	1	2	20	0	6	3	2	1	4	39
Pleural effusion	102	102	44	94	81	102	99	97	94	815
Pleural thickening	0	0	1	0	0	0	0	0	0	1
Pneumonia	8	7	3	0	1	1	0	7	0	27
Pneumothorax	30	31	28	29	26	30	30	30	25	259
Sarcoidosis	1	1	0	0	1	1	0	1	1	6
Soft tissue	0	0	0	0	0	0	1	0	0	1
Stasis/edema	82	81	51	80	63	77	76	78	72	660
Subcutaneous emphysema	2	2	2	0	2	2	1	2	2	15

Table A2. *Cont.*

	Annotators									
	Radiologist, Inter-Mediate	Radiologist, Novice	Radiographer, Experienced	Radiographer, Novice	Physician, Non-Radiologist	Senior Medical Student	Senior Radiologist 3	Senior Radiologist 2	Senior Radiologist 1	All
Support devices	0	0	1	1	0	0	0	2	0	4
Tuberculosis	2	2	0	0	1	1	0	2	2	10
Vascular changes	3	0	0	2	0	10	4	0	0	19

Table A3. Number of unmatched labels of both positive and negative findings after subtraction of matched labels by individual annotators, majority of annotators, and gold standard annotations.

	Number of Unmatched Labels (by Annotator)								
Compared to annotator	Radiologist, Intermediate	Radiologist, Novice	Radiographer, Experienced	Radiographer, Novice	Physician, Non-Radiologist	Senior Medical Student	Majority	Majority excl. Intermed. Radiologist	Gold Standard
Radiologist, intermediate		101	144	128	121	114	30	75	32
Radiologist, novice	118		169	150	130	135	45	70	58
Radiographer, experienced	288	296		271	277	277	180	205	209
Radiographer, novice	182	187	181		164	155	71	84	88
Physician, non-radiologist	214	206	226	203		205	110	139	133
Senior medical student	135	139	154	122	133		41	62	57
Majority	173	171	179	160	160	163		61	96
Majority excl. Intermed. Radiologist	157	135	143	112	128	123	0		75
Gold Standard	201	210	234	203	209	205	122	162	

Fewest unmatched (best)   50% fractile   Most unmatched (worst)

Table A4. Number of matched cases (accumulated) on specific labels in the labeling scheme for all labels except labels in the "lung tissue findings" category and the "cardiomediastinum" category. * Rows and columns belonging to the parent nodes "lung tissue finding" or "cardiomediastinal findings" and that did not have any label disagreements have been pruned and thus number of rows does not match number of columns.

		Gold Standard *							
	Bone	Correct Placement	Fracture	Non-Correct Placement	Operation and Implants	Other Bone Pathology	Stasis/Edema	Subcutaneous Emphysema	Support Devices
Bone	11		10			10			13
Correct placement		115							
Differential diagnosis							1		
Foreign object					1				
Fracture	2		29						
Non-correct placement				6					1
Operation and implants					38	38			
Other bone pathology	3							1	
Soft tissue							576		
Stasis/edema								28	
Subcutaneous emphysema									
Support devices		48							24

Annotators *

0 labels matched — 100+ labels matched

References

1. Performance Analysis Team. *Diagnostic Imaging Dataset Statistical Release*; NHS: London, UK, 2022/2023. Available online: https://www.england.nhs.uk/statistics/statistical-work-areas/diagnostic-imaging-dataset/diagnostic-imaging-dataset-2022-23-data/ (accessed on 7 February 2022).
2. Li, D.; Pehrson, L.M.; Lauridsen, C.A.; Tottrup, L.; Fraccaro, M.; Elliott, D.; Zajac, H.D.; Darkner, S.; Carlsen, J.F.; Nielsen, M.B. The Added Effect of Artificial Intelligence on Physicians' Performance in Detecting Thoracic Pathologies on CT and Chest X-ray: A Systematic Review. *Diagnostics* **2021**, *11*, 2206. [CrossRef]
3. Kim, T.S.; Jang, G.; Lee, S.; Kooi, T. Did You Get What You Paid For? Rethinking Annotation Cost of Deep Learning Based Computer Aided Detection in Chest Radiographs. In Proceedings of the International Conference on Medical Image Computing and Computer-Assisted Intervention, Singapore, 18–22 September 2022; pp. 261–270.
4. Willemink, M.J.; Koszek, W.A.; Hardell, C.; Wu, J.; Fleischmann, D.; Harvey, H.; Folio, L.R.; Summers, R.M.; Rubin, D.L.; Lungren, M.P. Preparing medical imaging data for machine learning. *Radiology* **2020**, *295*, 4–15. [CrossRef]
5. Bustos, A.; Pertusa, A.; Salinas, J.-M.; de la Iglesia-Vayá, M. Padchest: A large chest x-ray image dataset with multi-label annotated reports. *Med. Image Anal.* **2020**, *66*, 101797. [CrossRef]
6. Irvin, J.; Rajpurkar, P.; Ko, M.; Yu, Y.; Ciurea-Ilcus, S.; Chute, C.; Marklund, H.; Haghgoo, B.; Ball, R.; Shpanskaya, K. Chexpert: A large chest radiograph dataset with uncertainty labels and expert comparison. In Proceedings of the Proceedings of the AAAI Conference on Artificial Intelligence, Honolulu, HI, USA, 27 January–1 February 2019; pp. 590–597.
7. Putha, P.; Tadepalli, M.; Reddy, B.; Raj, T.; Chiramal, J.A.; Govil, S.; Sinha, N.; KS, M.; Reddivari, S.; Jagirdar, A. Can artificial intelligence reliably report chest X-rays?: Radiologist validation of an algorithm trained on 2.3 million X-rays. *arXiv* **2018**, arXiv:1807.07455.
8. Li, D.; Pehrson, L.M.; Tottrup, L.; Fraccaro, M.; Bonnevie, R.; Thrane, J.; Sorensen, P.J.; Rykkje, A.; Andersen, T.T.; Steglich-Arnholm, H.; et al. Inter- and Intra-Observer Agreement When Using a Diagnostic Labeling Scheme for Annotating Findings on Chest X-rays-An Early Step in the Development of a Deep Learning-Based Decision Support System. *Diagnostics* **2022**, *12*, 3112. [CrossRef]
9. Mehrotra, P.; Bosemani, V.; Cox, J. Do radiologists still need to report chest x rays? *Postgrad. Med. J.* **2009**, *85*, 339. [CrossRef]
10. Peng, Y.; Wang, X.; Lu, L.; Bagheri, M.; Summers, R.; Lu, Z. NegBio: A high-performance tool for negation and uncertainty detection in radiology reports. *AMIA Summits Transl. Sci. Proc.* **2018**, *2018*, 188.
11. McDermott, M.B.; Hsu, T.M.H.; Weng, W.-H.; Ghassemi, M.; Szolovits, P. Chexpert++: Approximating the chexpert labeler for speed, differentiability, and probabilistic output. In Proceedings of the Machine Learning for Healthcare Conference, Durham, NC, USA, 7–8 August 2020; pp. 913–927.
12. Wang, S.; Cai, J.; Lin, Q.; Guo, W. An Overview of Unsupervised Deep Feature Representation for Text Categorization. *IEEE Trans. Comput. Soc. Syst.* **2019**, *6*, 504–517. [CrossRef]
13. Thangaraj, M.; Sivakami, M. Text classification techniques: A literature review. *Interdiscip. J. Inf. Knowl. Manag.* **2018**, *13*, 117. [CrossRef]
14. Calderon-Ramirez, S.; Giri, R.; Yang, S.; Moemeni, A.; Umaña, M.; Elizondo, D.; Torrents-Barrena, J.; Molina-Cabello, M.A. Dealing with Scarce Labelled Data: Semi-supervised Deep Learning with Mix Match for Covid-19 Detection Using Chest X-ray Images. In Proceedings of the 2020 25th International Conference on Pattern Recognition (ICPR), Milan, Italy, 10–15 January 2021; pp. 5294–5301.
15. Munappy, A.; Bosch, J.; Olsson, H.H.; Arpteg, A.; Brinne, B. Data Management Challenges for Deep Learning. In Proceedings of the 2019 45th Euromicro Conference on Software Engineering and Advanced Applications (SEAA), Kallithea-Chalkidiki, Greece, 28–30 August 2019; pp. 140–147.
16. Brady, A.P. Radiology reporting-from Hemingway to HAL? *Insights Imaging* **2018**, *9*, 237–246. [CrossRef]
17. Ogawa, M.; Lee, C.H.; Friedman, B. Multicenter survey clarifying phrases in emergency radiology reports. *Emerg. Radiol.* **2022**, *29*, 855–862. [CrossRef]
18. Klobuka, A.J.; Lee, J.; Buranosky, R.; Heller, M. When the Reading Room Meets the Team Room: Resident Perspectives From Radiology and Internal Medicine on the Effect of Personal Communication After Implementing a Resident-Led Radiology Rounds. *Curr. Probl. Diagn. Radiol.* **2019**, *48*, 312–322. [CrossRef]
19. Hansell, D.M.; Bankier, A.A.; MacMahon, H.; McLoud, T.C.; Muller, N.L.; Remy, J. Fleischner Society: Glossary of terms for thoracic imaging. *Radiology* **2008**, *246*, 697–722. [CrossRef]
20. Chicco, D.; Jurman, G. The Matthews correlation coefficient (MCC) should replace the ROC AUC as the standard metric for assessing binary classification. *BioData Min.* **2023**, *16*, 4. [CrossRef]
21. McKinney, W. Data Structures for Statistical Computing in Python. 2010, pp. 56–61. Available online: https://conference.scipy.org/proceedings/scipy2010/pdfs/mckinney.pdf (accessed on 7 February 2022).
22. Harris, C.R.; Millman, K.J.; van der Walt, S.J.; Gommers, R.; Virtanen, P.; Cournapeau, D.; Wieser, E.; Taylor, J.; Berg, S.; Smith, N.J.; et al. Array programming with NumPy. *Nature* **2020**, *585*, 357–362. [CrossRef]
23. Asch, V.V. Macro-and Micro-Averaged Evaluation Measures [BASIC DRAFT]. 2013. Available online: https://cupdf.com/document/macro-and-micro-averaged-evaluation-measures-basic-draft.html?page=1 (accessed on 7 February 2022).
24. Hagberg, A.A.; Schult, D.A.; Swart, P.J. Exploring Network Structure, Dynamics, and Function Using NetworkX. In Proceedings of the 7th Python in Science Conference, Pasadena, CA, USA, 19–24 August 2008; pp. 11–15.

25. Wigness, M.; Draper, B.A.; Ross Beveridge, J. Efficient label collection for unlabeled image datasets. In Proceedings of the IEEE Conference on Computer Vision and Pattern Recognition, Boston, MA, USA, 8–10 June 2015; pp. 4594–4602.
26. Lee, B.; Whitehead, M.T. Radiology Reports: What YOU Think You're Saying and What THEY Think You're Saying. *Curr. Probl. Diagn. Radiol.* **2017**, *46*, 186–195. [CrossRef]
27. Lacson, R.; Odigie, E.; Wang, A.; Kapoor, N.; Shinagare, A.; Boland, G.; Khorasani, R. Multivariate Analysis of Radiologists' Usage of Phrases that Convey Diagnostic Certainty. *Acad. Radiol.* **2019**, *26*, 1229–1234. [CrossRef]
28. Shinagare, A.B.; Lacson, R.; Boland, G.W.; Wang, A.; Silverman, S.G.; Mayo-Smith, W.W.; Khorasani, R. Radiologist Preferences, Agreement, and Variability in Phrases Used to Convey Diagnostic Certainty in Radiology Reports. *J. Am. Coll. Radiol.* **2019**, *16*, 458–464. [CrossRef]
29. Berlin, L. Medicolegal: Malpractice and ethical issues in radiology. Proofreading radiology reports. *AJR Am. J. Roentgenol.* **2013**, *200*, W691–W692. [CrossRef]
30. Mylopoulos, M.; Woods, N.N. Having our cake and eating it too: Seeking the best of both worlds in expertise research. *Med. Educ.* **2009**, *43*, 406–413. [CrossRef]
31. Winder, M.; Owczarek, A.J.; Chudek, J.; Pilch-Kowalczyk, J.; Baron, J. Are We Overdoing It? Changes in Diagnostic Imaging Workload during the Years 2010-2020 including the Impact of the SARS-CoV-2 Pandemic. *Healthcare* **2021**, *9*, 1557. [CrossRef]
32. Sriram, V.; Bennett, S. Strengthening medical specialisation policy in low-income and middle-income countries. *BMJ Glob. Health* **2020**, *5*, e002053. [CrossRef]
33. Mylopoulos, M.; Regehr, G.; Ginsburg, S. Exploring residents' perceptions of expertise and expert development. *Acad. Med.* **2011**, *86*, S46–S49. [CrossRef]
34. Farooq, F.; Mahboob, U.; Ashraf, R.; Arshad, S. Measuring Adaptive Expertise in Radiology Residents: A Multicenter Study. *Health Prof. Educ. J.* **2022**, *5*, 9–14. [CrossRef]
35. Grant, S.; Guthrie, B. Efficiency and thoroughness trade-offs in high-volume organisational routines: An ethnographic study of prescribing safety in primary care. *BMJ Qual. Saf.* **2018**, *27*, 199–206. [CrossRef]
36. Croskerry, P. Adaptive expertise in medical decision making. *Med. Teach.* **2018**, *40*, 803–808. [CrossRef]
37. Lafortune, M.; Breton, G.; Baudouin, J.L. The radiological report: What is useful for the referring physician? *Can. Assoc. Radiol. J.* **1988**, *39*, 140–143.
38. Branstetter, B.F.t.; Morgan, M.B.; Nesbit, C.E.; Phillips, J.A.; Lionetti, D.M.; Chang, P.J.; Towers, J.D. Preliminary reports in the emergency department: Is a subspecialist radiologist more accurate than a radiology resident? *Acad. Radiol.* **2007**, *14*, 201–206. [CrossRef]
39. Clinger, N.J.; Hunter, T.B.; Hillman, B.J. Radiology reporting: Attitudes of referring physicians. *Radiology* **1988**, *169*, 825–826. [CrossRef]
40. Kruger, P.; Lynskey, S.; Sutherland, A. Are orthopaedic surgeons reading radiology reports? A Trans-Tasman Survey. *J. Med. Imaging Radiat. Oncol.* **2019**, *63*, 324–328. [CrossRef]
41. Lin, C.; Bethard, S.; Dligach, D.; Sadeque, F.; Savova, G.; Miller, T.A. Does BERT need domain adaptation for clinical negation detection? *J. Am. Med. Inf. Assoc.* **2020**, *27*, 584–591. [CrossRef]
42. van Es, B.; Reteig, L.C.; Tan, S.C.; Schraagen, M.; Hemker, M.M.; Arends, S.R.S.; Rios, M.A.R.; Haitjema, S. Negation detection in Dutch clinical texts: An evaluation of rule-based and machine learning methods. *BMC Bioinform.* **2023**, *24*, 10. [CrossRef]
43. Rokach, L.; Romano, R.; Maimon, O. Negation recognition in medical narrative reports. *Inf. Retr.* **2008**, *11*, 499–538. [CrossRef]
44. Zhang, J. Knowledge Learning With Crowdsourcing: A Brief Review and Systematic Perspective. *IEEE/CAA J. Autom. Sin.* **2022**, *9*, 749–762. [CrossRef]
45. Li, J.; Zhang, R.; Mensah, S.; Qin, W.; Hu, C. Classification-oriented dawid skene model for transferring intelligence from crowds to machines. *Front. Comput. Sci.* **2023**, *17*, 175332. [CrossRef]
46. Whitehill, J.; Ruvolo, P.; Wu, T.; Bergsma, J.; Movellan, J. Whose vote should count more: Optimal integration of labels from labelers of unknown expertise. In Proceedings of the Advances in Neural Information Processing Systems 22-Proceedings of the 2009 Conference, Vancouver, BC, Canada, 7–9 December 2009; pp. 2035–2043.
47. Sheng, V.S.; Zhang, J.; Gu, B.; Wu, X. Majority Voting and Pairing with Multiple Noisy Labeling. *IEEE Trans. Knowl. Data Eng.* **2019**, *31*, 1355–1368. [CrossRef]
48. Schmidt, H.G.; Boshuizen, H.P.A. On acquiring expertise in medicine. *Educ. Psychol. Rev.* **1993**, *5*, 205–221. [CrossRef]
49. Yavas, U.S.; Calisir, C.; Ozkan, I.R. The Interobserver Agreement between Residents and Experienced Radiologists for Detecting Pulmonary Embolism and DVT with Using CT Pulmonary Angiography and Indirect CT Venography. *Korean J. Radiol.* **2008**, *9*, 498–502. [CrossRef]
50. Wang, X.; Peng, Y.; Lu, L.; Lu, Z.; Bagheri, M.; Summers, R. ChestX-ray14: Hospital-scale Chest X-ray Database and Benchmarks on Weakly-Supervised Classification and Localization of Common Thorax Diseases. In Proceedings of the IEEE Conference on Computer Vision and Pattern Recognition, Honolulu, HI, USA, 21–26 July 2017.
51. Frénay, B.; Verleysen, M. Classification in the Presence of Label Noise: A Survey. *Neural Netw. Learn. Syst. IEEE Trans.* **2014**, *25*, 845–869. [CrossRef]
52. Callen, A.L.; Dupont, S.M.; Price, A.; Laguna, B.; McCoy, D.; Do, B.; Talbott, J.; Kohli, M.; Narvid, J. Between Always and Never: Evaluating Uncertainty in Radiology Reports Using Natural Language Processing. *J. Digit. Imaging* **2020**, *33*, 1194–1201. [CrossRef]

53. Wootton, D.; Feldman, C. The diagnosis of pneumonia requires a chest radiograph (X-ray)-yes, no or sometimes? *Pneumonia* **2014**, *5*, 1–7. [CrossRef]
54. Loeb, M.B.; Carusone, S.B.; Marrie, T.J.; Brazil, K.; Krueger, P.; Lohfeld, L.; Simor, A.E.; Walter, S.D. Interobserver reliability of radiologists' interpretations of mobile chest radiographs for nursing home-acquired pneumonia. *J. Am. Med. Dir. Assoc.* **2006**, *7*, 416–419. [CrossRef]
55. Byrt, T.; Bishop, J.; Carlin, J.B. Bias, prevalence and kappa. *J. Clin. Epidemiol.* **1993**, *46*, 423–429. [CrossRef]
56. Chicco, D.; Jurman, G. The advantages of the Matthews correlation coefficient (MCC) over F1 score and accuracy in binary classification evaluation. *BMC Genom.* **2020**, *21*, 6. [CrossRef]
57. Hight, S.L.; Petersen, D.P. Dissent in a Majority Voting System. *IEEE Trans. Comput.* **1973**, *100*, 168–171. [CrossRef]

Disclaimer/Publisher's Note: The statements, opinions and data contained in all publications are solely those of the individual author(s) and contributor(s) and not of MDPI and/or the editor(s). MDPI and/or the editor(s) disclaim responsibility for any injury to people or property resulting from any ideas, methods, instructions or products referred to in the content.

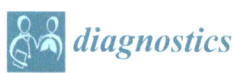

Article

Cross Dataset Analysis of Domain Shift in CXR Lung Region Detection

Zhiyun Xue *, Feng Yang, Sivaramakrishnan Rajaraman, Ghada Zamzmi and Sameer Antani

Computational Health Research Branch, National Library of Medicine, National Institutes of Health, Bethesda, MD 20894, USA
* Correspondence: zhiyun.xue@nih.gov

Abstract: Domain shift is one of the key challenges affecting reliability in medical imaging-based machine learning predictions. It is of significant importance to investigate this issue to gain insights into its characteristics toward determining controllable parameters to minimize its impact. In this paper, we report our efforts on studying and analyzing domain shift in lung region detection in chest radiographs. We used five chest X-ray datasets, collected from different sources, which have manual markings of lung boundaries in order to conduct extensive experiments toward this goal. We compared the characteristics of these datasets from three aspects: information obtained from metadata or an image header, image appearance, and features extracted from a pretrained model. We carried out experiments to evaluate and compare model performances within each dataset and across datasets in four scenarios using different combinations of datasets. We proposed a new feature visualization method to provide explanations for the applied object detection network on the obtained quantitative results. We also examined chest X-ray modality-specific initialization, catastrophic forgetting, and model repeatability. We believe the observations and discussions presented in this work could help to shed some light on the importance of the analysis of training data for medical imaging machine learning research, and could provide valuable guidance for domain shift analysis.

Keywords: domain shift; lung region detection; chest X-ray datasets; catastrophic forgetting; modality-specific initialization

Citation: Xue, Z.; Yang, F.; Rajaraman, S.; Zamzmi, G.; Antani, S. Cross Dataset Analysis of Domain Shift in CXR Lung Region Detection. *Diagnostics* **2023**, *13*, 1068. https:// doi.org/10.3390/diagnostics13061068

Academic Editor: Dechang Chen

Received: 9 February 2023
Revised: 3 March 2023
Accepted: 7 March 2023
Published: 11 March 2023

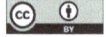

Copyright: © 2023 by the authors. Licensee MDPI, Basel, Switzerland. This article is an open access article distributed under the terms and conditions of the Creative Commons Attribution (CC BY) license (https:// creativecommons.org/licenses/by/ 4.0/).

1. Introduction

Chest radiography is an important imaging tool for the examination, identification, and diagnosis of cardiothoracic and pulmonary abnormalities. Radiological findings are frequently used for triage, screening, and diagnosis. The computer-aided diagnosis (CAD) of chest X-rays using deep learning (DL) and image processing techniques has been actively studied in the literature. A very recent comprehensive survey on publications using DL on chest radiographs can be found in [1]. However, despite this extensive research, very few methods have been translated into real-world clinical use.

Domain shift is a significant challenge that machine learning (ML) algorithms often face when models are deployed for real-world use. It refers to the phenomenon of unreliable prediction performance when the distribution of the data used to train and evaluate ML models in the development stage is different from that of the data seen by the deployed models. Because of the existence of domain shift, the performance of models during deployment may be significantly worse than what was observed during developmental experiments. This issue can be more substantial for medical imaging applications due to several factors: (i) training data size-medical images are often available either in small quantities, especially for abnormal cases; (ii) limited number of annotations due to the shortage of medical experts as well as the required intensity of labor efforts; (iii) lack of diversity in the distribution of patient population as data may be sourced from a single site; (iv) lack of variety in severity and type of disease manifestations; and (v) lack of multiple imaging modalities. Furthermore, the images obtained from different clinical providers are often taken by different imaging devices with varying manufacturer sensor designs and on-device post-processing, image acquisition parameters/protocols, and illumination conditions for optical imagery. As a result, the characteristics of images from different sources can be considerably different, which may create domain shift issues and low generalization performance of models on target. Therefore, it is of high value to study the problem of domain shift in medical applications and develop methods to provide necessary controls or, ideally, remedy it.

As summarized by [1], there have been limited works on domain adaptation for automated chest X-ray analysis [2–4]. In this work, we focus on an important pre-processing step in chest X-ray analysis—lung region detection to analyze domain shift problems in localizing lung region-of-interest (ROI). The problem of extracting the bounding box that encloses two lungs, as shown in Figure 1, can reduce the interference of irrelevant areas in the image for cardiopulmonary diseases and lessen the challenge of learning data-driven DL models in the succeeding steps, especially when the data are limited.

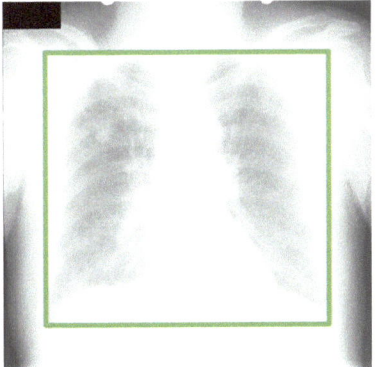

Figure 1. Lung ROI detection.

To investigate the domain shift for lung region localization, we used five chest X-ray datasets. Each dataset contains images in a range of a few hundred or less. These datasets were collected from different sources, and they vary from each other in multiple aspects, including patient population, disease manifestation, imaging devices, clinical providers, and the number of images. DLs are data-driven. Therefore, the characteristics of data have a significant impact on the performance of DL models and play a key role in explaining and understanding the model behavior. Domain shift, also called distributional shift, in essence, is due to the changes in data characteristics. Hence, to obtain some insights into model explanation and analysis, we need to analyze and compare the data characteristics among these datasets first. We conducted the comparison and analysis from three aspects: information obtained from metadata or image header, image appearance, and feature extracted from a pretrained model. Through these three complementary approaches, we evaluated the datasets for homogeneity, diversity, and variability.

To examine the effect of domain shift on DL models, we carried out extensive experiments in four scenarios. We trained lung region detection models using individual datasets as well as combinations of datasets. We evaluated and compared the intra/inter-dataset performances among all models. We observed and discussed interesting results. We also experimented with modality-specific initialization, i.e., the model to be trained on one CXR dataset is initialized with the weights from the model that has been trained on another

CXR dataset. We evaluated the additional effects that are often encountered in medical AI applications, viz., catastrophic forgetting and model repeatability.

It is very important to understand and explain the reasons behind such observations of performance variations, that is, why does a certain model work better than another model on a certain dataset? To this end, we proposed a new and simple approach that converts the multi-scale feature maps extracted from several stages in the applied object detection network into a feature vector, and generated feature embeddings in a 2D plot to show the feature representation characteristics of the network for images from different datasets.

To summarize, our main contributions include the following:

- We designed and carried out extensive experiments using five small chest X-ray datasets to study the cross-dataset performance and domain shift issue on lung detection in CXRs.
- We proposed to use three complementary approaches (at text, image, and feature level, respectively) for data analysis and understanding, a key prerequisite step that needs to be carried out before DL design and implementation but is often paid insufficient attention to in the literature.
- We considered and compared four scenarios in the experiments, using or not using the dataset combination, as well as different model initializations.
- We proposed a new method to extract and visualize the features from the object detection models which were shown to be helpful for providing insights into explaining the obtained detection performances on datasets.

Although our methods were developed and evaluated for lung region detection, a vital step in a CAD system for CXR analysis, they can be applied and adapted to other medical image analysis applications. We hope the observations and discussion of the experimental results presented in this work help shed some light on the importance of data analysis for medical imaging machine learning research, especially when the dataset at hand is small, and provide valuable input for domain shift analysis. In the following Sections 2 and 3, we present detailed descriptions of the analysis and comparison of dataset characteristics, the methods for detecting lung ROI, the approach for analyzing domain shift across datasets, the design of the experimental tests, and the discussion of the results. We conclude the paper and provide suggestions for future work in Section 4.

2. Methods

2.1. Datasets

We used five deidentified chest X-ray datasets in this work that were collected from different sources and have manual lung masks: (1) Montgomery; (2) Shenzhen; (3) JSRT; (4) Pediatric; and (5) Indiana. The bounding boxes of manual lung masks were used as ground truth for this detection work.

Both Montgomery and Shenzhen datasets are made publicly available by the U.S. National Library of Medicine (NLM) [5]. The Montgomery set was sampled from images acquired by the Department of Health and Human Services, Montgomery County, Maryland, under its Tuberculosis (TB) Control program over many years. It consists of 138 posterior-anterior (PA) X-rays (80 controls and 58 TB cases with manifestations of tuberculosis), left and right lung lobe binary masks for each image, as well as patient age and gender information. The consensus annotations of regions of manifestations from two radiologists and their radiology readings were also added to the dataset later [6]. The Shenzhen set was collected and provided by Shenzhen No.3 Hospital in Shenzhen, Guangdong providence, China. It contains 326 normal chest X-rays and 336 abnormal chest X-rays showing various TB-consistent manifestations. The dataset also includes consensus annotations of regions of manifestations from two radiologists. The use and sharing of both the Montgomery and Shenzhen sets were reviewed and exempted from IRB review by the NIH Office of Human Research Protections Programs. The manual binary lung masks of a subset (566 images) of the Shenzhen dataset were provided through Kaggle by another research group [7]. JSRT [8] is a public chest radiograph dataset released by the

Japanese Society of Radiological Technology (JSRT) two decades ago. There are 247 scanned chest radiographs in the dataset, 154 of which have malignant or benign nodules and 93 have normal lungs. The manual binary masks of the lungs for each chest X-ray are also available [9]. Associated textual information includes patient age, gender, nodule diagnosis, and coordinates of nodule location. The pediatric dataset was acquired from a private clinic in India. It contains 161 pediatric chest radiographs. Each image has a corresponding manual lung segmentation mask. We also used a very small subset (55 frontal images) of the Indiana University hospital network image collection, made available through Open-i [10], that have manual lung masks. Each image in this subset has a clinical report that included information on findings and impressions but no patient demographic information such as age and gender.

Pre-Processing

The image formats in the five datasets may be different from set to set, although PNG and DICOM are two of the main formats. For example, the images in the Pediatric dataset are in both formats, where the PNG images have 12-bit gray-scale color depth, while the JSRT has PNG images of 12-bit gray-scale (also converted to TIF images of 8-bit gray-scale [11]) and the PNG images in Indiana set are with 8-bit gray scale (were contrast-enhanced for the convenience of lung mask lineation). The ground truth lung segmentation mask images may be in TIF, GIF, and PNG formats, respectively. We converted the images of all the datasets to the JPG format of 8-bit gray scale. It should be noted that special attention needs to be given when converting images [11]. We generated the ground truth lung region bounding boxes from the manual lung segmentation masks provided in each dataset. For the Shenzhen dataset, since only 566 images have lung segmentation masks available, we manually drew the bounding boxes of lungs for all the remaining 96 images (using the Matlab ImageLaber tool). The dimensions of images vary across datasets and within some individual datasets. For example, the Montgomery dataset has two distinctive sizes (4020 × 4892 or 4892 × 4020 pixels), and the Pediatric dataset images are in varied resolutions (2446 × 2010, 1772 × 1430, and 2010 × 1572 pixels). The lung masks may be of different sizes to the corresponding images. We resized all the images (and corresponding masks) to be on the same scale. In addition to the whole images, we also generated the so-called cropped lung images where the images were cropped to the lung region box.

2.2. Data Analysis and Comparison

The DL models are data-driven such that their performance can be significantly influenced by their data characteristics. However, the robustness, reliability, and accuracy of models can be improved through better DL architecture design, hyperparameter optimization, and training strategy. Therefore, the step of analyzing the training data itself is very important and can provide valuable information and insights toward robust and effective DL algorithm design, implementation, and evaluation. As a result, we first examined and compared the data characteristics among the datasets at three levels: text, image, and feature.

2.2.1. Analysis of Textual Information Obtained from Metadata or Image Header

These datasets vary from each other with respect to geographical regions, populations, diseases, imaging devices, providers, views, dataset size, image formats, image size, and gray scale depth. A summary of the information on these aspects of each dataset is provided in Table 1. We extracted some text information from the DICOM header if the dataset did not directly provide related information in their description or through the papers. We put "N/A" in the table if we did not find relevant information. Since all the images input to the DL network were resized to have the same scale in dimension and their intensity pixel values were converted to have the same depth (8-bit) in a JPG image format, these three attributes of intensity depth, image dimension, and image format were not included in the table. For easy visual comparison, we generated the pie charts with respect to the ratio of disease, gender, and age category in the datasets in which such information is available. They are displayed in Figure 2, respectively.

Table 1. Comparison of datasets.

Dataset	No. of Images	Disease	Country	Gender	Age	Device	View
Montgomery	138	Normal/TB	USA	Male, Female	Adult, Pediatric	Konica Minolta	PA
Shenzhen	662	Normal/TB	China	Male, Female	Adult, Pediatric	N/A	PA, AP
JSRT	247	With/without Nodule	Japan	Male, Female	Adult, Pediatric	Konica LD 4500 & 5500	N/A
Pediatric	161	N/A	India	Male, Female	Pediatric	Konica Minolta	PA, AP
Indiana	55	Normal	USA	N/A	Adult	N/A	PA, AP

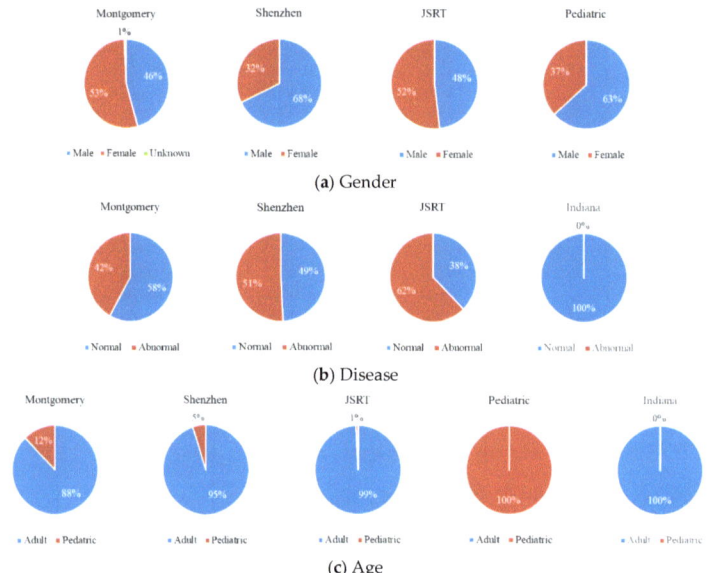

Figure 2. Comparison of datasets with respect to the percentage of gender, age, and disease categories.

2.2.2. Analysis of Image Appearance

Besides comparing the datasets using textual information, comparing images themselves in different datasets is also highly desirable as they are the data directly input to and used by the DL networks. Although manually browsing the images in each dataset can help to provide some extent of understanding and perception of what the images in each dataset look like, it is appealing and vital to have a general representative picture that can show the characteristics of the images in each set (at least to some degree) as it can be perceived promptly. To this end, we used a simple approach which was to create the average image of the whole images [12], as well as the cropped lung images of each set. This approach was carried out by finding the mean width and the mean height of all images first, then resizing all images to have the width and the height equal to the calculated mean width and mean height, respectively, and then adding the resized images all together and taking the average value at each pixel. Figure 3 shows the average whole image and the average cropped lung image calculated from each dataset, respectively. As demonstrated by Figure 3, the shape, intensity, and size of the lung areas as well as the whole upper body are different from one average image to another; although, there are similarities due to the intrinsic anatomical structure of body and organs. Among the five datasets, the average image of the Pediatric dataset is the most distinguished from that of other datasets regarding body and lung shapes, which is consistent with clinical observations [13].

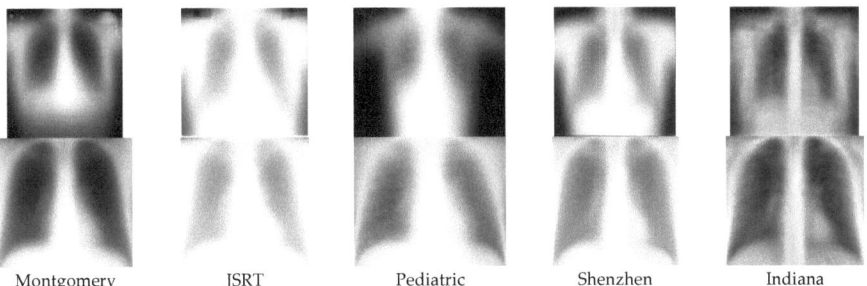

Figure 3. Average image of each dataset (1st row: whole image; 2nd row: cropped image).

2.2.3. Analysis of Features Extracted from the Pretrained Model

To obtain more insight into the lung region differences across datasets, we also extracted the feature vectors from the whole images as well as the cropped lung region images in each dataset using a DL classification network and visualized those features in a 2D space. For the DL classification model, we used an ImageNet trained Swin Transformer. Swin Transformer [14] was developed by aiming to make the transformer architecture designed originally for Natural Language Processing (NLP) more suitable for vision applications. It constructs hierarchical feature maps based on the key idea of utilizing shifted window partitioning for calculating self-attention locally, and achieves linear computational complexity w. r. t. image size. In our work, we used the Swin-B model which uses 384×384 pixels as input image size, 4×4 pixels as patch size, and 12×12 pixels as window size. The feature vector at the average pooling layer before the classification head layer was extracted. The feature has a length of 1024. For dimension reduction and feature visualization, we used UMAP (Uniform Manifold Approximation and Projection) [15]. UMAP, like tSNE, generates a low-dimensional graph which is optimized to be as structurally similar as possible to the high-dimensional graph representation of the data it has constructed, but may be faster and may preserve global structure better [15]. The UMAP plots of the ImageNet Swin-B model features of the five datasets obtained from using the whole image as the model input are displayed in Figure 4a. The whole image features of the five datasets are separated very well from each other (with the exception of only a few images from one dataset falling in the cluster of another dataset). We also extracted the same types of features for cropped images. As seen in its UMAP plot, shown in Figure 4b, the cropped image features among Montgomery, JSRT, Pediatric, and Shenzhen sets are well separated from each other, but the Indiana cluster blends with the Shenzhen cluster, indicating these two datasets have high similarity w. r. t. this specific type of features. Another observation is that there is a small number of Shenzhen images that are closer to the Pediatric cluster. We checked these Shenzhen images and found that they are pediatric images contained in the Shenzhen set. Although it should be noted that observations are dependent on what specific kind of features are used for analysis, they demonstrate that there are differences existing between the images in these datasets to a degree.

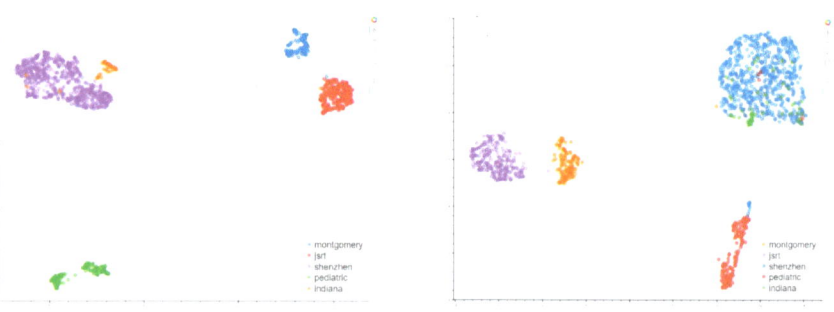

(a) original images   (b) cropped images

Figure 4. UMAPs of ImageNet Swin-B classification model features extracted from (**a**) original and (**b**) cropped images.

2.3. Lung ROI Detection Network

Object detection networks can be generally categorized into two types: one-stage detectors and two-stage detectors. One-stage detectors omit the step of region candidate proposal, a key component in two-stage detectors, and have object classification and bounding box regression performed directly using anchors extracted from the feature maps obtained from the entire image. Representative detection networks include Faster RCNN [16], YOLO [17], RetinaNet [18], SSD [19], DETR [20], etc. For a comprehensive literature review of object detection networks, please refer to a very recent survey paper in [21]. To localize the lung ROI, we applied a recent variant in the one-stage detector family of YOLO algorithms, that is, YOLOv5 [22]. Since the proposal of the original network version in 2016, YOLO has gone through multiple versions with various changes and improvements regarding backbone network, loss function, feature aggregation, data augmentation, activation function, normalization methods, regularization methods, optimization methods, among others [23]. On the shoulders of previous versions of YOLO (v1–v4), YOLOv5 was developed in Pytorch and is available in GitHub as an open-source package [22]. It is actively maintained and constantly improved by Ultralytics. Innovative and practical engineering maneuvers as well as algorithm bells and whistles have been applied, implemented, added, and adapted regularly. YOLOv5 itself has four variants of model structures that have different memory storage sizes. The general architecture of YOLOv5 models consists of three modules: (1) backbone—for extracting features of various sizes from the input image; (2) neck—for generating feature pyramids and performing feature fusion; and (3) head—for performing the final detection which consists of both bounding box regression and class prediction. The specific model structures, training strategies, loss functions, augmentation methods, as well as other up-to-date implementation and algorithm details of YOLOv5 can be found in its repository [22].

2.4. Feature Visualization of Lung ROI Detection Network

Besides evaluating the detection performance within a single dataset or across different datasets, we were also interested in understanding why a certain detection model works well/better on a certain dataset but not on another dataset, and explaining the generalization discrepancy across datasets. To this end, we proposed a new method for analyzing the features extracted from the YOLOv5 network. Different from other detection networks that contain fully connected layers, such as Faster RCNN, the YOLOv5 network consists of convolutional layers whose outputs are three-dimensional feature maps before the head module. To generate UMAP plots, as shown in Figure 4, which require the use of feature vectors, we first selected the three groups of feature maps (having different scales) that are the inputs to the head module in the network. Then, we applied the global average pooling to the feature maps in each group by which those feature maps in each group were converted into one feature vector. Next, we concatenated the feature vectors of all three groups to generate the final feature vector for each image. Last, we used the feature vectors extracted from all the images of interest to create a corresponding UMAP plot. Based on our best knowledge, there is no such work reported in the literature on generating feature visualization 2D plots for YOLOv5 models.

3. Experimental Results and Discussion

3.1. Experiment Settings

We split each dataset randomly (at the patient level) into training, validation, and test sets using a ratio of 70/10/20. The specific number of images in each set of each dataset is listed in Table 2, respectively. As shown in Table 2, except for the Shenzhen dataset which has the largest number of images with 463 in the training set, the size of the training set is quite small for all the other datasets, especially the Indiana dataset.

Table 2. The number of images in the training/validation/test set in each dataset.

Datasets	Training	Validation	Test	Total
Montgomery	97	14	27	138
Shenzhen	463	67	132	662
JSRT	173	25	49	247
Pediatric	113	16	32	161
Indiana	39	6	10	55
Total	1263	885	128	250

To alleviate over-fitting, we used the YOLOv5s model structure (which has the smallest storage size among the four YOLOv5 structures) and initialized the weights using a COCO pretrained model. YOLOv5 also utilizes several types of image augmentation such as color modification, scaling, translating, flipping, and mosaic augmentation. Mosaic augmentation, a novel augmentation method proposed by YOLOv5, generates a new training image that consists of four tiles with a random ratio obtained by combining one original image and three other randomly selected images. The specific software version setting we used was YOLOv5s 6.0. The backbone, neck, and head parts of its model structure are based on CSP-Darknet53 [24], SPPF [22] and PAnet [25], and YOLOv3 head layers, respectively. It uses binary cross entropy loss for calculating both classification loss and objectiveness loss, and CIoU [26] loss for computing bounding box regression loss. A summary of information on this specific version including employed training strategies can be found in [27]. For training, the batch size was 16, the number of epochs was 100, and the input image size was 640 × 640 pixels. For other hyperparameters and arguments (such as optimizer, initial learning rate, momentum, weight decay, warmup epochs, augmentation methods, etc.), the default values were used. For testing and evaluating, we set the image size as the same as that in training, the confidence threshold to be 0.25, the IoU threshold to be 0.45, the maximum number of output detections to be 1, and kept the other parameters to be the same as default values. The models were trained on a Lambda server with 8 GeForce RTX 2080 Ti GPUs. Unless specifically pointed out, the parameters, software (dependency library versions) and hardware settings remained the same for all the experiments presented and discussed in this paper.

For feature extraction, we converted the multi-scale feature maps at the stage 23, 20, and 17 of the YOLOv5 model, respectively, into a feature vector using global average pooling, and then concatenated the feature vectors obtained from the three stages (with the order of stage 23, 20, and 17). For example, at the stage 23, the global average pooling takes the average of the 17 × 20 feature map at each of the 512 channels and outputs a feature vector with a length of 512. The final feature vector obtained by concatenating feature vectors of all three stages has a length of 896 (=512 + 256 + 128). The feature vectors of all the images of interest were extracted from a model and then used to generate a UMAP plot.

3.2. Experiments in Four Scenarios

To investigate and analyze domain shift across datasets, we considered and carried out experiments in the following scenarios: (1) models trained using each individual dataset; (2) models trained using a combination of all the datasets except one; and (3) models trained using a combination of all the datasets. For all the above three scenarios, the models were initialized using the weights of the model pretrained with the COCO dataset. To check and verify the existence and extent of catastrophic forgetting and the effectiveness of modality-specific initialization, we also examined another scenario: (4) models trained using each individual dataset but initialized using weights from another model that was trained with a different dataset. Figure 5 shows the example workflow diagrams in the above four scenarios, respectively. All the models were evaluated and compared using the test set of each individual dataset. We used mAP@0.5:0.95 as the evaluation metric.

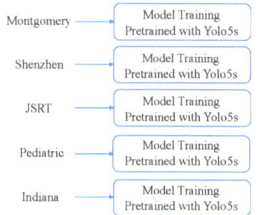

Scenario 1: models trained using each individual dataset

Scenario 2: models trained using all datasets but one

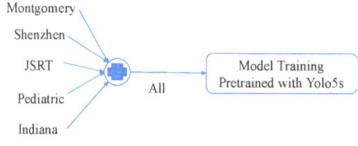

Scenario 3: model trained using all datasets

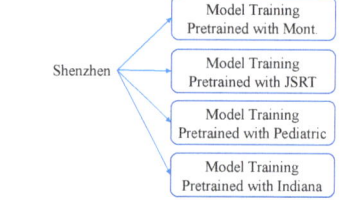

Scenario 4: models with modality-specific initialization

Figure 5. Diagrams of four experiments scenarios.

To check the repeatability of the model performance (i.e., to see if the model produces the same result for the same experiment and the same setup), we re-trained some models several times on the same GPU server using the same training/validation set, while keeping the settings of software environment, network hyperparameters, code version, and arguments the same, and examined testing performance on the same test set. The performances of all runs in each repeatability experiment were observed to remain the same. Table 3 lists the test performance of models trained in the first three scenarios and Table 4 lists the test performance of models trained in the fourth scenario.

Table 3. The performance (mAP0.5:0.95) of models on the test set of each individual dataset for scenarios 1–3.

Model	Test Set (mAP0.5:0.95)				
	Mont.	Shenzhen	JSRT	Pediatric	Indiana
Scenario 1: models trained using each individual dataset					
Mont.	0.908	0.875	0.500	0.681	0.813
Shenzhen	0.953	0.953	0.938	0.889	0.925
JSRT	0.817	0.883	0.964	0.723	0.583
Pediatric	0.829	0.872	0.451	0.904	0.831
Indiana	0.883	0.847	0.425	0.777	0.938
Scenario 2: models trained using all datasets but one					
All-Mont.	0.964	0.959	0.982	0.939	0.941
All-Shenzhen	0.963	0.946	0.977	0.943	0.953
All-JSRT	0.980	0.960	0.954	0.937	0.940
All-Ped.	0.987	0.959	0.990	0.903	0.979
All-Indiana	0.987	0.954	0.986	0.953	0.936
Scenario 3: model trained using all datasets					
All	0.976	0.958	0.978	0.932	0.955

Table 4. Trained with individual dataset but initialized with weights from models trained with another dataset.

Montgomery Model and Test Set			Shenzhen Model and Test Set		
Pretrained Model	Test on Montgomery	Test on the Dataset Used in the Pretrained Model	Pretrained Model	Test on Shenzhen	Test on the Dataset Used in the Pretrained Model
Yolo5s	0.908		Yolo5s	0.953	
Shenzhen	0.980	0.943	Montgomery	0.953	0.956
JSRT	0.943	0.938	JSRT	0.951	0.921
Pediatric	0.948	0.899	Pediatric	0.951	0.891
Indiana	0.965	0.893	Indiana	0.957	0.886
All-Montgomery	0.979	0.941	All-Shenzhen	0.958	0.939
JSRT model and test set			Pediatric model and test set		
Pretrained model	Test on JSRT	Test on the dataset used in the pretrained model	Pretrained model	Test on Pediatric	Test on the dataset used in the pretrained model
Yolo5s	0.964		Yolo5s	0.904	
Montgomery	0.945	0.742	Montgomery	0.896	0.852
Shenzhen	0.976	0.929	Shenzhen	0.926	0.931
Pediatric	0.946	0.819	JSRT	0.921	0.806
Indiana	0.961	0.586	Indiana	0.929	0.815
All-JSRT	0.987	0.934	All-Pediatric	0.930	0.939
Indiana model and test set					
Pretrained model	Test on Indiana	Test on the dataset used in the pretrained model			
Yolo5s	0.938				
Montgomery	0.931	0.897			
Shenzhen	0.964	0.926			
JSRT	0.908	0.709			
Pediatric	0.903	0.844			
All-Indiana	0.977	0.933			

3.2.1. Scenario 1: Models Trained Using Each Individual Dataset

The Scenario 1 section in Table 3 shows the results of testing the model trained with each individual dataset on the test set of each of the five datasets. The mAP@0.5:0.95 values in this section indicate that the within-dataset performance is higher than any of its cross-dataset performances for all the models except the Shenzhen model. For example, the JSRT model (the third row in the Scenario 1 section) achieves 0.964 on its own test set but 0.583, 0.723, 0.817, and 0.883 on the test sets of Indiana, Pediatric, Montgomery, and Shenzhen datasets, respectively. The cross-dataset performances of these individual dataset models vary considerably from model to model on the same test set. The Shenzhen model obtained the best cross-dataset performance among all models. It is the second-best performing model for the test set of Pediatric, JSRT, and Indiana datasets, and is even significantly better than the Montgomery model on the Montgomery test set. We hypothesize that one key factor contributing to this performance gain is that the size of Shenzhen dataset is significantly larger than that of the other four datasets. As a result of having a larger volume, its data diversity can also be increased, which boosts its chance to better represent the data of other datasets and reduce the extent of domain shift. This hypothesis seems to be backed up by UMAP plots in Appendix A Figure A1 (showing features of images in all test sets extracted from these individual dataset models). Except the UMAP plot for the Shenzhen model (Appendix A Figure A1b) where the feature cluster of the Shenzhen training set seems to be mixing well or close with that of test images in the other four datasets, the features of the training dataset in all the other four UMAPs (Appendix A Figure A1a,c–e) look generally well separated from those of test datasets, unless the test set is from the same dataset as the training set. The UMAP plots in Appendix A Figure A1 can also shed some light on why a certain model performs significantly worse on a certain dataset. For example, for the JSRT model (Appendix A Figure A1c), the features of Pediatric and Indiana test images are far from those of the JSRT training/test images. This observation aligns with the detection performance comparison between different test datasets for this model, which is indicated by the mAP@0.5:0.95 values in Table 3. The agreement between the observations from these UMAPs and the quantitative evaluation results demonstrates the usefulness of the proposed YOLOv5 feature analysis method.

3.2.2. Scenario 2: Models Trained Using All Datasets but One

One approach that can reduce domain shift issues across datasets is to combine the labeled training images from all available sources. It is based on the expectation that the data from different sources may be complementary to each other and by combining them, the diversity of source data can be increased, which, in turn, could lead to the improvement in the feature representation capability and the network generalization ability with respect to the data distribution in the target domain. In Scenario 2, we wanted to examine the performance of models trained using all datasets except one, especially on the dataset that was excluded from the training process. As shown in the Scenario 2 section of Table 3, the cross-domain performance was indeed substantially improved for all the models with this simple approach of combining datasets. For example, the "All-Pediatric" model (trained with the combination of all datasets but the Pediatric dataset) achieved 0.903 on the Pediatric test set, while all the other non-Pediatric individual models (shown in the "Pediatric" column of the Scenario 1 section in the Table 3) obtained 0.681, 0.889, 0.723, and 0.777, respectively, on the same test set. Appendix A Figure A2 displays the UMAP plots for each model in Scenario 2, where the features of images from the training datasets and the target test dataset are visualized. For example, regarding the All-Montgomery model, the embeddings of features from the Shenzhen, JSRT, Pediatric, and Indiana training sets and the features from the Montgomery test set are shown in Appendix A Figure A2a with different colors, respectively. It can be observed that for the same test set, the feature space of training images covers that of test images much better than that of the individual training set. This demonstrates the effectiveness of combining training datasets that are obtained from different sources for our specific datasets and task, even though the combined training dataset does not contain any images from the target source. As shown by comparison to Appendix A Figure A1, in general, the feature space of training images in Appendix A Figure A2 becomes more spread, has a larger overlapping area with, or is closer to that of, test images due to the increase in data volume and diversity. Besides the significant improvement on cross-domain prediction performance, the models remain working well on the test images that are from the same source as the training images. For example, the mAP0.5:0.95 values of the All-Indiana model are 0.987, 0.954, 0.986, 0.953 on Montgomery,

Shenzhen, JSRT, and Pediatric test sets, respectively. Similarly, by comparing the values in each column in the Scenario 2 section in Table 3, we can observe that among all five All-1 models, the models trained with images including those from the target dataset have either better or comparable performance than the model trained without such images.

3.2.3. Scenario 3: Model Trained Using All Datasets

In this scenario, we trained a model using the combination of training images from all five datasets. We then checked and evaluated its performance on each dataset's test set. The results are given in the last row of Table 3. As expected, including the training images from the target dataset increases model performance on the target dataset. That is, the mAP0.5:0.95 value in each column of the last row (for the All model) is significantly larger than that in the diagonal line of the Scenario 2 section in Table 3. For example, the performance on the JSRT test set is improved from 0.954 (All-JSRT model) to 0.978 (All model) by adding JSRT training images to the training set. One interesting observation exhibited by comparing the results of Scenario 3 and Scenario 2 is that although increasing data volume and diversity increases the chance of making the source domain data represent the target domain data better, it may not always be the case. For example, for the Montgomery test set, the All model is markedly outperformed by the All-Pediatric model and the All-Indiana model (0.976 vs. 0.987 and 0.987). It indicates, for this case, that using training images from four of the five datasets can produce better performance than using images from all five datasets. Therefore, adding more data may not necessarily produce better results and alleviate domain shift issues, even if the quality of the added data is good. The characteristics of the data to be added and how similar it is to that of the target domain play an important role as well. We tried to see if we could obtain some explanations and insights for this phenomenon by comparing the UMAPs of these models (Appendix A Figure A3b–d), but it seems that we are unable to draw a conclusive decision from those UMAPs regarding it. This demonstrates the challenges of explanation and analysis for network prediction, as well as the complicated factors contributing to network generalization capability, signifying the need to make more efforts on such kinds of research and experimental evaluations.

3.2.4. Scenario 4: Models with Modality-Specific Initialization

To train a deep network with a small medical dataset, one commonly used technique is applying transfer learning, that is, initializing the model architecture with weights from a model pretrained with a huge dataset, such as ImageNet. Recently, there have been studies showing that using modality-specific initialization, that is, a model pretrained with the same modality of medical images (with annotations from a task different from the one at hand), can produce better performance for the medical imaging applications than the one pretrained with the frequently used general-domain image dataset (ImageNet) [28]. In this experiment scenario, we were interested in checking if this observation holds when the model is initialized, using the weights of models trained with a different dataset in our five datasets. Such experiments also allow us to examine another issue caused by the existence of domain shift-catastrophic forgetting, i.e., the model forgets what it has learned from the previous dataset after fine-tuning on the new dataset. Table 4 lists the performance comparison of each individual model that was trained using different initialization weights. For example, in the sub-section of the Shenzhen model in Table 4, the first column lists the name of the pretrained model, the second column shows the performance on the Shenzhen test set of the model fine-tuned with Shenzhen training set, and the third column shows the performance of the fine-tuned model on the test set of the dataset that was used in the pretraining. From Table 4, we observed that only for the Montgomery model, the modality-specific initialization with any of the five pretrained models (Shenzhen, JSRT, Pediatric, Indiana, and All-Montgomery) outperforms the general-image initialization (Yolo5s which was trained with COCO dataset) considerably. For the other four individual dataset models, using modality-specific pretrained models is not always beneficial. For example, for the Indiana model, using the model pretrained with the Pediatric dataset performed markedly worse (0.903) than that with Yolo5s (0.938), while using the Shenzhen pretrained model accomplished a significant gain in performance (0.964). We also noticed that using the All-1 pretrained model to initialize the model achieved better results than using the Yolo5s for all the individual dataset models, suggesting the modality-specific initialization can be of an advantage when using a larger dataset with more variety and diversity. By comparing the third column in each sub-section in Table 4 (performance of models on the old dataset after fine-tuning on a new dataset) and the diagonal value of the Scenario 1 section in Table 3 (original performance of the models on the same dataset before fine-tuning), we found that there was forgetting for all the individual dataset models except the Montgomery model fine-tuned with the Shenzhen dataset (the fine-tuned model obtained 0.956 on Montgomery test set, while the original model obtained 0.908).

3.3. Discussion

Data characteristics can have a great impact on the design and prediction performance of ML algorithms, especially for medical applications. The key characteristics for medical data include *Volume*, *Veracity*, *Validity*, *Variety*, and *Velocity* [29] which refer to the amount of data, the truthfulness of data, the quality and consistency of data, the diversity of data, and the generation duration of data, respectively. Analyzing these data characteristics can not only facilitate ML researchers to develop better and more suitable architectures/methods for the goal of increasing model reliability and robustness, but also help to obtain more information from data which is also of value to clinicians. Given that the volume of medical image data (especially labeled data) is generally small and image data from different clinical centers are usually different, it is important to investigate and examine the domain shift issue across small datasets from different sources. The presented work is mainly related to the study of data volume and variety, and their impact on domain shift for the specific task of lung region detection in X-ray images. Our analysis of the data in the five datasets indicated the existence of cross-dataset differences exhibited in image appearance due to multiple contributing factors, such as variabilities in sensors, populations, disease manifestations, on-device processing, and imaging conditions. It is desirable that ML models can tolerate the data variability across different clinical centers well and be reliable when deployed in a new center, even though no data from the new center were available in the training stage of the models. Generally speaking, it is expected that increasing the volume and variety of the training data will reduce domain shift and increase the reliability of ML generalization in an unseen environment. However, our experimental results revealed that it may not always be the case when having notably limited data. That is, adding more data may not necessarily produce better results even if the data have good quality. It also depends on the characteristics of the added data and their similarity to those of the target domain. Similarly, the benefit of using modality-specific pretrained models over the ones pretrained with the frequently used general-domain image dataset is not observed for some models, although the modality-specific initialization can be of an advantage when using a larger dataset with more variety and diversity. Therefore, special attention and caution need to be paid when utilizing these techniques to mitigate domain shift issues among limited data. It is of great help, especially for high-risk situations such as clinical applications, to have effective tools that can predict and analyze the likely behaviors of models in the target domain. To this end, we developed a method to visualize the model features which can show the difference of data distributions. It can explain model behavior to a certain extent. However, it has limitations, as it cannot produce conclusive analysis results for some model predictions. In this work, we focused on studying the domain shift issue for lung region detection without specifically considering the normality or abnormality of lungs, an initial effort toward building a reliable and robust CXR AI system. In the future, we will expand the work to evaluate disease detection which would have more clinical impact and attract more interest. Nonetheless, our experiments demonstrate that modal behaviors and performance can be different from common expectations when datasets are small, and our analysis methods can be applied to other medical imaging applications.

4. Conclusions

One of the ML challenges in medical image analysis is domain shift. That is, the data distribution of the training dataset is different from that of the test dataset, which may lead to significant performance degradation of ML models in a real-world deployment. In this work, we aimed to study and analyze the domain shift issue across multiple datasets w. r. t. the task of detecting lung regions. Lung region detection in chest radiographs is an important early step in the ML pipeline for pulmonary disease screening and diagnosis. Like many other medical imaging applications, manual annotations of lung regions are limited. We had gathered five small such datasets that were collected from different sources. Using these datasets, we made efforts from several aspects in order to study domain shift issue. Specifically, we proposed to examine the characteristics of the datasets and their differences from three levels: text, image, and feature. We compared the information extracted from metadata, created an average image for each dataset, and checked features extracted using a pretrained CNN classifier. To evaluate and compare model performance under different situations, we designed four experimental scenarios including training with an individual dataset as well as a combination of multiple datasets. We also checked modality-specific initialization, catastrophic forgetting, and model repeatability. In addition, we developed a new visualization method for the applied detection network to obtain an explanation on the model performance variations. We found that there was generally a good alignment among feature distributions in the 2D plots and the obtained values of metrics for quantitatively evaluating the detection performance of different models. This demonstrates the usefulness of the proposed visualization method, although some observations cannot be explained by the feature visualization plots. We discussed the observations from the experimental results which demonstrate the complicated nature of both domain shift and the effects of data characteristics on model capacity for small datasets. From the experimental results, we noticed two key observations: (1) although increasing data volume and diversity increases the chance of making the source domain data representing the target domain data better, it may not always be the case; (2) using modality-specific pretrained models may not always be beneficial. The insights, analysis, and observations provided by our work can be valuable for the understanding and alleviation of domain shift in medical imaging applications in which a small amount of data are available from each of the different sources. In the future, we will explore techniques in semi-supervised learning and active learning to remedy the domain shift for lung region detection, and extend the current work and analysis for abnormality detection in the lungs.

Author Contributions: Conceptualization, Z.X., F.Y., S.R., G.Z. and S.A.; data curation, Z.X. and S.R.; formal analysis, Z.X., S.R. and F.Y.; funding acquisition, S.A.; investigation, S.A.; methodology, Z.X., F.Y., S.R. and G.Z.; project administration, S.A.; resources, S.A.; software, Z.X. and F.Y.; supervision, S.A.; validation, Z.X., F.Y. and S.A.; visualization, Z.X. and S.R.; writing—original draft, Z.X.; writing—review and editing, Z.X., S.R., G.Z., F.Y. and S.A. All authors have read and agreed to the published version of the manuscript.

Funding: This research was supported by the Intramural Research Program of the National Library of Medicine, National Institutes of Health.

Institutional Review Board Statement: Ethical review and approval were waived for this study because of the retrospective nature of the study and the use of anonymized patient data.

Informed Consent Statement: Patient consent was waived by the IRBs because of the retrospective nature of this investigation and the use of anonymized patient data.

Data Availability Statement: Montgomery dataset: https://data.lhncbc.nlm.nih.gov/public/Tuberculosis-Chest-X-ray-Datasets/Montgomery-County-CXR-Set/MontgomerySet/index.html (images and lung masks) (accessed on 6 March 2023). Shenzhen dataset: https://data.lhncbc.nlm.nih.gov/public/Tuberculosis-Chest-X-ray-Datasets/Shenzhen-Hospital-CXR-Set/index.html (images) (accessed on 27 January 2023). https://www.kaggle.com/datasets/yoctoman/shcxr-lung-mask (lung masks) (accessed on 27 January 2023). JSRT dataset: http://db.jsrt.or.jp/eng.php (accessed on 27 January 2023). Pediatric dataset: cannot be made public due to patient privacy constraints. Indiana lung mask subset: https://lhncbc.nlm.nih.gov/LHC-downloads/downloads.html (images and lung masks) (accessed on 6 March 2023).

Acknowledgments: We also want to thank Stefan Jaeger at NLM/NIH, Sema Candemir at Eskişehir Technical University in Turkey, and Alexandros Karargyris for their help with several datasets used in this work.

Conflicts of Interest: The authors declare no conflict of interest.

Appendix A

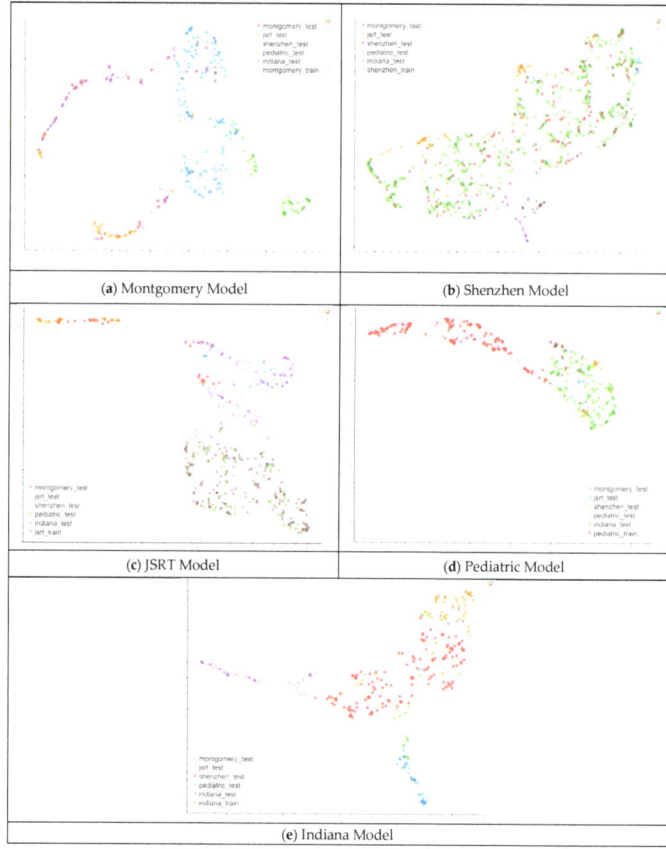

Figure A1. UMAP of YOLOv5 features extracted from individual dataset models.

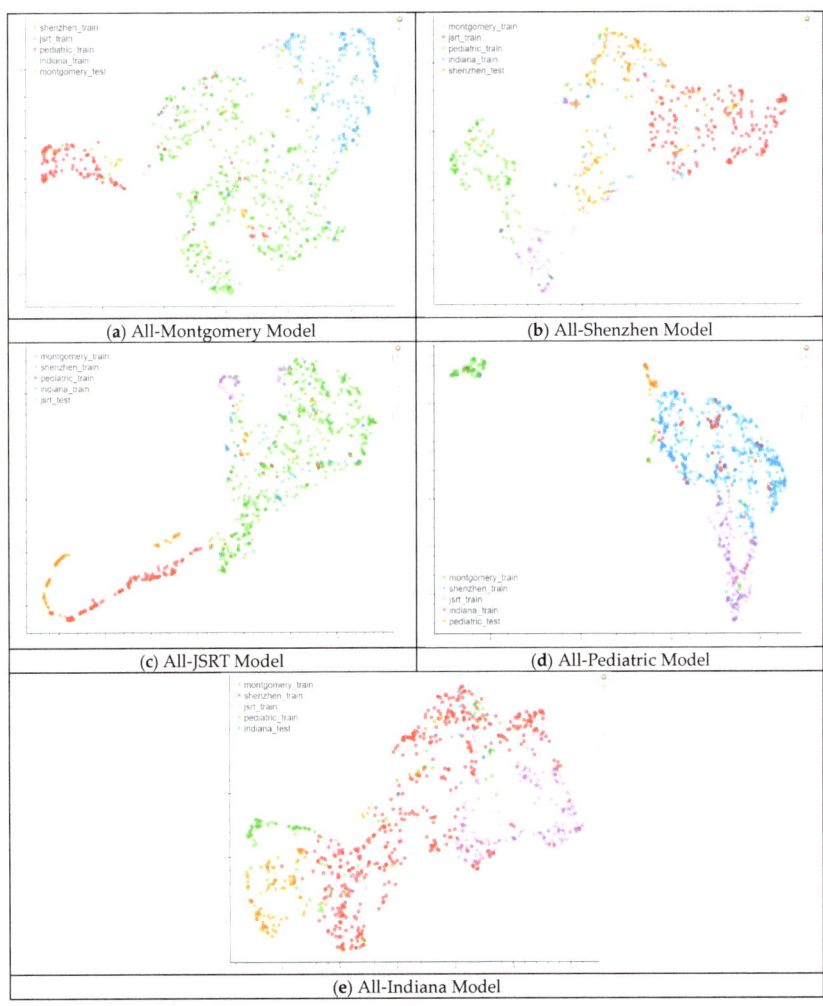

Figure A2. UMAP of YOLOv5 features extracted from All-one dataset models.

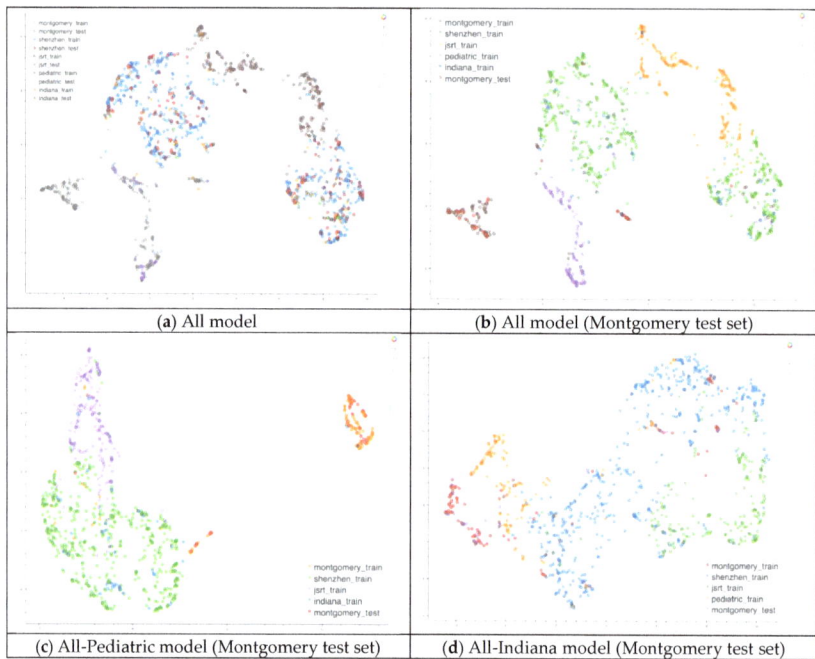

Figure A3. UMAP of YOLOv5 features extracted from the All model.

References

1. Çallı, E.; Sogancioglu, E.; van Ginneken, B.; van Leeuwen, K.G.; Murphy, K. Deep Learning for Chest X-Ray Analysis: A Survey. *Med. Image Anal.* **2021**, *72*, 102125. [CrossRef] [PubMed]
2. Tang, Y.; Tang, Y.; Sandfort, V.; Xiao, J.; Summers, R.M. TUNA-Net: Task-Oriented Unsupervised Adversarial Network for Disease Recognition in Cross-Domain Chest X-Rays. In *Medical Image Computing and Computer Assisted Intervention—MICCAI 2019*; Springer: Cham, Switzerland, 2019; Volume 11769, pp. 431–440. [CrossRef]
3. Lenga, M.; Schulz, H.; Saalbach, A. Continual Learning for Domain Adaptation In Chest X-Ray Classification. In Proceedings of the Third Conference on Medical Imaging with Deep Learning, PMLR (2020), Montreal, QC, Canada, 6–8 July 2020; Volume 121, pp. 413–423.
4. Sathitratanacheewin, S.; Sunanta, P.; Pongpirul, K. Deep Learning for Automated Classification of Tuberculosis-Related Chest X-Ray: Dataset Distribution Shift Limits Diagnostic Performance Generalizability. *Heliyon* **2020**, *6*, e04614. [CrossRef] [PubMed]
5. Jaeger, S.; Candemir, S.; Antani, S.; Wang, Y.X.; Lu, P.X.; Thoma, G. Two Public Chest X-Ray Datasets for Computer-Aided Screening of Pulmonary Diseases. *Quant. Imaging Med. Surg.* **2014**, *4*, 475–477. [CrossRef] [PubMed]
6. Rajaraman, S.; Folio, L.R.; Dimperio, J.; Alderson, P.O.; Antani, S.K. Improved Semantic Segmentation of Tuberculosis-Consistent Findings in Chest X-rays Using Augmented Training of Modality-Specific U-Net Models with Weak Localizations. *Diagnostics* **2021**, *11*, 616. [CrossRef] [PubMed]
7. Lung Masks for Shenzhen Hospital Chest X-ray Set. Available online: https://www.kaggle.com/datasets/yoctoman/shcxr-lung-mask (accessed on 27 January 2023).
8. Shiraishi, J.; Katsuragawa, S.; Ikezoe, J.; Matsumoto, T.; Kobayashi, T.; Komatsu, K.; Matsui, M.; Fujita, H.; Kodera, Y.; Doi, K. Development of A Digital Image Database for Chest Radiographs With And Without A Lung Nodule: Receiver Operating Characteristic Analysis Of Radiologists' Detection Of Pulmonary Nodules. *AJR Am. J. Roentgenol.* **2000**, *174*, 71–74. [CrossRef] [PubMed]
9. Ginneken, B.; Stegmann, M.; Loog, M. Segmentation of Anatomical Structures in Chest Radiographs Using Supervised Methods: A Comparative Study on A Public Database. *Med. Image Anal.* **2006**, *10*, 19–40. [CrossRef]

10. Open Access Biomedial Image Search Engine. Available online: https://openi.nlm.nih.gov/ (accessed on 27 January 2023).
11. Candemir, S.; Jaeger, S.; Palaniappan, K.; Musco, J.P.; Singh, R.K.; Xue, Z.; Karargyris, A.; Antani, S.; Thoma, G.; McDonald, C.J. Lung Segmentation in Chest Radiographs Using Anatomical Atlases with Nonrigid Registration. *IEEE Trans. Med. Imaging.* **2014**, *33*, 577–590. [CrossRef] [PubMed]
12. Candemir, S.; Antani, S.; Jaeger, S.; Browning, R.; Thoma, G. Lung Boundary Detection in Pediatric Chest X-Rays. *SPIE Med. Imaging PACS Imaging Inform. Next Gener. Innov.* **2015**, *9418*, 94180Q. [CrossRef]
13. Schneider, K. Specific characteristics of chest X-ray in childhood: Basics for radiologists. *Radiologe* **2018**, *58*, 359–376. [CrossRef] [PubMed]
14. Liu, Z.; Lin, Y.; Cao, Y.; Hu, H.; Wei, Y.; Zhang, Z.; Lin, S.; Guo, B. Swin Transformer: Hierarchical Vision Transformer Using Shifted Windows. In Proceedings of the IEEE/CVF International Conference on Computer Vision (ICCV), Montreal, QC, Canada, 10–17 October 2021; pp. 9992–10002. [CrossRef]
15. McInnes, L.; Healy, J.; Saul, N.; Großberger, L. UMAP: Uniform Manifold Approximation and Projection. *J. Open Source Softw.* **2018**, *3*, 861. [CrossRef]
16. Ren, S.; He, K.; Girshick, R.; Sun, J. Faster R-CNN: Towards Real-Time Object Detection with Region Proposal Networks. *IEEE Trans. Pattern Anal. Mach. Intell.* **2017**, *39*, 1137–1149. [CrossRef] [PubMed]
17. Redmon, J.; Divvala, S.; Girshick, R.; Farhadi, A. You Only Look Once: Unified, Real-Time Object Detection. In Proceedings of the IEEE Conference on Computer Vision and Pattern Recognition (CVPR), Las Vegas, NV, USA, 27–30 June 2016; pp. 779–788. [CrossRef]
18. Lin, T.; Goyal, P.; Girshick, R.B.; He, K.; Dollár, P. Focal Loss for Dense Object Detection. In Proceedings of the IEEE International Conference on Computer Vision (ICCV), Venice, Italy, 22–29 October 2017; pp. 2999–3007.
19. Liu, W.; Anguelov, D.; Erhan, D.; Szegedy, C.; Reed, S.; Fu, C.; Berg, A.C. SSD: Single Shot MultiBox Detector. In *Computer Vision—ECCV 2016*; Lecture Notes in Computer Science; Leibe, B., Matas, J., Sebe, N., Welling, M., Eds.; Springer: Cham, Switzerland, 2016; Volume 9905. [CrossRef]
20. Zhu, X.; Su, W.; Lu, L.; Li, B.; Wang, X.; Dai, J. Deformable DETR: Deformable Transformers for End-to-End Object Detection. In Proceedings of the International Conference on Learning Representations, Virtual Event, 3–7 May 2021.
21. Zaidi, S.S.A.; Ansari, M.S.; Aslam, A.; Kanwal, N.; Asghar, M.; Lee, B. A Survey of Modern Deep Learning Based Object Detection Models. *Digit. Signal Process.* **2022**, *126*, 103514. [CrossRef]
22. YOLOv5. Available online: https://github.com/ultralytics/yolov5/ (accessed on 27 January 2023).
23. Diwan, T.; Anirudh, G.; Tembhurne, J.V. Object Detection Using YOLO: Challenges, Architectural Successors, Datasets and Applications. *Multimed. Tools Appl.* **2023**, *82*, 9243–9275. [CrossRef] [PubMed]
24. Bochkovskiy, A.; Wang, C.; Liao, H.M. YOLOv4: Optimal Speed and Accuracy of Object Detection. *arXiv* **2020**, arXiv:2004.10934.
25. Liu, S.; Qi, L.; Qin, H.; Shi, J.; Jia, J. Path Aggregation Network for Instance Segmentation. In Proceedings of the IEEE Conference on Computer Vision and Pattern Recognition (CVPR), Salt Lake City, UT, USA, 18–23 June 2018; pp. 8759–8768.
26. Zheng, Z.; Wang, P.; Liu, W.; Li, J.; Ye, R.; Ren, D. Distance-IoU Loss: Faster and Better Learning for Bounding Box Regression. In Proceedings of the AAAI Conference on Artificial Intelligence (AAAI), New York, NY, USA, 7–12 February 2020.
27. YOLOv5 (6.0/6.1) Brief Summary. Available online: https://github.com/ultralytics/yolov5/issues/6998 (accessed on 27 January 2023).
28. Rajaraman, S.; Antani, S. Modality-Specific Deep Learning Model Ensembles Toward Improving TB Detection in Chest Radiographs. *IEEE Access.* **2020**, *8*, 27318–27326. [CrossRef] [PubMed]
29. Rajaraman, S.; Zamzmi, G.; Yang, F.; Xue, Z.; Antani, S. Data Characterization for Reliable AI in Medicine. In *Recent Trends in Image Processing and Pattern Recognition*; Springer: Cham, Switzerland, 2023; Volume 1704, pp. 3–11, PMCID: PMC9912175. [CrossRef] [PubMed]

Disclaimer/Publisher's Note: The statements, opinions and data contained in all publications are solely those of the individual author(s) and contributor(s) and not of MDPI and/or the editor(s). MDPI and/or the editor(s) disclaim responsibility for any injury to people or property resulting from any ideas, methods, instructions or products referred to in the content.

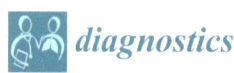

Article

Assessing the Impact of Image Resolution on Deep Learning for TB Lesion Segmentation on Frontal Chest X-rays

Sivaramakrishnan Rajaraman *, Feng Yang, Ghada Zamzmi, Zhiyun Xue and Sameer Antani

Computational Health Research Branch, National Library of Medicine, National Institutes of Health, Bethesda, MD 20894, USA
* Correspondence: sivaramakrishnan.rajaraman@nih.gov

Abstract: Deep learning (DL) models are state-of-the-art in segmenting anatomical and disease regions of interest (ROIs) in medical images. Particularly, a large number of DL-based techniques have been reported using chest X-rays (CXRs). However, these models are reportedly trained on reduced image resolutions for reasons related to the lack of computational resources. Literature is sparse in discussing the optimal image resolution to train these models for segmenting the tuberculosis (TB)-consistent lesions in CXRs. In this study, we investigated the performance variations with an Inception-V3 UNet model using various image resolutions with/without lung ROI cropping and aspect ratio adjustments and identified the optimal image resolution through extensive empirical evaluations to improve TB-consistent lesion segmentation performance. We used the Shenzhen CXR dataset for the study, which includes 326 normal patients and 336 TB patients. We proposed a combinatorial approach consisting of storing model snapshots, optimizing segmentation threshold and test-time augmentation (TTA), and averaging the snapshot predictions, to further improve performance with the optimal resolution. Our experimental results demonstrate that higher image resolutions are not always necessary; however, identifying the optimal image resolution is critical to achieving superior performance.

Keywords: aspect ratio; chest X-ray; deep learning; image resolution; segmentation; tuberculosis; test-time augmentation; threshold selection

1. Introduction

Mycobacterium tuberculosis (MTB) is the cause of pulmonary tuberculosis (TB) [1]; however, it can also affect other body organs including the brain, spine, and kidneys. TB infection can be categorized into latent and active types. Latent TB refers to cases where the MTB remains inactive and causes no symptoms. Active TB is contagious and can spread to others. The Centers for Disease Control and Prevention recommends people having an increased risk of acquiring TB infection including those with HIV/AIDS, using intravenous drugs, and from countries with a high prevalence, be screened for the disease [2]. Chest X-ray (CXR) is the most commonly used radiographic technique to screen for cardiopulmonary abnormalities, particularly TB [3]. Some of the TB-consistent abnormal manifestations in the lungs include apical thickening; calcified, non-calcified, and clustered nodules; infiltrates; cavities; linear densities; adenopathy; miliary patterns; and retraction, among others [1]. These manifestations can be observed anywhere in the lungs and may vary in size, shape, and density.

While CXRs are widely adopted for TB infection screening, human expertise is scarce [4], particularly in low and middle-resourced regions, for reading the CXRs. The development of machine learning-based (ML) artificial intelligence (AI) tools could aid in the screening through automated segmentation of disease-consistent regions of interest (ROIs) in the images.

Citation: Rajaraman, S.; Yang, F.; Zamzmi, G.; Xue, Z.; Antani, S. Assessing the Impact of Image Resolution on Deep Learning for TB Lesion Segmentation on Frontal Chest X-rays. *Diagnostics* 2023, 13, 747. https://doi.org/10.3390/diagnostics13040747

Academic Editor: Costin Teodor Streba

Received: 27 January 2023
Revised: 10 February 2023
Accepted: 15 February 2023
Published: 16 February 2023

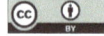

Copyright: © 2023 by the authors. Licensee MDPI, Basel, Switzerland. This article is an open access article distributed under the terms and conditions of the Creative Commons Attribution (CC BY) license (https://creativecommons.org/licenses/by/4.0/).

2. Related Literature and Contributions of the Study

Currently, deep learning (DL) models, a subset of ML algorithms, are observed to perform on par with human experts in segmenting body organs such as the lungs, heart, clavicles [5,6], and other cardiopulmonary disease manifestations including brain tumor [7–9], COVID-19 [10], pneumonia [11], and TB [12] in CXRs. These CXRs are made publicly available at high resolutions. Digital CXRs typically have a full resolution of approximately 2000 × 2500 pixels [13]; however, these may vary based on the sensor matrix. For instance, the CXRs in the Shenzhen CXR data collection [14] have an average resolution of 2644-pixel width × 2799-pixel height. However, a majority of current segmentation studies [15–17] are conducted using CXRs that are down-sampled to 224 × 224 pixel resolution due to GPU constraints. An extensive reduction in image resolution may eliminate subtle or weakly-expressed disease-relevant information. This important information may be hidden in small details, such as the surface and contour of the lesion, and other patterns in findings. As the details preserved in the visual information can drastically vary with the changes in image resolution and the type of subsampling method used, we believe the choice of image resolution should not depend on the computational hardware availability, but rather on the characteristics of the data.

Our review of the literature revealed the importance of image resolution and its impact on performance. For example, the authors in [18] found that changes in endoscopy image resolution impact classification performance. Another study [19] reported an improved disease classification performance at lower CXR image resolutions. The authors observed that the overfitting issues were resolved at lower input image resolutions. Our review of the literature also revealed that identifying the optimal image resolution for the task under study remains an open avenue for research. Until the writing of this manuscript, we have not found any study that discussed the impact of image resolution on a CXR-based segmentation task, particularly for segmenting TB-consistent lesions. To close this gap in the literature, this work aims to study the impact of training a model on varying image resolutions with/without lung ROI cropping and aspect ratio adjustments to find the optimal resolution that improves fine-grained TB-consistent lesion segmentation. Further, this work proposes to improve performance at the optimal resolution through a combinatorial approach consisting of storing model snapshots, optimizing the test-time augmentation (TTA) methods, optimizing the segmentation threshold, and averaging the predictions of the model snapshots.

Section 3 discusses the materials and methods. Section 4 elaborates on the results, and Section 5 discusses and concludes this study.

3. Materials and Methods

3.1 Data Characteristics

This study uses the Shenzhen CXR dataset [14] collected at the Shenzhen No. 3 hospital, in Shenzhen, China. The CXRs were de-identified at the source and are made available by the National Library of Medicine (NLM). The dataset contains 336 CXRs collected from microbiologically confirmed TB cases and 326 CXRs showing normal lungs. Table 1 shows the dataset characteristics.

Table 1. Dataset characteristics. The age of the population of men and women, image width, and image height are given in terms of mean ± standard deviation.

# TB CXRs	# Men	# Women	Age of Men (in Years)	Age of Women (in Years)	# Lung Masks	# TB Masks	Image Width (in Pixels)	Image Height (in Pixels)
336	228	108	38.29 ± 15.12	36.5 ± 14.75	287	336	2644 ± 253	2799 ± 206

# denotes the number of images.

The CXRs manifesting TB were annotated by two radiologists from the Chinese University of Hong Kong. The labeling was initially conducted by a junior radiologist, and then the labels were all checked by a senior radiologist, with a consensus reached for all cases. The annotations were stored as both binarized masks as well as pixel boundaries stored in JSON format [1]. The authors of [20] manually segmented the lung regions and made them available as lung masks. These masks are available for 287 CXRs manifesting TB-consistent abnormalities and 279 CXRs showing normal lungs. We used these 287 TB CXRs out of 336 TB CXRs that have both lung masks and TB lesion-consistent masks. Figure 1 shows the following: (a) The binarized TB masks of men and women were resized to 256 × 256 to maintain uniformity in scale. Then, the masks were averaged, normalized to the range [0, 1], and displayed using the "jet" colormap. (b) Pie chart showing the proportion and distribution of TB in men and women. (c) Age-wise distribution of the normal and TB-infected population of men and women.

These 287 CXRs were further divided at the patient level into 70% for training ($n = 201$), 10% for validation ($n = 29$), and 20% for hold-out testing ($n = 57$). The masks were thresholded and binarized to separate the foreground lung/TB-lesion pixels from the background pixels.

3.2. Model Architecture

We used the Inception-V3 UNet model architecture that we have previously demonstrated [12] to deliver superior TB-consistent lesion segmentation performance. The Inception-V3-based encoder [21] was initialized with ImageNet weights. The model was trained for 128 epochs at various image resolutions and is discussed in Section 3.3. We used an Adam optimizer with an initial learning rate of 1×10^{-3} to minimize the boundary-uncertainty augmented focal Tversky loss [8]. The learning rate was reduced if the validation loss ceased to improve after 5 epochs. This is called the *patience* parameter; its value was chosen from pilot evaluations. We stored the model weights whenever the validation loss decreased. The best-performing model with the validation data was used to predict the test data. The models were trained using Keras with Tensorflow backend (*ver. 2.7*) using a single NVIDIA GTX 1080 Ti GPU and CUDA dependencies.

3.3. Image Resolution

We empirically identified the optimal image resolution at which the Inception-V3 UNet model delivered superior performance toward the TB-consistent lesion segmentation task. The model was trained using various image/mask resolutions, viz., 32 × 32, 64 × 64, 128 × 128, 256 × 256, 512 × 512, 768 × 768, and 1024 × 1024. We used a batch size of 128, 64, 32, 16, 8, 4, and 2, respectively. We used bicubic interpolation to down-sample the 287 CXR images and their associated TB masks to the aforementioned resolutions, as shown in Figure 2. As expected, the visual details improved with increasing resolution.

We evaluated the model performance under the following conditions:

(i) The 287 CXRs and their associated TB masks were directly down-sampled using bi-cubic interpolation to the aforementioned resolutions. The OpenCV package (*ver. 4.5.4*) was used in this regard.
(ii) The lung masks were overlaid on the CXRs and their associated TB masks to delineate the lung boundaries. The lung ROI was cropped to the size of a bounding box and also down-sampled to the aforementioned resolutions.
(iii) Based on performance, the data from step (i) or step (ii) was corrected for aspect ratio, the details are discussed in Section 3.4. The corrected aspect-ratio CXRs/masks were further down-sampled to the aforementioned resolutions.

3.4. Aspect Ratio Correction

The aspect ratio is defined as the ratio of width to height [22]. To find the aspect ratio, the mean and standard deviation of the widths and heights of the CXRs manifesting TB-consistent abnormalities were computed. For the original CXRs, we observed that the width and height are 2644 ± 253 pixels and 2799 ± 206 pixels, respectively. For the lung-cropped CXRs, we observed that the width and height are 1929 ± 151 pixels and 1999 ± 231 pixels, respectively. For the original CXRs, the computed aspect ratio is 0.945.

For the lung-cropped CXRs, the computed aspect ratio is 0.965. We maintained the larger dimension (i.e., height) as constant at various image resolutions and modified the smaller dimension (i.e., width) to adjust the aspect ratio. We constrained the width and height of the images/masks to be divisible by 32 to be compatible with the UNet architecture [23]. For this, we padded the images such that the width was to the nearest lower value that is divisible by 32.

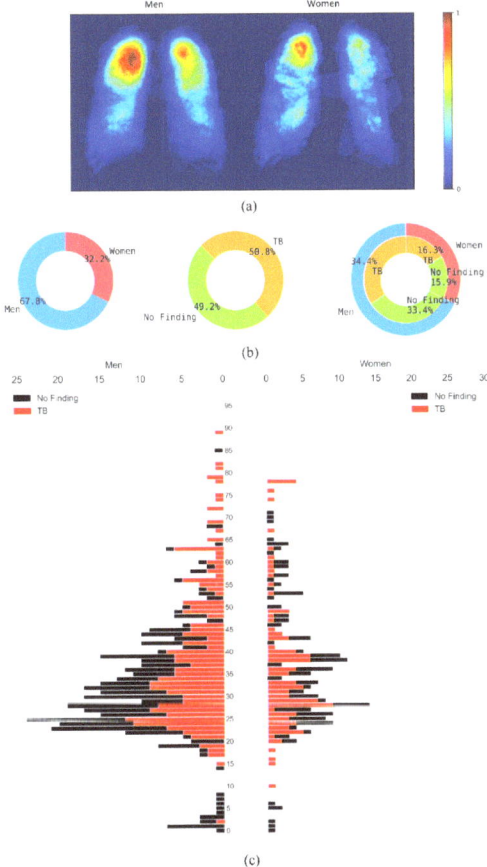

Figure 1. Data characteristics are shown as a proportion of men and women in the Shenzhen CXR collection. (**a**) Heatmaps showing regions of TB infestation in men and women. (**b**) Pie chart showing the proportion and distribution of TB in men and women, and (**c**) Age-wise distribution of the normal and TB-infected population in men and women.

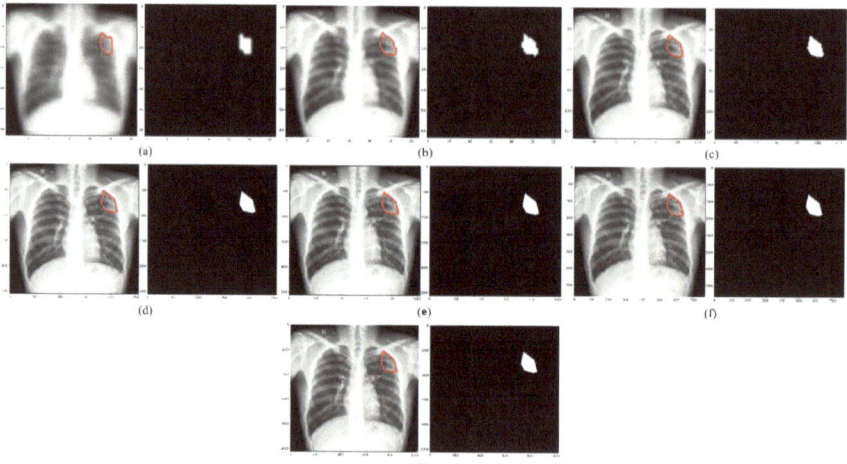

Figure 2. CXRs and their corresponding TB-consistent lesion masks at various image resolutions. (**a**) 32 × 32; (**b**) 64 × 64; (**c**) 128 × 128; (**d**) 256 × 256; (**e**) 512 × 512; (**f**) 768 × 768; and (**g**) 1024 × 1024. All images and masks are rescaled to 256 × 256 to compare quality. The red contours indicate ground truth annotations.

3.5. Performance Evaluation

The trained models were evaluated using (i) pixel-wise metrics [24], consisting of the intersection of union (IoU) and Dice score, and (ii) image-wise metrics, consisting of structural similarity index measure (SSIM) [25,26] and signal-to-reconstruction error ratio (SRE) [27]. While IoU and Dice are the most commonly used metrics to evaluate segmentation performance, a study of the literature [28] reveals that pixel-wise metrics ignore the dependencies among the neighboring pixels. The authors of [29] minimized a loss function derived from SSIM to segment ROIs in the Cityscapes and PASCAL VOC 2012 datasets. It was found that the masks predicted by the model that was trained to minimize the SSIM loss were more structurally similar to the ground truth masks compared to the model trained using the conventional cross-entropy loss. Motivated by this study, we used the SSIM metric to evaluate the structural similarity between the ground truth and predicted TB masks.

The SSIM of a pair of images (a, b) is given by a multiplicative combination of the structure (s), contrast (c), and luminance (l) factors, as given in Equation (1):

$$SSIM(a, b) = [l(a, b)]^{\alpha} \cdot [c(a, b)]^{\beta} \cdot [s(a, b)]^{\gamma} \tag{1}$$

The luminance (l) is measured by averaging over all the image pixel values. It is given by Equation (2). The luminance comparison between a pair of images (a, b) is given by a function of μ_a and μ_b, as shown in Equation (3):

$$\mu_a = \frac{1}{N} \sum_{i=1}^{N} a_i \tag{2}$$

$$l(a, b) = \frac{2\mu_a \mu_b + C_1}{\mu_a^2 + \mu_b^2 + C_1} \tag{3}$$

The contrast (c) is measured by taking the square root of the variance of all the image pixel values. The comparison of contrast between two images (a, b) is given by Equations (4) and (5):

$$\sigma_a = \left(\frac{1}{N-1}\sum_{i=1}^{N}(a_i - \mu_a)^2\right)^{1/2} \quad (4)$$

$$c(a,b) = \frac{2\sigma_a\sigma_b + C_2}{\sigma_a^2 + \sigma_b^2 + C_2} \quad (5)$$

The structural (s) comparison is given by dividing the input by its standard deviation, as shown in Equations (6) and (7):

$$s(a,b) = \frac{\sigma_{ab} + C_3}{\sigma_a\sigma_b + C_3} \quad (6)$$

$$\sigma_{ab} = \frac{1}{N-1}\sum_{i=1}^{N}((a_i - \mu_a)(b_i - \mu_b)) \quad (7)$$

The constants C_1, C_2, C_3 ensure numerical stability when the denominator becomes 0. The value of IoU, Dice, and SSIM range from [0, 1].

We visualized the SSIM quality map (using "jet" colormap) to interpret the quality of the predicted masks. The quality map is identical in size to the corresponding scaled version of the image. Small values of SSIM appear as dark blue activations, denoting regions of poor similarity to the ground truth. Large values of SSIM appear as dark red activations, denoting regions of high similarity.

The authors of [27] proposed a metric called signal-to-reconstruction error ratio (SRE) that measures the error relative to the mean image intensity. The authors discussed that the SRE metric is robust to brightness changes while measuring the similarity between the predicted image and ground truth. The SRE metric is measured in decibels (dB) and is given by Equation (8):

$$SRE = 10\,log_{10}\left(\frac{\mu_a^2}{\frac{||\hat{a}-a||^2}{n}}\right) \quad (8)$$

where, μ_a denotes the average value of the image a and n denotes the number of pixels in image a.

3.6. Optimizing the Segmentation Threshold

Studies in the literature [15,30,31] used a threshold of 0.5 by default in segmentation tasks. However, the process of selecting the segmentation threshold should be driven by the data under study. An arbitrary threshold of 0.5 is not guaranteed to be optimal, particularly considering imbalanced data, as in our case, where the number of foreground TB-consistent lesion pixels is considerably smaller compared to the background pixels. It is therefore important to perform a threshold tuning, in which we iterate among different segmentation threshold values in the range of [0, 1] and find the optimal threshold that would maximize performance. In our case, we generated 200 equally spaced samples in the closed interval [0, 1] and used a looping mechanism to find the optimal segmentation threshold that maximized the IoU metric for the validation data. This threshold was used to binarize the predicted masks using the test data and the performance was measured in terms of the evaluation metrics discussed in Section 3.5.

3.7. Storing Model Snapshots at the Optimal Resolution

After we empirically identified the optimal resolution, we further improved performance at this resolution as follows: (i) we adopted a method called "snapshot ensembling" [32], which involves using an aggressive cyclic learning rate to train and store diversified model snapshots (i.e., the model weights) during a single training run; (ii) we initialized the training process with a high learning rate of 1×10^{-2}, defined the number of training epochs as 320, and the number of training cycles as 8 so that each training cycle is composed of 40 epochs; (iii) the learning rate was rapidly decreased to the minimum value of 1×10^{-8} at the end of each training cycle before being drastically increased during the next cycle. This acts similar to a simulated restart, resulting in using good weights as the initialization for the subsequent cycle, thereby allowing the model to converge to different local optima; (iv) the weights at the bottom of each cycle are stored as snapshots (with 8 training cycles, we stored 8 model snapshots); (v) we evaluated the validation performance of each of these snapshots at their optimal segmentation threshold identified as discussed in Section 3.6. This threshold was further used to binarize the predicted test data and the performance was measured.

3.8. Test-Time Augmentation (TTA)

Test-time augmentation (TTA) refers to the process of augmenting the test set [33]. That is, the trained model predicts the original and transformed versions of the test set, and the predictions are aggregated to produce the final result. One advantage of performing TTA is that no changes are required to be made to the trained model. TTA ensures diversification and helps the model with improved chances of better capturing the target shape, thereby improving model performance and eliminating overconfident predictions. However, these studies [33–35] are observed to perform multiple random image augmentations without identifying the optimal augmentation method(s) that would help improve performance. A possible negative effect of destroying/degrading visual information with non-optimal augmentation(s) might outweigh the benefit of augmentation while also resulting in increased computational load.

After storing the model snapshots as discussed in Section 3.7, we performed TTA with the validation data using each model snapshot. In addition to the original input, we used the augmentation methods consisting of horizontal flipping, pixel-wise width, height shifting ($-5, 5$), and rotation in degrees ($-5, 5$) individually and in combination, as shown in Table 2.

Table 2. TTA combinations.

Method	TTA Combinations
M1	Original + horizontal flipping
M2	Original + width shifting
M3	Original + height shifting
M4	Original + width shifting + height shifting
M5	Original + horizontal flipping + width shifting + height shifting
M6	Original + rotation
M7	Original + width shifting + height shifting + rotation
M8	Original + horizontal flipping + width shifting + height shifting + rotation

For each TTA combination shown in Table 2, an aggregation function takes the set of predictions and averages them to produce the final prediction. We identified the optimal segmentation threshold that maximized the IoU for each model snapshot and every TTA combination. With the identified optimal TTA augmentation combination and the segmentation threshold, we augmented the test data, recorded the predictions, binarized them, and evaluated performance. This process is illustrated in Figure 3. We further constructed an ensemble of the top-K (K = 2, 3, ..., 6) by averaging their predictions. We call this *snapshot averaging*. The pseudocode explaining our proposal is shown in Figure 4.

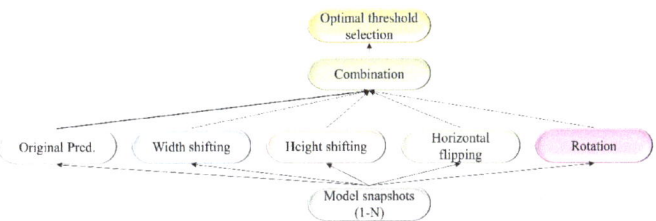

Figure 3. A combinatorial workflow showing the storage of model snapshots and identifying the optimal TTA combination at the optimal segmentation threshold for each snapshot. The term "Original pred." refers to the model predicting the original, non-augmented data.

```
# Divide 287 CXRs into training, validation, and testing sets
CXRs = 287
training_set_size = 201
validation_set_size = 29
testing_set_size = 57
training_set = CXRs * 70%
validation_set = CXRs * 10%
testing_set = CXRs * 20%

# Threshold and binarize masks
for each mask in training_set + validation_set + testing_set:
    threshold_mask(mask)
    binarize_mask(mask)

# Use InceptionV3-UNet architecture
model = InceptionV3-UNet()

# Train model at various image/mask resolutions
resolutions = [32x32, 64x64, 128x128, 256x256, 512x512, 768x768, 1024x1024]
for resolution in resolutions:
    train_model(model, training_set, resolution)

# Evaluate model performance using the validation set
for resolution in resolutions:
    for CXR, mask in validation_set:
        down_sample_CXR_and_mask(CXR, mask, resolution)
        correct_aspect_ratio(CXR, mask)
        down_sample_corrected_CXR_and_mask(CXR, mask, resolution)
        optimal_resolution(CXR, mask)
        optimal_threshold(CXR, mask)
        store_model_snapshot(model, optimal_resolution, optimal_threshold)
        evaluate_model_snapshot(model, validation_set, optimal_resolution, optimal_threshold)

# Evaluate model performance using the test set
for resolution in resolutions:
    for CXR, mask in test_set:
        test_time_augmentation(CXR, mask, optimal_resolution, optimal_threshold)
        evaluate_model_snapshot(model, test_set, optimal_resolution, optimal_threshold)

# Construct ensemble of top-K model snapshots
K = 2 to 6
ensemble = average_predictions(top_K_model_snapshots)

# Evaluate ensemble using the test set
for CXR, mask in test_set:
    evaluate_ensemble(ensemble, CXR, mask)
```

Figure 4. Pseudocode of our proposal.

3.9. Statistical Analysis

We measured the 95% binomial Clopper–Pearson confidence intervals (CIs) for the IoU metric obtained at various stages of our empirical analyses.

4. Results

Table 3 shows the performance achieved through training the Inception-V3 UNet model using the CXRs/TB masks of varying image resolutions, viz., 32 × 32, 64 × 64, 128 × 128, 256 × 256, 512 × 512, 768 × 768, and 1024 × 1024. Figure 5 shows the sample predictions at these resolutions. The performances are reported for each image resolution at its optimal segmentation threshold. The term O and CR denote the original and lung-cropped CXRs/masks, respectively. We observed poor performance at 32 × 32 resolution with both original and lung-cropped data.

Table 3. Performance achieved by the Inception-V3-UNet model with original and lung-cropped CXRs and TB-lesion-consistent masks. The term SRE, O, CR, and Opt. T denotes signal-to-reconstruction error ratio, original CXRs and TB-lesion-consistent masks, lung-ROI-cropped CXRs and TB-lesion-consistent masks, and the optimal segmentation threshold. Values in parenthesis denote the 95% CIs as the Exact measure of the Clopper–Pearson interval for the IoU metric. The bold numerical values denote superior performance for the respective columns.

Resolution	IoU	Dice	SSIM	SRE	Opt. T
32 × 32 (O)	0.2183 (0.1110, 0.3256)	0.3583	0.3725	19.9014	0.9548
32 × 32 (CR)	0.2934 (0.1751, 0.4117)	0.4537	0.4414	22.5763	0.6332
64 × 64 (O)	0.3105 (0.1903, 0.4307)	0.4739	0.5548	20.5444	0.3719
64 × 64 (CR)	0.3789 (0.2529, 0.5049)	0.5496	0.5584	24.4192	0.1005
128 × 128 (O)	0.4298 (0.3012, 0.5584)	0.6012	0.6694	23.1622	0.2663
128 × 128 (CR)	0.4652 (0.3357, 0.5947)	0.6350	0.7028	30.1203	0.0704
256 × 256 (O)	0.4567 (0.3273, 0.5861)	0.6271	0.7456	25.3184	0.9900
256 × 256 (CR)	**0.4859 (0.3561, 0.6157)**	**0.6540**	0.7720	29.1329	0.9950
512 × 512 (O)	0.4435 (0.3145, 0.5725)	0.6144	0.8327	27.6090	0.9799
512 × 512 (CR)	0.4799 (0.3502, 0.6096)	0.6485	0.8788	31.7887	0.9950
768 × 768 (O)	0.4428 (0.3138, 0.5718)	0.6138	0.8683	29.3264	0.9899
768 × 768 (CR)	0.4512 (0.3220, 0.5804)	0.6219	0.9073	33.3214	0.9899
1024 × 1024 (O)	0.2746 (0.1587, 0.3905)	0.4309	0.8545	28.4218	0.9796
1024 × 1024 (CR)	0.3387 (0.2158, 0.4616)	0.5060	0.8796	33.3320	0.9950

The performance kept improving until 256 × 256-pixel resolution where the model achieved the best IoU of 0.4859 (95% CI: (0.3561, 0.6157)) and superior values for Dice, SSIM, and SRE metrics. The performance then kept decreasing from 256 × 256 to 1024 × 1024 resolution. The performance achieved with the lung-cropped data is superior compared to the original counterparts at all resolutions. These observations highlighted that 256 × 256 is the optimal resolution and using lung-cropped CXRs/masks gave a superior performance.

Figure 6 shows the SSIM quality maps achieved by the Inception-V3 UNet model for a sample test CXR at varying image resolutions. The quality maps are identical in size to the corresponding scaled version of the images/masks. We observed high activations, shown as red pixels, in regions where the predicted masks were highly similar to the ground truth masks. Blue pixel activations denote regions of poor similarity. We observed the following: (i) The predicted masks exhibited poor similarity to the ground truth masks along the mask edges for all image resolutions. (ii) The SSIM value obtained with the lung-cropped data was superior compared to the original counterparts.

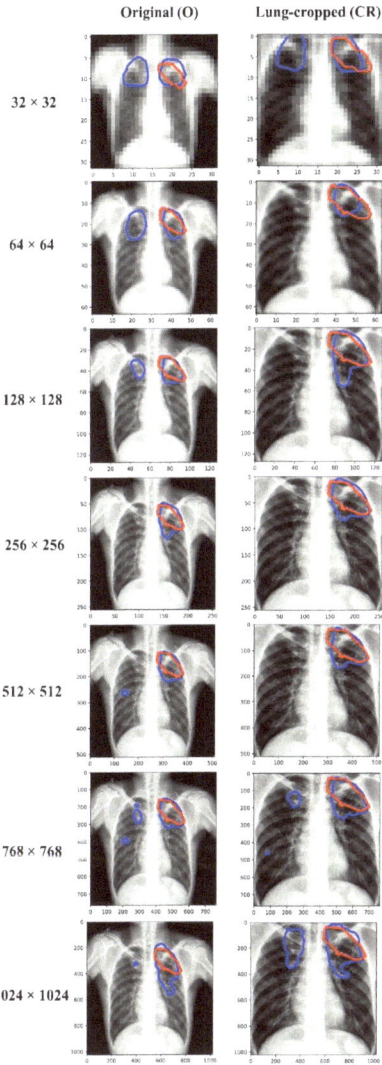

Figure 5. Visualizing and comparing the segmentation predictions of the Inception-V3 UNet model trained at various image resolutions, using a sample original, and its corresponding lung-cropped CXR/mask from the test set. The red and blue contours denote ground truth and predictions, respectively.

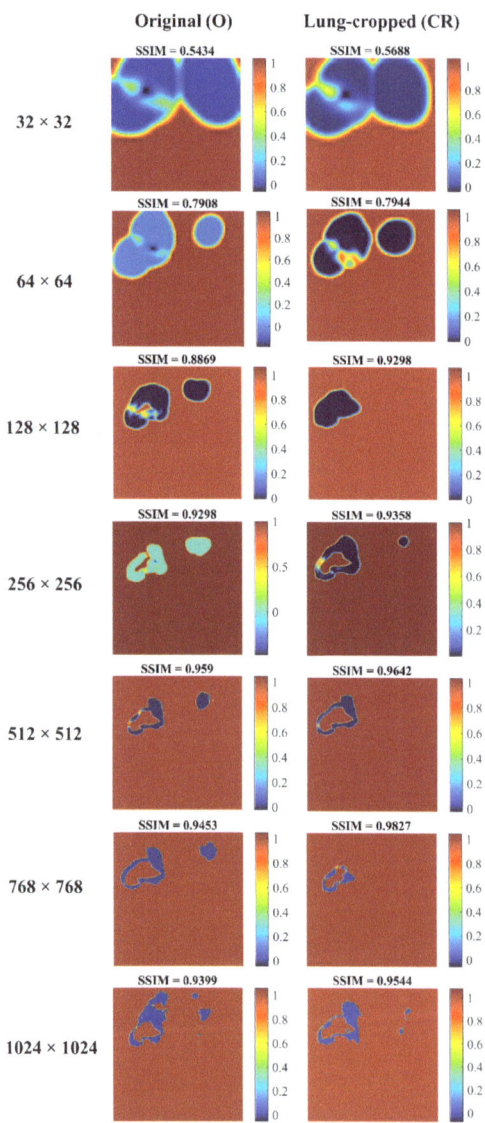

Figure 6. SSIM quality maps are shown for the predictions achieved by the Inception-V3 UNet model trained on various CXR/mask resolutions using a sample original and its corresponding lung-cropped data from the test set.

Table 4 shows the performance achieved by the Inception-V3 UNet model with aspect-ratio corrected (*AR-CR*) lung-cropped CXRs/masks for varying image resolutions. We observed no improvement in performance with aspect-ratio corrected data at any given image resolution compared to the results reported in Table 3.

Table 4. Performance achieved by the Inception-V3-UNet model with the aspect-ratio corrected lung-cropped (*AR-CR*) CXRs and TB-lesion-consistent masks. The image resolutions are given in terms of height × width.

Resolution (AR-CR)	IoU	Dice	SSIM	SRE	Opt. T
64 × 32	0.1583 (0.0635, 0.2531)	0.2734	0.1884	21.5695	0.9950
128 × 96	0.3474 (0.2237, 0.4711)	0.5157	0.5175	25.2175	0.9950
256 × 224	0.4447 (0.3156, 0.5738)	0.6151	0.7336	28.8964	0.9698
512 × 480	0.4815 (0.3517, 0.6113)	0.6500	0.8333	31.7451	0.9796
768 × 736	0.4200 (0.2918, 0.5482)	0.5916	0.8544	32.8540	0.9796
1024 × 960	0.3259 (0.2042, 0.4476)	0.4915	0.8710	33.6026	0.0204

To improve performance at the optimal image resolution, i.e., 256 × 256, we stored the model snapshots, as discussed in Section 3.7, and performed TTA augmentation for each recorded snapshot, as discussed in Section 3.8. Table 5 shows the optimal TTA combinations that delivered superior performance for each model snapshot at its optimal segmentation threshold identified from the validation data.

Table 5. Optimal test-time augmentation combination for each model snapshot.

Snapshot	Opt. TTA Combination
S1	Original+ width shifting + height shifting + rotation
S2	Original + height shifting
S3	Original+ horizontal flipping + width shifting + height shifting + rotation
S4	Original+ horizontal flipping + width shifting + height shifting + rotation
S5	Original+ horizontal flipping + width shifting + height shifting + rotation
S6	Original+ width shifting + height shifting
S7	Original+ horizontal flipping + width shifting + height shifting + rotation
S8	Original+ horizontal flipping + width shifting + height shifting + rotation

The terms S1, S2, S3, S4, S5, S6, S7, and S8 denote the 1st, 2nd, 3rd, 4th, 5th, 6th, 7th, and 8th model snapshot, respectively. The TTA combination that aggregates (averages) the predictions of the original test data with those obtained from other augmentations consisting of horizontal flipping, width shifting, height shifting, and rotation, delivered superior performance for the S3, S4, S5, S7, and S8 model snapshots. The aggregation of the original predictions with height-shifting augmentation delivered superior performance for the S2 snapshot. The S6 snapshot delivered superior performance while aggregating the original predictions with those obtained from the width and height-shifted images. Aggregating the predictions of the original test data with those augmented by width, height shifting, and rotation, delivered superior test performance while using the S1 model snapshot. The first row of Table 6 shows the performance achieved by the model trained with the 256 × 256 lung-cropped CXRs/masks, denoted as *CR-baseline* (from Table 3).

Table 6. Performance achieved by each model snapshot before and after applying the optimal TTA and averaging the snapshots after TTA. Bold numerical values denote superior performance in respective columns.

Model	IoU	Dice	SSIM	SRE	Opt. T
256 × 256 (CR-Baseline)	0.4859 (0.3561, 0.6157)	0.6540	0.7720	29.1329	0.9950
S1	0.4880 (0.3582, 0.6178)	0.6559	0.7676	29.0406	0.9950
S2	0.5090 (0.3792, 0.6388)	0.6746	0.7937	29.4457	0.9698
S3	0.5024 (0.3725, 0.6323)	0.6688	0.7900	29.4709	0.9749
S4	0.4935 (0.3637, 0.6233)	0.6609	0.7872	29.4803	0.9296
S5	0.4974 (0.3675, 0.6273)	0.6643	0.7906	29.4893	0.4271
S6	0.4939 (0.3641, 0.6237)	0.6612	0.7876	29.4833	0.6683
S7	0.4970 (0.3671, 0.6269)	0.6640	0.7887	29.5248	0.9296
S8	0.4780 (0.3483, 0.6077)	0.6469	0.7772	29.4381	0.0100
S1-TTA	0.4947 (0.3649, 0.6245)	0.6620	0.7788	29.2889	0.7959
S2-TTA	0.5107 (0.3809, 0.6405)	0.6762	0.7943	29.4858	0.6633
S3-TTA	0.5110 (0.3812, 0.6408)	0.6764	0.7950	29.5209	0.4975
S4-TTA	0.5000 (0.3701, 0.6299)	0.6667	0.7926	29.5162	0.4975
S5-TTA	0.5031 (0.3732, 0.6330)	0.6694	0.7952	29.5535	0.4975
S6-TTA	0.5020 (0.3721, 0.6319)	0.6684	0.7920	29.5307	0.4271
S7-TTA	0.5083 (0.3785, 0.6381)	0.6740	0.7944	29.5845	0.4925
S8-TTA	0.4872 (0.3574, 0.6170)	0.6552	0.7888	29.5341	0.3878
S2, S3-TTA	0.5174 (0.3876, 0.6472)	0.6819	0.7997	29.6055	0.5779
S2, S3, S5-TTA	0.5182 (0.3884, 0.6480)	0.6827	0.8002	29.6076	0.5126
S2, S3, S5, S7-TTA	**0.5200 (0.3902, 0.6498)**	**0.6842**	0.8007	29.6174	0.4925
S2, S3, S5, S7, S6-TTA	**0.5200 (0.3902, 0.6498)**	**0.6842**	**0.8018**	**29.6408**	0.4874
S2, S3, S5, S7, S6, S4-TTA	0.5193 (0.3895, 0.6491)	0.6836	0.8009	29.6186	0.4925

Rows 2–9 denote the performance achieved by the model snapshots S1–S8. Rows 10–17 show the performances achieved by the model snapshots at their optimal TTA combination (Table 5). We observed that TTA improved segmentation performance for the recorded model snapshot in terms of all metrics compared to the model snapshots without TTA and the "CR baseline".

We ranked the model snapshots S1–S8 in terms of their IoU. We observed the S2 snapshot delivered the best IoU, followed by S3, S5, S7, S6, and S4 model snapshots. We constructed an ensemble of the top-K snapshots (K = 2, 3, ..., 6), as discussed in Section 3.8, by averaging their predictions obtained using their optimal TTA combination. Rows 18–22 show the performances achieved by the ensemble of the top-2, top-3, top-4, top-5, and top-6 model snapshots, respectively. We observed that the snapshot averaging ensemble constructed using the top-4 and top-5 model snapshots delivered superior performance in terms of the IoU and Dice metrics while the top-5 snapshot ensemble delivered superior values also in terms of the SSIM and SRE metrics. The segmentation performance improved in terms of all evaluation metrics at the optimal 256 × 256 resolution by constructing an averaging ensemble of the top-5 model snapshots compared to the *CR-baseline*.

Figure 7 shows the predictions achieved by the baseline (i.e., the Inception-V3 UNet model trained with the lung-cropped CXRs/masks at the 256 × 256 resolution), and snapshot averaging of the top-5 model snapshots with TTA for a couple of CXRs from the test set. In the first row, we could observe that snapshot averaging removed the false positives (predictions shown with blue contours). In the second row, we could observe that the predicted masks were increasingly similar to the ground truth masks (shown with red contours), compared to the baseline.

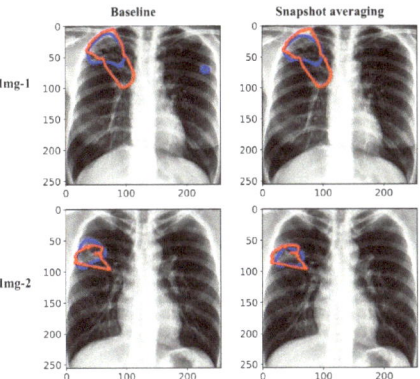

Figure 7. Visualizing and comparing the segmentation predictions of the baseline (i.e., Inception-V3 UNet model trained with lung-cropped CXRs/masks at the 256 × 256 resolution), and the snapshot averaging of the top-5 model snapshots. The red and blue contours denote ground truth and predictions, respectively.

Figure 8 shows the SSIM quality maps achieved with the baseline and snapshot averaging for a couple of CXR instances from the test set.

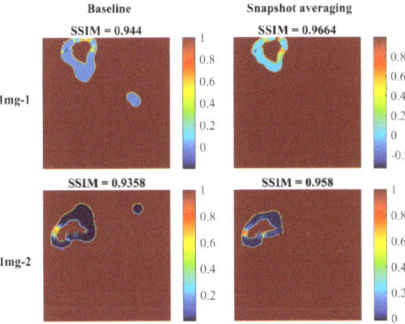

Figure 8. SSIM quality maps shown for the predictions achieved for a couple of test CXRs, by the baseline (Inception-V3 UNet model trained with lung-cropped CXRs/masks at the 256 × 256 resolution), and the snapshot averaging of the top-5 model snapshots with their optimal TTA combination. We observed higher values for the SSIM using the snapshot averaged predictions compared to the baseline, signifying that the predicted masks were increasingly similar to the ground truth masks. Snapshot averaging removed the false positives, and demonstrated improved prediction similarity to the ground truth, with a higher SSIM value, compared to the baseline.

5. Discussion and Conclusions

We observed that the segmentation performance improved with increasing image resolution from 32 × 32 up to 256 × 256. The performance achieved with the lung-cropped

CXRs/TB-lesion masks was superior compared to their original counterparts. These findings are consistent with [31,36–38], in which lung cropping was reported to improve performance in medical image segmentation and classification tasks. We observed that increasing the resolution beyond 256 × 256 decreased segmentation performance. This can be attributed to the fact that (i) increasing resolution also increased the feature space to be learned by the models, and (ii) increased parameter count might have led to model overfitting to the training data because of limited data availability.

We observed that the SSIM value decreased with decreasing resolution. The possible reasons for this reduction are as follows: the SSIM index is based on three components, the luminance component, which compares the average pixel intensity of the two images, the contrast component, which compares the standard deviation of the pixel intensities, and the structural component, which compares the similarity of patterns in the two images. When the resolution of an image is decreased, the number of pixels in the image is reduced, which can lead to a loss of detail in the image. This loss of detail can result in lower values for the luminance and contrast components, which in turn can lead to a lower overall SSIM score. In addition, the structural component of the SSIM index compares the similarity of patterns in the two images using a windowed function, which is sensitive to the resolution of the image. When the resolution is reduced, the window function captures less information and thus, the structural component becomes less effective in capturing the similarities between the two images. However, the SSIM metrics achieved with the lung-cropped images were superior to the original images, and the performance further improved with snapshot averaging.

We did not observe a considerable performance improvement with aspect ratio corrections. We were constrained by the UNet architecture [23], which requires that the length and width of the images/masks should be divisible by 32. This limitation did not allow us to make precise aspect ratio corrections. However, the study of literature [22] revealed that DL models trained on medical images are robust to changes in the aspect ratio. Abnormalities manifesting TB do not have a precise shape and they exhibit a high degree of variabilities such as nodules, effusions, infiltrations, cavitations, miliary patterns, and consolidations, among others. These manifestations would appear with their inherent characteristics that provide diversified features to learn for a segmentation model.

We identified the optimal image resolution and further improved performance at that resolution through a combinatorial approach consisting of storing model snapshots, optimizing the TTA and segmentation threshold, and averaging the snapshot predictions. These findings are consistent with the literature in which storing model snapshots and performing TTA considerably improved performance in natural and medical computer vision tasks [33,39–42]. We further emphasize that identifying the optimal TTA method(s) is indispensable to achieve superior performance compared to randomly augmenting the test data. We underscore the importance of using the optimal segmentation threshold compared to the conventional threshold of 0.5, as widely discussed in the literature [43,44].

Another limitation is that our experiments and conclusions are based on the Shenzhen CXR dataset where we observed that segmenting TB-consistent lesions using an UNet model trained on lung-cropped CXRs/masks delivers optimal performance at the 256 × 256 image resolution. These observations could vary across the datasets. We, therefore, emphasize that the characteristics of the data under study, the model performances at varying image resolutions with/without ROI cropping, and aspect ratio adjustments should be discussed in all studies.

Due to GPU constraints, we were not able to train high-resolution models at larger batch sizes. However, with the advent of high-performance computing, this can be made feasible. High-resolution datasets might require newer model architecture and hardware advancements. Nevertheless, although the full potential of high-resolution datasets is not explored yet, it is indispensable to collect data at the highest resolution possible. Additionally, irrespective of the image resolution, adding more experts to the annotation process may reduce the variation in the ground truth, which we believe may improve segmentation performance.

Author Contributions: Conceptualization, S.R., F.Y., G.Z., Z.X. and S.A.; Data curation, S.R. and F.Y.; Formal analysis, S.R. and F.Y.; Funding acquisition, S.A.; Investigation, S.A.; Methodology, S.R. and F.Y.; Project administration, S.A.; Resources, S.A.; Software, S.R. and F.Y.; Supervision, S.A.; Validation, S.R., F.Y. and S.A.; Visualization, S.R.; Writing—original draft, S.R.; Writing—review & editing, S.R., F.Y., G.Z., Z.X. and S.A. All authors have read and agreed to the published version of the manuscript.

Funding: This research was supported by the Intramural Research Program of the National Library of Medicine, National Institutes of Health. The funders had no role in the study design, data collection, analysis, decision to publish, or preparation of the manuscript.

Institutional Review Board Statement: Ethical review and approval were waived for this study because of the retrospective nature of the study and the use of anonymized patient data.

Informed Consent Statement: Patient consent was waived by the IRBs because of the retrospective nature of this investigation and the use of anonymized patient data.

Data Availability Statement: The data required to reproduce this study is publicly available and cited in the manuscript.

Conflicts of Interest: The authors declare no conflict of interest.

References

1. Yang, F.; Lu, P.X.; Deng, M.; Xi, Y.; W, J.; Rajaraman, S.; Xue, Z.; Folio, L.R.; Antani, S.K.; Jaeger, S. Annotations of Lung Abnormalities in the Shenzhen Chest Pulmonary Diseases. *MDPI Data* **2022**, *7*, 95. [CrossRef]
2. Geng, E.; Kreiswirth, B.; Burzynski, J.; Schluger, N.W. Clinical and Radiographic Correlates of Primary and Reactivation Tuberculosis: A Molecular Epidemiology Study. *J. Am. Med. Assoc.* **2005**, *293*, 2740–2745. [CrossRef] [PubMed]
3. Demner-Fushman, D.; Kohli, M.D.; Rosenman, M.B.; Shooshan, S.E.; Rodriguez, L.; Antani, S.; Thoma, G.R.; McDonald, C.J. Preparing a Collection of Radiology Examinations for Distribution and Retrieval. *J. Am. Med. Inform. Assoc.* **2016**, *23*, 304–310. [CrossRef] [PubMed]
4. Kwee, T.C.; Kwee, R.M. Workload of Diagnostic Radiologists in the Foreseeable Future Based on Recent Scientific Advances: Growth Expectations and Role of Artificial Intelligence. *Insights Imaging* **2021**, *12*, 1–12. [CrossRef] [PubMed]
5. Hesamian, M.H.; Jia, W.; He, X.; Kennedy, P. Deep Learning Techniques for Medical Image Segmentation: Achievements and Challenges. *J. Digit. Imaging* **2019**, *32*, 582–596. [CrossRef] [PubMed]
6. Narayanan, B.N.; De Silva, M.S.; Hardie, R.C.; Ali, R. Ensemble Method of Lung Segmentation in Chest Radiographs. *Proc. IEEE Natl. Aerosp. Electron. Conf. NAECON* **2021**, *2021-Augus*, 382–385. [CrossRef]
7. Khan, A.R.; Khan, S.; Harouni, M.; Abbasi, R.; Iqbal, S.; Mehmood, Z. Brain Tumor Segmentation Using K-Means Clustering and Deep Learning with Synthetic Data Augmentation for Classification. *Microsc. Res. Tech.* **2021**, *84*, 1389–1399. [CrossRef]
8. Iqbal, S.; Ghani Khan, M.U.; Saba, T.; Mehmood, Z.; Javaid, N.; Rehman, A.; Abbasi, R. Deep Learning Model Integrating Features and Novel Classifiers Fusion for Brain Tumor Segmentation. *Microsc. Res. Tech.* **2019**, *82*, 1302–1315. [CrossRef]
9. Sadad, T.; Rehman, A.; Munir, A.; Saba, T.; Tariq, U.; Ayesha, N.; Abbasi, R. Brain Tumor Detection and Multi-Classification Using Advanced Deep Learning Techniques. *Microsc. Res. Tech.* **2021**, *84*, 1296–1308. [CrossRef] [PubMed]
10. Saqib, M.; Anwar, A.; Anwar, S.; Petersson, L.; Sharma, N.; Blumenstein, M. COVID-19 Detection from Radiographs: Is Deep Learning Able to Handle the Crisis? *Signals* **2022**, *3*, 296–312. [CrossRef]
11. Kermany, D.S.; Goldbaum, M.; Cai, W.; Valentim, C.C.S.; Liang, H.; Baxter, S.L.; McKeown, A.; Yang, G.; Wu, X.; Yan, F.; et al. Identifying Medical Diagnoses and Treatable Diseases by Image-Based Deep Learning. *Cell* **2018**, *172*, 1122–1131.e9. [CrossRef] [PubMed]
12. Rajaraman, S.; Yang, F.; Zamzmi, G.; Xue, Z.; Antani, S.K. A Systematic Evaluation of Ensemble Learning Methods for Fine-Grained Semantic Segmentation of Tuberculosis-Consistent Lesions in Chest Radiographs. *Bioengineering* **2022**, *9*, 413. [CrossRef] [PubMed]
13. Huda, W.; Brad Abrahams, R. X-ray-Based Medical Imaging and Resolution. *Am. J. Roentgenol.* **2015**, *204*, W393–W397. [CrossRef] [PubMed]
14. Jaeger, S.; Candemir, S.; Antani, S.; Wang, Y.-X.J.; Lu, P.-X.; Thoma, G. Two Public Chest X-ray Datasets for Computer-Aided Screening of Pulmonary Diseases. *Quant. Imaging Med. Surg.* **2014**, *4*, 475–477. [CrossRef] [PubMed]
15. Zamzmi, G.; Rajaraman, S.; Hsu, L.-Y.; Sachdev, V.; Antani, S. Real-Time Echocardiography Image Analysis and Quantification of Cardiac Indices. *Med. Image Anal.* **2022**, *80*, 102438. [CrossRef] [PubMed]
16. Van Ginneken, B.; Katsuragawa, S.; Ter Haar Romeny, B.M.; Doi, K.; Viergever, M.A. Automatic Detection of Abnormalities in Chest Radiographs Using Local Texture Analysis. *IEEE Trans. Med. Imaging* **2002**, *21*, 139–149. [CrossRef]

17. Tang, P.; Yang, P.; Nie, D.; Wu, X.; Zhou, J.; Wang, Y. Unified Medical Image Segmentation by Learning from Uncertainty in an End-to-End Manner. *Knowl. Based Syst.* **2022**, *241*, 108215. [CrossRef]
18. Thambawita, V.; Strümke, I.; Hicks, S.A.; Halvorsen, P.; Parasa, S.; Riegler, M.A. Impact of Image Resolution on Deep Learning Performance in Endoscopy Image Classification: An Experimental Study Using a Large Dataset of Endoscopic Images. *Diagnostics* **2021**, *11*, 2183. [CrossRef]
19. Sabottke, C.F.; Spieler, B.M. The Effect of Image Resolution on Deep Learning in Radiography. *Radiol. Artif. Intell.* **2020**, *2*, e190015. [CrossRef]
20. Gordienko, Y.; Gang, P.; Hui, J.; Zeng, W.; Kochura, Y.; Alienin, O.; Rokovyi, O.; Stirenko, S. Deep Learning with Lung Segmentation and Bone Shadow Exclusion Techniques for Chest X-ray Analysis of Lung Cancer. In *ICCSEEA 2018: Advances in Computer Science for Engineering and Education*; Hu, Z., Petoukhov, S., Dychka, I., He, M., Eds.; Advances in Intelligent Systems and Computing; Springer: Cham, Switzerland, 2018; Volume 754. [CrossRef]
21. Pavel Yakubovskiy Segmentation Models. Available online: https://github.com/qubvel/segmentation_models (accessed on 2 May 2021).
22. Liu, W.; Li, C.; Rahaman, M.M.; Jiang, T.; Sun, H.; Wu, X.; Hu, W.; Chen, H.; Sun, C.; Yao, Y.; et al. Is the aspect ratio of cells important in deep learning? A robust comparison of deep learning methods for multi-scale cytopathology cell image classification: From convolutional neural networks to visual transformers. *Comput. Biol. Med.* **2022**, *141*, 105026. [CrossRef]
23. Ronneberger, O.; Fischer, P.; Brox, T. U-Net: Convolutional Networks for Biomedical Image Segmentation. In *Medical Image Computing and Computer-Assisted Intervention—MICCAI 2015*; Navab, N., Hornegger, J., Wells, W., Frangi, A., Eds.; Lecture Notes in Computer Science(LNCS); Springer: Cham, Switzerland; Volume 9351. [CrossRef]
24. Sagar, A. Uncertainty Quantification Using Variational Inference for Biomedical Image Segmentation. In Proceedings of the 2022 IEEE/CVF Winter Conference on Applications of Computer Vision Workshops (WACVW), Waikoloa, HI, USA, 4–8 January 2022; pp. 44–51. [CrossRef]
25. Rajaraman, S.; Zamzmi, G.; Folio, L.; Alderson, P.; Antani, S. Chest X-ray Bone Suppression for Improving Classification of Tuberculosis-Consistent Findings. *Diagnostics* **2021**, *11*, 840. [CrossRef] [PubMed]
26. Brunet, D.; Vrscay, E.R.; Wang, Z. On the Mathematical Properties of the Structural Similarity Index. *IEEE Trans. Image Process.* **2012**, *21*, 1488–1499. [CrossRef] [PubMed]
27. Lanaras, C.; Bioucas-Dias, J.; Galliani, S.; Baltsavias, E.; Schindler, K. Super-Resolution of Sentinel-2 Images: Learning a Globally Applicable Deep Neural Network. *ISPRS J. Photogramm. Remote Sens.* **2018**, *146*, 305–319. [CrossRef]
28. Jadon, S. SemSegLoss: A Python Package of Loss Functions for Semantic Segmentation [Formula Presented]. *Softw. Impacts* **2021**, *9*, 100079. [CrossRef]
29. Zhao, S.; Wu, B.; Chu, W.; Hu, Y.; Cai, D. Correlation Maximized Structural Similarity Loss for Semantic Segmentation. *arXiv* **2019**, arXiv:1910.08711.
30. Renard, F.; Guedria, S.; De Palma, N.; Vuillerme, N. Variability and Reproducibility in Deep Learning for Medical Image Segmentation. *Sci. Rep.* **2020**, *10*, 1–16. [CrossRef]
31. Candemir, S.; Antani, S. A Review on Lung Boundary Detection in Chest X-rays. *Int. J. Comput. Assist. Radiol. Surg.* **2019**, *14*, 563–576. [CrossRef]
32. Huang, G.; Li, Y.; Pleiss, G.; Liu, Z.; Hopcroft, J.E.; Weinberger, K.Q. Snapshot Ensembles: Train 1, Get M for Free. In Proceedings of the 5th International Conference on Learning Representations, ICLR 2017, Toulon, France, 24–26 April 2017.
33. Moshkov, N.; Mathe, B.; Kertesz-Farkas, A.; Hollandi, R.; Horvath, P. Test-Time Augmentation for Deep Learning-Based Cell Segmentation on Microscopy Images. *Sci. Rep.* **2020**, *10*, 1–7. [CrossRef]
34. Wang, G.; Li, W.; Aertsen, M.; Deprest, J.; Ourselin, S.; Vercauteren, T. Aleatoric Uncertainty Estimation with Test-Time Augmentation for Medical Image Segmentation with Convolutional Neural Networks. *Neurocomputing* **2019**, *338*, 34–45. [CrossRef]
35. Abedalla, A.; Abdullah, M.; Al-Ayyoub, M.; Benkhelifa, E. Chest X-ray Pneumothorax Segmentation Using U-Net with Efficient-Net and ResNet Architectures. *PeerJ Comput. Sci.* **2021**, *7*, 1–36. [CrossRef]
36. Rajaraman, S.; Folio, L.R.; Dimperio, J.; Alderson, P.O.; Antani, S.K. Improved Semantic Segmentation of Tuberculosis—Consistent Findings in Chest x-Rays Using Augmented Training of Modality-Specific u-Net Models with Weak Localizations. *Diagnostics* **2021**, *11*, 616. [CrossRef] [PubMed]
37. Li, H.; Han, H.; Li, Z.; Wang, L.; Wu, Z.; Lu, J.; Zhou, S.K. High-Resolution Chest X-ray Bone Suppression Using Unpaired CT Structural Priors. *IEEE Trans. Med. Imaging* **2020**, *39*, 3053–3063. [CrossRef] [PubMed]
38. Zamzmi, G.; Rajaraman, S.; Antani, S. UMS-Rep: Unified Modality-Specific Representation for Efficient Medical Image Analysis. *Inform. Med. Unlocked* **2021**, *24*, 100571. [CrossRef]
39. P, S.A.B.; Annavarapu, C.S.R. Deep Learning-Based Improved Snapshot Ensemble Technique for COVID-19 Chest X-ray Classification. *Appl. Intell.* **2021**, *51*, 3104–3120. [CrossRef] [PubMed]
40. Chowdhury, N.K.; Kabir, M.A.; Rahman, M.M.; Rezoana, N. ECOVNet: A Highly Effective Ensemble Based Deep Learning Model for Detecting COVID-19. *PeerJ Comput. Sci.* **2021**, *7*, 1–25. [CrossRef] [PubMed]
41. Nguyen, T.; Pernkopf, F. Lung Sound Classification Using Snapshot Ensemble of Convolutional Neural Networks. *Proc. Annu. Int. Conf. IEEE Eng. Med. Biol. Soc. EMBS* **2020**, *2020-July*, 760–763. [CrossRef]

42. Jha, D.; Smedsrud, P.H.; Johansen, D.; De Lange, T.; Johansen, H.D.; Halvorsen, P.; Riegler, M.A. A Comprehensive Study on Colorectal Polyp Segmentation with ResUNet++, Conditional Random Field and Test-Time Augmentation. *IEEE J. Biomed. Heal. Inform.* **2021**, *25*, 2029–2040. [CrossRef]
43. Lv, Z.; Wang, L.; Guan, Z.; Wu, J.; Du, X.; Zhao, H.; Guizani, M. An Optimizing and Differentially Private Clustering Algorithm for Mixed Data in SDN-Based Smart Grid. *IEEE Access* **2019**, *7*, 45773–45782. [CrossRef]
44. Decencière, E.; Zhang, X.; Cazuguel, G.; Laÿ, B.; Cochener, B.; Trone, C.; Gain, P.; Ordóñez-Varela, J.R.; Massin, P.; Erginay, A.; et al. Feedback on a Publicly Distributed Image Database: The Messidor Database. *Image Anal. Stereol.* **2014**, *33*, 231–234. [CrossRef]

Disclaimer/Publisher's Note: The statements, opinions and data contained in all publications are solely those of the individual author(s) and contributor(s) and not of MDPI and/or the editor(s). MDPI and/or the editor(s) disclaim responsibility for any injury to people or property resulting from any ideas, methods, instructions or products referred to in the content.

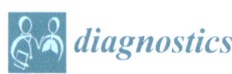

Article

Analysis of Chest X-ray for COVID-19 Diagnosis as a Use Case for an HPC-Enabled Data Analysis and Machine Learning Platform for Medical Diagnosis Support

Chadi Barakat [1,2,3,*,†], Marcel Aach [1,2], Andreas Schuppert [3,4], Sigurður Brynjólfsson [1], Sebastian Fritsch [2,3,5,‡] and Morris Riedel [1,2,3,‡]

1 School of Engineering and Natural Science, University of Iceland, 107 Reykjavik, Iceland
2 Jülich Supercomputing Centre, Forschungszentrum Jülich, 52428 Jülich, Germany
3 SMITH Consortium of the German Medical Informatics Initiative, 07747 Leipzig, Germany
4 Joint Research Centre for Computational Biomedicine, University Hospital RWTH Aachen, 52074 Aachen, Germany
5 Department of Intensive Care Medicine, University Hospital RWTH Aachen, 52074 Aachen, Germany
* Correspondence: c.barakat@fz-juelich.de
† Current address: Jülich Supercomputing Centre, Forschungszentrum Jülich, 52428 Jülich, Germany.
‡ These authors contributed equally to this work.

Citation: Barakat, C.; Aach, M.; Schuppert, A.; Brynjólfsson, S.; Fritsch, S.; Riedel, M. Analysis of Chest X-ray for COVID-19 Diagnosis as a Use Case for an HPC-Enabled Data Analysis and Machine Learning Platform for Medical Diagnosis Support. *Diagnostics* **2023**, *13*, 391. https://doi.org/10.3390/diagnostics13030391

Academic Editors: Sivaramakrishnan Rajaraman, Zhiyun Xue and Sameer Antani

Received: 20 December 2022
Revised: 14 January 2023
Accepted: 18 January 2023
Published: 20 January 2023

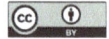

Copyright: © 2022 by the authors. Licensee MDPI, Basel, Switzerland. This article is an open access article distributed under the terms and conditions of the Creative Commons Attribution (CC BY) license (https://creativecommons.org/licenses/by/4.0/).

Abstract: The COVID-19 pandemic shed light on the need for quick diagnosis tools in healthcare, leading to the development of several algorithmic models for disease detection. Though these models are relatively easy to build, their training requires a lot of data, storage, and resources, which may not be available for use by medical institutions or could be beyond the skillset of the people who most need these tools. This paper describes a data analysis and machine learning platform that takes advantage of high-performance computing infrastructure for medical diagnosis support applications. This platform is validated by re-training a previously published deep learning model (COVID-Net) on new data, where it is shown that the performance of the model is improved through large-scale hyperparameter optimisation that uncovered optimal training parameter combinations. The per-class accuracy of the model, especially for COVID-19 and pneumonia, is higher when using the tuned hyperparameters (healthy: 96.5%; pneumonia: 61.5%; COVID-19: 78.9%) as opposed to parameters chosen through traditional methods (healthy: 93.6%; pneumonia: 46.1%; COVID-19: 76.3%). Furthermore, training speed-up analysis shows a major decrease in training time as resources increase, from 207 min using 1 node to 54 min when distributed over 32 nodes, but highlights the presence of a cut-off point where the communication overhead begins to affect performance. The developed platform is intended to provide the medical field with a technical environment for developing novel portable artificial-intelligence-based tools for diagnosis support.

Keywords: deep learning; COVID-19; high-performance computing; image-based diagnostics; medical diagnosis support

1. Introduction

As the COVID-19 pandemic threatened to break down medical infrastructure all over the world, it became evident that effective and efficient methods of diagnosis are necessary in order to improve outcomes and save the lives of hospital patients [1]. Especially during the early phase of the pandemic, when antigen-based rapid tests were not yet available, there was an urgent need for alternative diagnostic procedures. The standard approach using reverse-transcription polymerase chain-reaction (RT-PCR) required a lot of time, trained staff, and laboratory capacity and showed, especially at the beginning of the pandemic, very heterogeneous accuracy [2,3]. Since pulmonary involvement in particular posed a risk to patients with COVID-19, it was reasonable to examine conventional chest-X-ray (CXR) images, which are a rapid and widely available diagnostic tool for COVID-19-specific changes [4]. Thus, early publications had already reported the presence of specific changes in thoracic imaging before a laboratory test yielded a positive result [5]. Focusing on readily available and inexpensive diagnostic procedures is especially meaningful as research predicts that such large-scale contagion events will happen at an increasing rate [6].

However, given the current advancements in high-performance computing (HPC) technology and the availability of commercial cloud computing (CC) resources to the general public, as well as large increases in online data storage and sharing capabilities, an increasing interest in machine learning (ML) and deep learning (DL) applications that put these resources to use in order to solve common problems can be observed [7–9]. Similarly, these techniques and resources are being employed towards extracting information from Big Data repositories that would otherwise require hundreds of researchers over several thousand hours [10,11]. More recently, the combination of HPC, Big Data, and ML have made headlines in the scientific community with the publication of two DL models, AlphaFold from DeepMind and RoseTTAFold from Baek et al., which match or even outperform existing methods for protein structure prediction [12,13].

It follows that several research groups have developed ML and DL methods for detecting COVID-19 from sonographic [14] and X-ray images of the thorax [15–17], or for predicting the mortality of COVID-19 patients from medical data [18], with all of the results highlighting how effective these models might be for quick triaging. In a similar application field, Rajaraman et al. merged several trained DL models to improve the diagnosis of pneumonia from CXR images with a higher success rate than conventional image recognition models [19]. Other researchers have made use of cutting-edge HPC resources, namely the Jülich Wizard for European Leadership Science (JUWELS) (https://www.fz-juelich.de/en/ias/jsc/systems/supercomputers/juwels (accessed on 19 December 2022)) cluster, one of Europe's fastest supercomputers to train advanced DL networks on Big Data from different fields, thus highlighting the need to make use of modular supercomputing architecture (MSA) to advance the field of artificial intelligence (AI) [20]. Furthermore, advanced automated hyperparameter tuning methods such as KerasTuner (https://keras.io/keras_tuner/ (accessed on 19 December 2022)) and Ray Tune (https://docs.ray.io/en/latest/tune/index.html (accessed on 19 December 2022)) have been developed, which simplify the parameter search process needed to fine-tune the training of neural networks, thus yielding the best performing model without major interventions from ML researchers [21].

Application of the available HPC resources in the medical field, thus contributing to the analysis of medical data and a timely and precise diagnosis, has the potential to reduce the amount of stress that medical personnel are exposed to during their work [22,23]. Similarly, the medical field presents a fertile ground for setting up frameworks that can be easily loaded, modified, and deployed where needed to help mitigate the effects of future epidemics and pandemics [24]. In the present paper, these approaches are thus validated in the application of the COVID-Net developed by Wang et al. on newly obtained CXR images that were provided by healthcare partner E*HealthLine (EHL) as part of the European Open Science Cloud (EOSC) Fast-Track grants for COVID-19 research.

The work presented in this article describes the culmination of work performed towards setting up a platform within which medical data can be stored, cleaned, and analysed, and easily used to train ML and DL models [25,26]. The platform makes use of highly specialised hardware and software available at the Jülich Supercomputing Centre (JSC) to develop and train these models in the most efficient manner. These include firstly the DEEP and JUWELS supercomputing clusters, and the storage made available through the related projects. Advanced hyperparameter tuning methods are also used to fine-tune the models to produce the best results.

The following sections go into the details of (a) training COVID-Net on newly acquired data, (b) performing large-scale hyperparameter tuning on the model in order to extract the parameter combinations that produce the best trained models, and (c) re-training the model to highlight the improvement achieved in per-class accuracy for each of these combinations.

Furthermore, resource scale-up is also performed in order to gauge the speed-up that can be achieved through the established platform.

Re-training the COVID-Net model in such a way serves as a preliminary proof-of-concept for the platform. Due to its easy adaptability to new use-cases and its portability on other academic or commercially available CC resources, this platform can support researchers in the medical field to create more complex models with better performance that would otherwise be impossible to develop due to a lack of computational resources and missing expertise in usage of HPC systems. Additionally, the models built and pre-trained within the platform rely on open-source data and software, making them easy to deploy on local machines in hospitals intensive care units (ICUs).

It is worth noting that several groups have applied hyperparameter optimisation to improve the results of DL-based COVID-19 diagnosis models [27–29]. However, comparison with these works cannot easily be undertaken, as the concept and specific innovation described in the present paper lies within scaling up the data storage, the model training, and the hyperparameter tuning processes through efficient use of HPC resources in order to cover more ground.

2. Materials and Methods

This section describes the hardware and software implemented within the developed data analysis and machine learning platform, as well as the methods and data through which the COVID-Net model, developed by Wang et al. [15], is re-trained on new data and its prediction performance is improved through large-scale hyperparameter tuning. Figure 1 presents a general overview of the re-training process and model improvement steps performed as part of the platform validation, and highlights how computationally expensive the hyperparameter tuning step is.

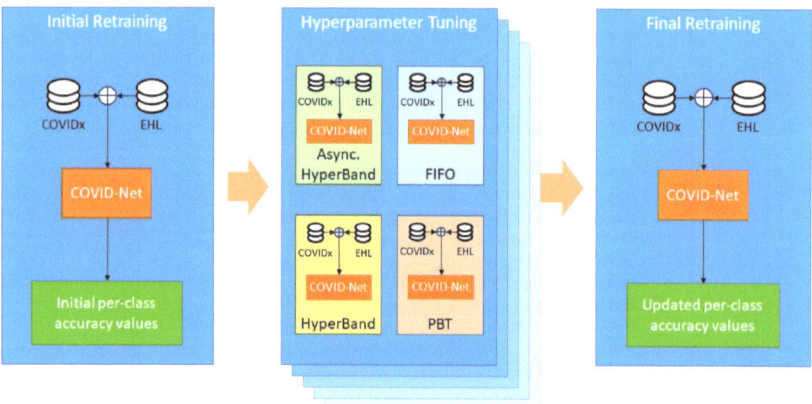

Figure 1. Block diagram representing the experimental process within the data analysis and machine learning platform. The different schedulers are represented as boxes within the hyperparameter tuning step. Due to the large amount of computations that it needs to perform, the hyperparameter tuning step requires significantly more resources than the remaining steps.

2.1. HPC Resources

In their presentation of a novel approach to build and organise HPC resources, Suarez et al. provide a thorough technical description of the hardware set up at JSC, with an emphasis on its modular aspects [30]. This is true in terms of the hardware dedicated to computation as well as that used for communication and for storage. In essence, the MSA allows for efficient scale-up as required by HPC researchers according to the tasks at hand.

The hardware is supported by the open-source scheduling software Simple Linux Utility for Resource Management (SLURM) (https://slurm.schedmd.com/(accessed on 19 December 2022)), which manages the workload over the available resources and leverages the scalability aspect of the modular system, but also reduces wasted computing time through intelligent prioritisation of tasks. Furthermore, aside from terminal access through SSH, users can directly access resources through an integrated Jupyter (https://jupyter-jsc.fz-juelich.de/ (accessed on 19 December 2022)) development environment, which can be adapted to the specific needs of the task at hand through pre-packaged data analytics and ML modules as well as personalised kernels and virtual environments.

2.1.1. DEEP

The DEEP series of projects has been setting up the path towards exascale computing since 2016, focusing on scaling available HPC resources through boosters [31]. These projects have received funding granted by the European Commission under the Horizon 2020 program and have so far had three iterations under the titles "DEEP", "DEEP-Extended Reach" (DEEP-ER), and "DEEP-Extreme Scale Technologies" (DEEP-EST). A fourth iteration upcoming as "DEEP-Software for Exascale Architectures" (DEEP-SEA) was launched in 2021 with the aim of delivering a standardised programming environment for exascale computing for the European HPC systems.

At the hardware level, DEEP-EST introduced the concept of MSA, making the cluster-booster architecture more attuned for data analytics tasks [32]. Accordingly, the system itself is divided into several modules, each sporting the necessary hardware for specific tasks (i.e., numerical data processing, image processing, hyperspectral image processing). These modules are presented in Table 1.

Table 1. Partitions on the DEEP prototype.

Partition	Nodes	CPUs/Node	GPU
DEEP-Data Analytics Module	16	96	NVIDIA V100 + Intel Stratix10 FGPA
DEEP-Extreme Scale Booster	75	16	NVIDIA V100
DEEP-Cluster Module	50	48	n/a

2.1.2. JUWELS

The JUWELS supercomputer consists of two main parts: a cluster module and a booster module, commissioned in 2018 and 2020, respectively. The cluster module is a BullSequana X1000 system (https://atos.net/en/solutions/high-performance-computing-hpc/bullsequana-x-supercomputers/bullsequana-x1000 (accessed on 19 December 2022)) with 2583 nodes totalling 122,768 CPUs. Furthermore, several nodes are specialised for visualisation, large-memory, and accelerated computing tasks (https://apps.fz-juelich.de/jsc/hps/juwels/configuration.html (accessed on 19 December 2022)). The booster module, a Bullsequana XH2000 system (https://atos.net/wp-content/uploads/2020/07/BullSequana XH2000_Features_Atos_supercomputers.pdf (accessed on 19 December 2022)), expands on the available computing power by adding a total of 940 nodes totalling 3744 GPUs.

In essence, the cluster module is intended for general-purpose computation tasks while the booster module allows for scalable computing, making large-scale simulation and visualisation tasks more possible [20]. By making use of the available high-speed network connections and available storage, the booster module has reached a peak performance of 73 petaflop per second. Kesselheim et al. validated its performance for large-scale AI research on several DL network training tasks across different fields. Their results and the recorded peak performance earned the JUWELS booster the top position on the fastest supercomputers in Europe in 2021 as well as the 7th spot on the international TOP500 list and the 3rd spot on the Green500 list.

For the purposes described in this manuscript, the development phase is performed on the DEEP-EST cluster and the usage of the JUWELS cluster and booster is reserved for large-scale production applications of the developed models.

2.2. Datasets

To validate the established platform, two separate datasets were used in order to train a pre-built classification model. The first dataset is the open-source COVIDx dataset (https://github.com/lindawangg/COVID-Net/blob/master/docs/COVIDx.md (accessed on 19 December 2022)), which was compiled by Wang et al. from a collection of open repositories as listed in Table 2 [15]. At the time of preparing the data, the most current version was COVIDx V8A. This dataset is subdivided into 3 main classes: Healthy, Non-COVID-19 Pneumonia, and COVID-19.

Table 2. COVIDx V8A dataset sources.

Title	URL
Cohen	https://github.com/ieee8023/covid-chestxray-dataset
Figure 1	https://github.com/agchung/Figure1-COVID-chestxray-dataset
Actualmed	https://github.com/agchung/Actualmed-COVID-chestxray-dataset
Sirm	https://www.kaggle.com/tawsifurrahman/covid19-radiography-database/version/3
RSNA	https://www.kaggle.com/c/rsna-pneumonia-detection-challenge/data
RICORD	https://wiki.cancerimagingarchive.net/pages/viewpage.action?pageId=70230281

The second dataset was pre-compiled by industry partner EHL and made available through file transfer protocol (FTP). The dataset is subdivided into training and testing sets, each of which is further divided into different conditions including Healthy, Pneumonia, COVID-19, Atelectasis, and Cardiomegaly, among others. Further details about the dataset constitutions are presented in later sections of this manuscript, though it is worth mentioning that there was a considerable difference in the image resolutions between the two datasets as can be seen in Figure 2. Additionally, Table 3 describes the class distribution of images within each dataset.

Table 3. Number of images within each dataset.

Dataset	Healthy	Non-COVID-19 Pneumonia	COVID-19
COVIDx	8066	5575	2358
EHL	1898	118	187
Fusion	9964	5693	2542

Finally, in order to increase the robustness of the model to be re-trained, the two datasets were merged into a Fusion dataset, preserving the split structures shown in Tables 4 and 5. The Fusion dataset represents the relatively heterogeneous data usually received from different medical institutions in special circumstances [33]. The applicability of the platform and its intended use on heterogeneous data represents one of the most important advantages.

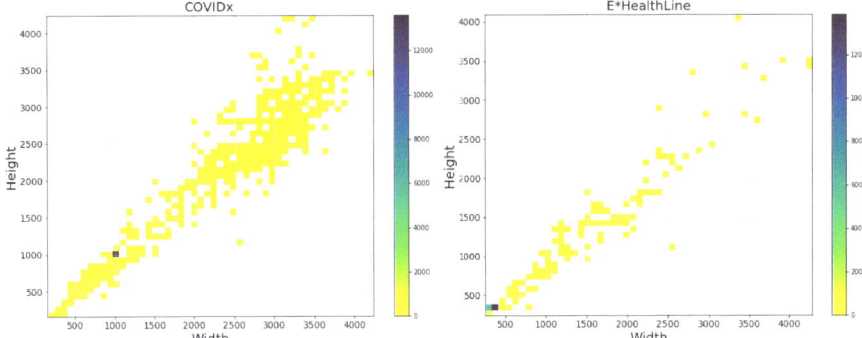

Figure 2. Range of image resolutions of the COVIDx (**left**) and EHL (**right**) datasets. A high concentration of images in the COVIDx dataset is centered around 1000 × 1000 pixels, but the majority of EHL images is below 480 × 480 pixels.

2.2.1. COVIDx Dataset

The process to obtain the COVIDx dataset is provided in detail as part of the COVID-Net Github (https://github.com/lindawangg/COVID-Net (accessed on 19 December 2022)) repository as it was compiled by Wang et al. [15]. The dataset was loaded into the online storage available at JSC and an analysis of the images was performed using the Open-Source Computer Vision Library (OpenCV) python package in order to verify that the dataset contains no duplicates or corruptions. The majority of the data provided in the COVIDx dataset are in the portable network graphics (PNG) image format. Table 4 presents the train-test split of the COVIDx dataset.

Table 4. COVIDx V8A dataset training and testing split.

Set	Healthy	Non-COVID-19 Pneumonia	COVID-19
Training	7966 (98.8%)	5475 (98.2%)	2158 (91.5%)
Testing	100 (1.2%)	100 (1.8%)	200 (8.5%)
Total	8066	5575	2358

2.2.2. EHL Dataset

The EHL dataset was made available through secure FTP and, similarly to the COVIDx dataset, loaded onto the online storage at JSC. The dataset is subdivided into several pulmonary and chest-related conditions, though for the purposes described in this manuscript solely the images within the Healthy, Non-COVID-19 Pneumonia, and COVID-19 directories were used. The remainder of the data will be used in a future transfer learning application of the available ML model.

After performing some verification steps on the data using OpenCV, it became evident that some images were duplicates of those available in the COVIDx dataset, which was traced back to the fact that one of the participating hospitals had made their data available as part of the Cohen dataset. These images were removed and the resulting distribution of data is presented in Table 5. The EHL dataset is made available as part of the European Open Science Cloud fast-track grant project and can be accessed online for research purposes (https://b2share.fz-juelich.de/records/aef5d3b8aa044485b9620b95b60c47a2 (accessed on 19 December 2022)). Evaluation of the trained models was performed using only the EHL dataset in order to verify these models' ability to predict over the new data.

Table 5. E*HealthLine dataset training and testing split.

Set	Healthy	Non-COVID-19 Pneumonia	COVID-19
Training	198 (10.4%)	21 (17.8%)	189 (65.4%)
Testing	1700 (89.6%)	97 (82.2%)	100 (34.6%)
Total	1898	118	289

2.3. COVID-Net Model

The COVID-Net deep learning model was developed and released by Wang et al. in May of 2020 in response to the COVID-19 pandemic to screen patients for COVID-19 using chest radiographs [15]. The model follows the current DL standard for image analysis of using convolutional neural networks (CNNs) with intermittently varying kernel sizes, but expands on it by employing the residual architecture that was introduced by He et al. in their pioneering work on residual networks for object detection in images [34]. COVID-Net was built using TensorFlow (https://www.tensorflow.org/ (accessed on 19 December 2022)) version 1.13.

The initial approach with COVID-Net within the scope of this project involved running inference using the pre-trained model on both available datasets in order to highlight their differences, before moving forward with the re-training attempts, which also served the purpose of highlighting the potential speed-up that can be achieved using the available MSA.

2.3.1. Model Selection

The Git repository for COVID-Net lists a number of models each with varying input image sizes and performance markers. At the time of performing this analysis, the best performing model was labelled "COVIDNet-CXR4-A", which scales input images to a resolution of 480×480 pixels. Two other versions of the model exist that take inputs of lower resolution (224×224 pixels) with the best performing among them being "COVIDNet-CXR Large". Both models are available for download from links in the repository.

Selecting the appropriate model for this application required an analysis of the resolutions of the available images, and since the majority of the images within the EHL dataset are below the threshold of 480×480 pixel resolution as can be seen in Figure 2, it became evident that the "COVIDNet-CXR Large" model would perform best. This decision is further supported by the initial inference results that will be presented below in Section 3, but follows the logic that down-sampling image data produces far less noise than up-sampling, which is more likely to generate artefacts by magnifying limited visual information.

2.3.2. Model Training

The repository for COVID-Net provides scripts and terminal commands for training the network. These scripts define the training parameters (learning rate, number of epochs, batch size, location of the pre-defined network weights) and the location of the datasets for training and testing. Accordingly, the parameters are adapted to the updated datasets being used in this application, and a range is defined over which the training will be parallelised.

Additionally, the training script is updated in order to introduce the possibility of many concurrent parallelised training runs, thus making use of the available HPC resources. The initial approach for parallelised training was through performing a grid-search of pre-defined parameters to tune and iteratively populating a job-script that would then be submitted to the HPC scheduler. Instead, hyperparameter tuning is implemented, as described in the next subsection, which can streamline the parameter search and potentially uncover hyperparameter combinations that would otherwise have been missed. Finally, a set of parameters is selected to train the model with an increasing number of nodes, using the Horovod (https://horovod.ai/ (accessed on 19 December 2022)) distributed DL framework, in order to determine the extent to which training can be accelerated as more resources are made available.

2.4. Hyperparameter Tuning

Hyperparameters are parameters which influence an algorithm's behaviour. These values are typically set by the user manually before the training of an algorithm. Choosing an optimal set of hyperparameters can significantly improve the performance of a model [35]. In order to easily find the best performing combination of parameters for training the COVID-Net model on the new and the combined datasets, the hyperparameter tuning library Tune, developed under the Ray framework, was employed [21,36]. This tuner takes a model and selected tunable parameters as input and performs an optimisation that highlights the combination of parameters that produces the best results according to a selected metric. Due to compatibility issues related to the earlier version of TensorFlow used in constructing COVID-Net, it was necessary to use version 0.6.2 of the Ray module.

The Ray framework employs schedulers that take advantage of parallel computing to scale up and speed up the task at hand; of these schedulers, population-based training (PBT), HyperBand, and Asynchronous HyperBand [37–39] are considered and compared to the default first-in, first-out (FIFO) scheduler. The comparison was performed by running the hyperparameter tuning process with each of the selected schedulers over the same parameter search space. The best-performing scheduler was selected based on runtime and the COVID-Net model's performance when re-trained using the optimal parameter combination that the tuning process output.

3. Results

3.1. Pre-Optimisation Analysis

Running inference with COVID-Net on the available images highlighted the differences between the two datasets. The network performance on COVIDx was in line with the results published by the original authors. However, the images from EHL were more likely to be misclassified. In fact, the results presented in Figure 3a highlight a bias towards predicting COVID-19.

After re-training the network on a combination of the newly acquired images and the original COVIDx dataset, the results achieved are presented in Figure 3b, where classification accuracy is improved. In order to achieve these results, several training runs were performed in parallel where the class weights (CWs) were adjusted, as well as the learning rate (LR), the batch size, the COVID-19 percentages (CPs), and the number of training epochs. Through these training runs the range of these parameters that are tuned on a larger scale in the next step was narrowed down.

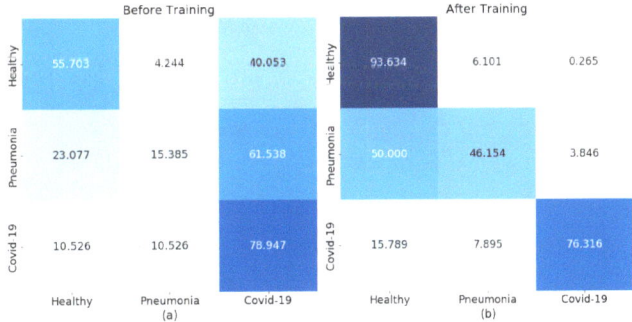

Figure 3. Prediction performance (in %) heatmaps for COVID-Net on the EHL dataset (**a**) before and (**b**) after initial re-training.

3.2. Hyperparameter Optimisation

The hyperparameter optimisation is performed on the DEEP-Extreme Scale Booster (ESB) partition, with 20 trials taking up 1 node each (see hardware configuration listed in Table 1). During these 20 trials the network is trained over 24 epochs, with each trial being assigned a different combination of the tunable parameters, in this case the COVID-19 percentage, the class weights, and the learning rate. The parameter values are chosen following a random uniform distribution in the case of the CWs and the CP, and a logarithmic uniform distribution for the LR. The selected schedulers distribute the tasks on the available nodes and in three of the four cases introduce further perturbations to the hyperparameters halfway through the training process. The specific experimental setup is further expanded in the below sections for each of the selected schedulers.

3.2.1. First-In First-Out

The default scheduling algorithm for the Ray library, first-in first-out (FIFO), performs the basic scheduling task of distributing the trials over the available nodes and does not update the tunable parameters during the training process. It is employed here as a benchmark to gauge the performance of the other schedulers.

Running all the trials in parallel took a total of 402 min to complete, after which the best performing combination of parameters was an LR of 0.00013, CWs of 1 for healthy, 1.38745 for pneumonia, and 6.1508 for COVID-19, and a CP value of 0.289. These parameters were used to re-train COVID-Net over 50 epochs and the prediction performance of the model re-trained using these parameters is highlighted in Figure 4a. The trained model in this case is very capable of detecting COVID-19 infections in CXRs, but pneumonia cases are almost always diagnosed as healthy.

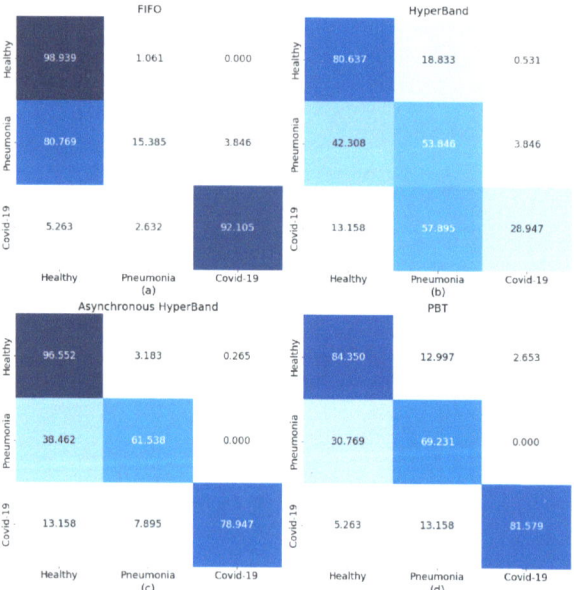

Figure 4. Prediction performance heatmaps for COVID-Net on the EHL dataset after re-training on the parameters chosen by (**a**) FIFO, (**b**) HyperBand, (**c**) Asynchronous HyperBand, and (**d**) PBT.

3.2.2. HyperBand

The HyperBand scheduler is activated in this case halfway through the training process, at which point it begins stopping tasks that underperform. The trials required a total of 421 min to complete, at which point stopped trials were discarded while the best performing trial was selected based on the overall accuracy, loss, and run time.

Interestingly, several of the trials that presented high accuracy at the end of tuning did not perform well when trained, showing a complete bias towards predicting one of the three conditions. The prediction performance of a model trained on the selected best parameters of LR = 0.0006, CW = [1, 5.0312, 3.4151], and CP = 0.081 is presented as a heatmap in Figure 4b. The trained model was unable to provide certain predictions when exposed to the images from the test set even after training for 50 epochs. The highest overall prediction accuracy is for healthy patients, but that is still at 80%.

3.2.3. Asynchronous HyperBand

Similarly to HyperBand, the Asynchronous HyperBand scheduler also implements early stopping, but does so while taking advantage of the available parallel processing power to distribute the tasks more efficiently.

Running the trials required a total of 422 min and the best performing model was chosen as having LR = 0.00012, CW = [1, 4.0981, 3.0387], and CP = 0.187. The outputs from the model trained on the best parameter combination from Asynchronous HyperBand are presented in Figure 4c. In this case, the generated parameters resulted in a trained model with improved results on the original re-trained COVID-Net presented in Figure 3b.

3.2.4. Population-Based Training

The PBT scheduler introduces perturbations to selected parameters at a set time during the tuning process. This introduces an extra layer of randomness to the hyperparameter tuning and potentially uncovers new combinations from the different trials running in parallel. In this case PBT is tasked to begin perturbing the LR halfway through the total training time.

The trials ran for a total of 419 min and from the results LR = 0.00024, CW = [1, 9.9599, 9.4996], and CP = 0.346 were selected to be used for re-training COVID-Net, the predictive performance of which is presented in Figure 4d. Similarly to the results obtained in the Asynchronous HyperBand trial, this model also presented an improved performance in detecting pneumonia and COVID-19 cases although the "Healthy" prediction was reduced to 84%.

Figure 5 compares the prediction performance of the original re-trained COVID-Net model with that of models retrained using the best performing hyperparameters from the tuning process with Asynchronous HyperBand and PBT.

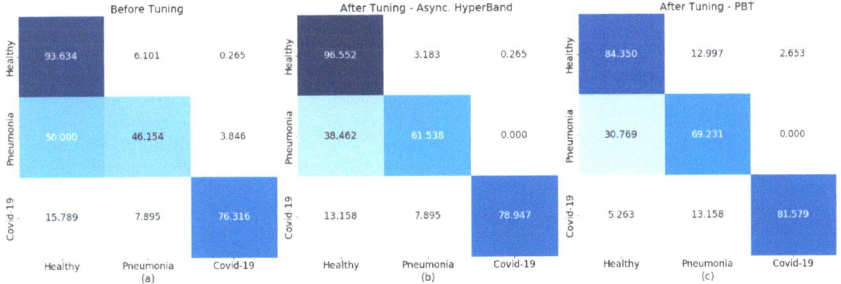

Figure 5. Comparison of trained COVID-Net prediction performance before (**a**) and after hyperparameter tuning with Asynchronous HyperBand (**b**) and PBT (**c**).

3.3. COVID-Net Re-Training

The Horovod framework was used to re-train the COVID-Net model based on parameters chosen from the previous results, while the resources available for training were iteratively increased. The graph presented in Figure 6a shows the change in training duration as more resources were made available.

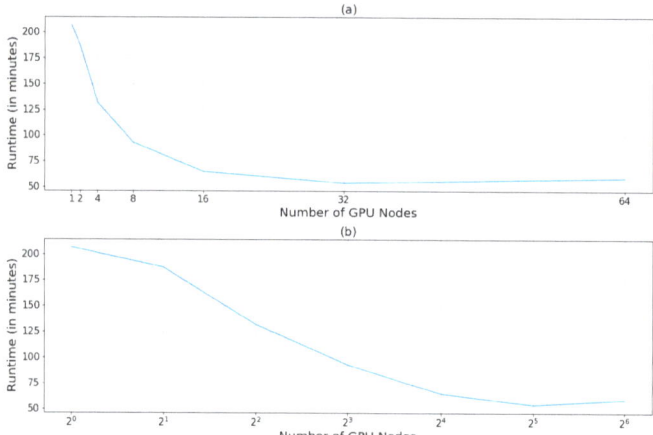

Figure 6. Training duration (in minutes) as more GPU nodes are recruited, (**a**) on a linear scale and (**b**) on a logarithmic scale.

The model trained significantly faster as the tasks were distributed among the increasing number of worker nodes. The time required to train over 25 epochs was reduced from 207 min on 1 node, to 54 min on 32 nodes. However, the rate of reduction decreased with resource increase as can be seen from the decreasing slope of Figure 6b. Ultimately, as the resources were increased to 64 nodes, the model training became slower and both curves switched to a positive slope, indicating that the cut-off point for speed-up had been reached.

4. Discussion

Through trial and error a set of parameters was selected to train the COVID-Net model on the Fusion dataset and the results obtained are shown in Figure 3b. In reality, several more parameters, including the batch size, the train-test split, the number of epochs, and freezing or unfreezing some layers from COVID-Net could have been tuned by hand in order to improve the results, but as the number of these parameters increases, so does the complexity of the optimisation problem. The results show that the model can be improved and highlight the fact that more effective tuning approaches are necessary.

Through four straightforward applications of a hyperparameter optimisation framework, it was possible to improve the predictive performance of COVID-Net on new data. The schedulers used for the optimisation took advantage of the available MSA and efficiently distributed the work over the available resources. In doing so, the framework was able to cover more ground and test more parameter combinations simultaneously in order to close in on the parameters with which the model would train more effectively. This process is not perfect, as can be seen from the results obtained from Hyperband, where the best-performing parameter combination yielded a model that underperformed, or through reducing the pneumonia class weights, the best performing parameters from the FIFO scheduler resulted in a model that was extremely good at finding COVID-19 patients, but completely incapable of predicting pneumonia. However, these results give insight into novel ways the parameters can be tuned and thus the model performance can be improved.

In the case of Asynchronous HyperBand and PBT, both resulting trained models performed more consistently than the original re-trained COVID-Net, with predictions trending towards true positives. The results also highlight the possibility of further improvement with longer training and further fine-tuning of the hyperparameters, both of which are made possible through the scale-up of the GPU resources on the compute clusters.

The reduction in training duration observed in Figure 6a is not infinite; in fact, as more nodes are recruited, the communication overhead between these nodes becomes more complex and more time-consuming, resulting in the flattening of the curve and ultimately the upward trend seen in Figure 6b. To counter this issue, it is important to understand the problem at hand and to recruit the appropriate hardware and software accordingly, while also performing many trials to pinpoint the cut-off at which training is the most efficient.

The work presented in this manuscript describes the large-scale re-training of COVID-Net as a use case to validate a modular medical diagnosis support platform built on an HPC infrastructure and taking advantage of novel and efficient ML algorithms. That is not to say that this work would not be possible without the specific HPC infrastructure used. In fact, the platform makes use of open-source software, making it easily portable onto commercially available cloud computing (CC) solutions. Similarly, the main aim is to develop the base infrastructure that takes advantage of the HPC resources to simplify the development of software that is lightweight enough to be easily deployed in most standard computers available in hospitals, making them a vital tool to support medical personnel.

Given that the medical field is regularly facing time-sensitive problems, this paper highlights the need for platforms that simplify access to cutting-edge resources for model training and development, and also for specially trained experts in the field of ML, data science, and HPC for medical applications, who would advise on applications, assist in setting up the problem solutions, and take part in the data analysis and the development of the diagnostic and treatment techniques of the future.

Finally, since the prototype platform described in this manuscript only used open-access data, there are no privacy risks and thus this issue was not addressed. As the platform moves towards production, and especially before dealing with restricted real-world data, its safety from outside threats will need to be assessed. Additionally, this process is still in its infancy and much work still needs to be done in order to test the robustness of this platform, and validate its performance in real-world use cases.

5. Conclusions

In the present manuscript, the re-training of a COVID-19 detection model was described as a use case through which an HPC-enabled data analysis and ML platform was validated. The MSA available at JSC, especially the scalable storage and computing resources, made it possible (1) to validate the performance of the COVID-Net model on the original COVIDx data as well as new data made available through research partners, (2) to perform large-scale hyperparameter tuning, through which the optimal training parameters for the model were uncovered, and (3) to re-train the model using the selected parameters and highlight the improvement that was achieved. Furthermore, the research also highlights the training speed-up that can be achieved using the platform.

The severity with which the COVID-19 pandemic struck worldwide, and research showing that such global phenomena may become more frequent, highlight the need for research platforms such as the one described in the present manuscript. These platforms would make use of highly efficient computing, communication, and storage technology, as well as open-source and interoperable software, and should be made available to assist the healthcare sector in order to simplify and accelerate the development of medical diagnosis support tools. This does not mean that medical institutions should be required to have access to HPC resources, which would put hospitals at a severe disadvantage, not only in developing countries. Rather, the models developed within these platforms ought to be more portable and easily implementable, while the communication channels between research institutions and medical centres ought to be strengthened, paving the way for effective medical and technological cooperation. Such platforms rely on the availability of data and the willingness of medical institutions to participate in the research, both of which are more likely to increase as the developed and validated models show beneficial effects in the field.

Author Contributions: Conceptualisation, C.B., M.R. and S.F.; methodology, C.B.; software, C.B. and M.A.; validation, C.B., M.A., M.R. and S.F.; formal analysis, C.B. and M.A.; investigation, C.B.; resources, M.R.; data curation, M.R.; writing—original draft preparation, C.B.; writing—review and editing, C.B., M.R. and S.F.; visualisation, M.A.; supervision, M.R., S.F., A.S. and S.B.; project administration, M.R. and S.F.; funding acquisition, M.R. All authors have read and agreed to the published version of the manuscript.

Funding: This work was performed in the Center of Excellence (CoE) Research on AI- and Simulation-Based Engineering at Exascale (RAISE), receiving funding from EU's Horizon 2020 Research and Innovation Framework Programme H2020-INFRAEDI-2019-1 under grant agreement no. 951733. The Icelandic HPC National Competence Center is funded by the EuroCC project that has received funding from the EU HPC Joint Undertaking (JU) under grant agreement no. 951732 and the EOSC COVID-19 Fast Track Grant under grant agreement no. 831644. This publication of the SMITH consortium was supported by the German Federal Ministry of Education and Research, grant no. 01ZZ1803M.

Institutional Review Board Statement: Not Applicable.

Informed Consent Statement: Not Applicable.

Data Availability Statement: The COVIDx dataset is available online at https://www.kaggle.com/datasets/andyczhao/covidx-cxr2 (accessed on 19 December 2022). The EHL dataset is available online at https://b2share.fz-juelich.de/records/aef5d3b8aa044485b9620b95b60c47a2 (accessed on 19 December 2022). COVID-Net is available at https://github.com/lindawangg/COVID-Net (accessed on 19 December 2022). The work described in this paper is available at https://github.com/c-barakat/covidnet_tune (accessed on 19 December 2022).

Acknowledgments: The authors acknowledge the support of E*HealthLine, who provided the data for re-training the COVID-Net model, as well as the Jülich Supercomputing Centre for providing access to the supercomputing resources including the DEEP-EST projects.

Conflicts of Interest: The authors declare no conflict of interest.

Abbreviations

The following abbreviations are used in this manuscript:

AI	artificial intelligence
CC	cloud computing
CNN	convolutional neural network
CP	COVID-19 percentage
CW	class weight
CXR	chest X-ray
DEEP	dynamic exascale entry platform
DL	deep learning
EHL	E*HealthLine
EOSC	European Open Science Cloud
ESB	extreme scale booster
FIFO	first-in, first-out
FTP	file transfer protocol
HPC	high-performance computing
ICU	intensive care unit
JSC	Jülich Supercomputing Centre
JUWELS	Jülich Wizard for European Leadership Science

LR	learning rate
ML	machine learning
MPI	message passing interface
MSA	modular supercomputing architecture
NumPy	Numerical Python
OpenCV	Open-Source Computer Vision Library
PBT	population-based training
PNG	portable network graphics
RT-PCR	reverse-transcription polymerase chain-reaction
SLURM	Simple Linux Utility for Resource Management
SSH	secure shell

References

1. French, G.; Hulse, M.; Nguyen, D.; Sobotka, K.; Webster, K.; Corman, J.; Aboagye-Nyame, B.; Dion, M.; Johnson, M.; Zalinger, B.; et al. Impact of Hospital Strain on Excess Deaths During the COVID-19 Pandemic—United States, July 2020–July 2021. *Morb. Mortal. Wkly. Rep.* **2021**, *70*, 1613–1616. [CrossRef] [PubMed]
2. Tahamtan, A.; Ardebili, A. Real-time RT-PCR in COVID-19 detection: Issues affecting the results. *Expert Rev. Mol. Diagn.* **2020**, *20*, 453–454. [CrossRef]
3. Teymouri, M.; Mollazadeh, S.; Mortazavi, H.; Naderi Ghale-noie, Z.; Keyvani, V.; Aghababaei, F.; Hamblin, M.R.; Abbaszadeh-Goudarzi, G.; Pourghadamyari, H.; Hashemian, S.M.R.; et al. Recent advances and challenges of RT-PCR tests for the diagnosis of COVID-19. *Pathol. Res. Pract.* **2021**, *221*, 153443. [CrossRef]
4. Roshkovan, L.; Chatterjee, N.; Galperin-Aizenberg, M.; Gupta, N.; Shah, R.; Barbosa Jr, E.M.; Simpson, S.; Cook, T.; Nachiappan, A.; Knollmann, F.; et al. The Role of Imaging in the Management of Suspected or Known COVID-19 Pneumonia. A Multidisciplinary Perspective. *Ann. Am. Thorac. Soc.* **2020**, *17*, 1358–1365. [CrossRef]
5. Ai, T.; Yang, Z.; Hou, H.; Zhan, C.; Chen, C.; Lv, W.; Tao, Q.; Sun, Z.; Xia, L. Correlation of chest CT and RT-PCR testing in coronavirus disease 2019 (COVID-19) in China: A report of 1014 cases. *Radiology* **2020**, *296*, E32–E40. [CrossRef]
6. Marani, M.; Katul, G.G.; Pan, W.K.; Parolari, A.J. Intensity and frequency of extreme novel epidemics. *Proc. Natl. Acad. Sci. USA* **2021**, *118*, e2105482118. [CrossRef]
7. Deng, J.; Dong, W.; Socher, R.; Li, L.J.; Li, K.; Fei-Fei, L. ImageNet: A Large-Scale Hierarchical Image Database. In Proceedings of the 2009 IEEE Conference on Computer Vision and Pattern Recognition, Miami, FL, USA, 20–25 June 2009; pp. 248–255. [CrossRef]
8. Huddar, V.; Desiraju, B.K.; Rajan, V.; Bhattacharya, S.; Roy, S.; Reddy, C.K. Predicting Complications in Critical Care Using Heterogeneous Clinical Data. *IEEE Access* **2016**, *4*, 7988–8001. [CrossRef]
9. Erlingsson, E.; Cavallaro, G.; Galonska, A.; Riedel, M.; Neukirchen, H. Modular supercomputing design supporting machine learning applications. In Proceedings of the 2018 41st International Convention on Information and Communication Technology, Electronics and Microelectronics (MIPRO), Opatija, Croatia, 21–25 May 2018; pp. 0159–0163. [CrossRef]
10. Sun, H.; Liu, Z.; Wang, G.; Lian, W.; Ma, J. Intelligent Analysis of Medical Big Data Based on Deep Learning. *IEEE Access* **2019**, *7*, 142022–142037. [CrossRef]
11. Sedona, R.; Cavallaro, G.; Jitsev, J.; Strube, A.; Riedel, M.; Benediktsson, J. Remote Sensing Big Data Classification with High Performance Distributed Deep Learning. *Remote. Sens.* **2019**, *11*, 3056. [CrossRef]
12. Jumper, J.; Evans, R.; Pritzel, A.; Green, T.; Figurnov, M.; Ronneberger, O.; Tunyasuvunakool, K.; Bates, R.; Žídek, A.; Potapenko, A.; et al. Highly accurate protein structure prediction with AlphaFold. *Nature* **2021**, *596*, 583–589. [CrossRef]
13. Baek, M.; DiMaio, F.; Anishchenko, I.; Dauparas, J.; Ovchinnikov, S.; Lee, G.R.; Wang, J.; Cong, Q.; Kinch, L.N.; Schaeffer, R.D.; et al. Accurate prediction of protein structures and interactions using a three-track neural network. *Science* **2021**, *373*, 871–876. [CrossRef] [PubMed]
14. Lugarà, M.; Tamburrini, S.; Coppola, M.G.; Oliva, G.; Fiorini, V.; Catalano, M.; Carbone, R.; Saturnino, P.P.; Rosano, N.; Pesce, A.; et al. The Role of Lung Ultrasound in SARS-CoV-19 Pneumonia Management. *Diagnostics* **2022**, *12*, 1856. [CrossRef] [PubMed]
15. Wang, L.; Lin, Z.Q.; Wong, A. COVID-Net: A tailored deep convolutional neural network design for detection of COVID-19 cases from chest X-ray images. *Sci. Rep.* **2020**, *10*, 19549. [CrossRef]
16. Lee, C.P.; Lim, K.M. COVID-19 Diagnosis on Chest Radiographs with Enhanced Deep Neural Networks. *Diagnostics* **2022**, *12*, 1828. [CrossRef] [PubMed]
17. Song, Y.; Liu, J.; Liu, X.; Tang, J. COVID-19 Infection Segmentation and Severity Assessment Using a Self-Supervised Learning Approach. *Diagnostics* **2022**, *12*, 1805. [CrossRef] [PubMed]
18. Elshennawy, N.M.; Ibrahim, D.M.; Sarhan, A.M.; Arafa, M. Deep-Risk: Deep Learning-Based Mortality Risk Predictive Models for COVID-19. *Diagnostics* **2022**, *12*, 1847. [CrossRef] [PubMed]
19. Rajaraman, S.; Guo, P.; Xue, Z.; Antani, S.K. A Deep Modality-Specific Ensemble for Improving Pneumonia Detection in Chest X-rays. *Diagnostics* **2022**, *12*, 1442. [CrossRef]

20. Kesselheim, S.; Herten, A.; Krajsek, K.; Ebert, J.; Jitsev, J.; Cherti, M.; Langguth, M.; Gong, B.; Stadtler, S.; Mozaffari, A.; et al. JUWELS Booster—A Supercomputer for Large-Scale AI Research. In *Proceedings of the High Performance Computing*; Jagode, H., Anzt, H., Ltaief, H., Luszczek, P., Eds.; Springer International Publishing: Cham, Switzerland, 2021; pp. 453–468.
21. Moritz, P.; Nishihara, R.; Wang, S.; Tumanov, A.; Liaw, R.; Liang, E.; Elibol, M.; Yang, Z.; Paul, W.; Jordan, M.I.; et al. Ray: A Distributed Framework for Emerging AI Applications. In Proceedings of the 13th USENIX Symposium on Operating Systems Design and Implementation (OSDI 18), Carlsbad, CA, USA, 8–10 October 2018; USENIX Association: Carlsbad, CA, USA, 2018; pp. 561–577.
22. Nijor, S.; Rallis, G.; Lad, N.; Gokcen, E. Patient safety issues from information overload in electronic medical records. *J. Patient Saf.* **2022**, *18*, e999–e1003. [CrossRef]
23. Manor-Shulman, O.; Beyene, J.; Frndova, H.; Parshuram, C.S. Quantifying the volume of documented clinical information in critical illness. *J. Crit. Care* **2008**, *23*, 245–250. [CrossRef]
24. Lundervold, A.S.; Lundervold, A. An overview of deep learning in medical imaging focusing on MRI. *Z. Med. Phys.* **2019**, *29*, 102–127. [CrossRef]
25. Barakat, C.; Fritsch, S.; Riedel, M.; Brynjólfsson, S. An HPC-Driven Data Science Platform to Speed-up Time Series Data Analysis of Patients with the Acute Respiratory Distress Syndrome. In Proceedings of the 2021 44th International Convention on Information, Communication and Electronic Technology (MIPRO), Opatija, Croatia, 24–28 May 2021; pp. 311–316. [CrossRef]
26. Barakat, C.; Fritsch, S.; Sharafutdinov, K.; Ingólfsson, G.; Schuppert, A.; Brynjólfsson, S.; Riedel, M. Lessons learned on using High-Performance Computing and Data Science Methods towards understanding the Acute Respiratory Distress Syndrome (ARDS). In Proceedings of the 2022 45th Jubilee International Convention on Information, Communication and Electronic Technology (MIPRO), Opatija, Croatia, 23–27 May 2022; pp. 368–373. [CrossRef]
27. Farag, H.H.; Said, L.A.A.; Rizk, M.R.M.; Ahmed, M.A.E. Hyperparameters optimization for ResNet and Xception in the purpose of diagnosing COVID-19. *J. Intell. Fuzzy Syst.* **2021**, *41*, 3555–3571. [CrossRef]
28. Adedigba, A.P.; Adeshina, S.A.; Aina, O.E.; Aibinu, A.M. Optimal hyperparameter selection of deep learning models for COVID-19 chest X-ray classification. *Intell.-Based Med.* **2021**, *5*, 100034. [CrossRef] [PubMed]
29. Arman, S.E.; Rahman, S.; Deowan, S.A. COVIDXception-Net: A Bayesian Optimization-Based Deep Learning Approach to Diagnose COVID-19 from X-Ray Images. *SN Comput. Sci.* **2021**, *3*, 115. [CrossRef] [PubMed]
30. Suarez, E.; Eickert, N.; Lippert, T. Modular Supercomputing architecture: From idea to production. In *Contemporary High Performance Computing: From Petascale toward Exascale*, 1st ed.; Vetter, J., Ed.; CRC Press: Boca Raton, FL, USA, 2019; Volume 3, pp. 223–251.
31. Eicker, N.; Lippert, T.; Moschny, T.; Suarez, E.; The DEEP Project. The DEEP Project An alternative approach to heterogeneous cluster-computing in the many-core era. *Concurr. Comput. Pract. Exp.* **2016**, *28*, 2394–2411. .: 10.1002/cpe.3562. [CrossRef]
32. Suarez, E.; Kreuzer, A.; Eicker, N.; Lippert, T. The DEEP-EST project. In *Porting Applications to a Modular Supercomputer-Experiences from the DEEP-EST Project*; Schriften des Forschungszentrums Jülich IAS Series; Forschungszentrum Jülich GmbH Zentralbibliothek, Verlag: Jülich, Germany, 2021; Volume 48, pp. 9–25.
33. Sharafutdinov, K.; Bhat, J.S.; Fritsch, S.J.; Nikulina, K.; Samadi, M.E.; Polzin, R.; Mayer, H.; Marx, G.; Bickenbach, J.; Schuppert, A. Application of convex hull analysis for the evaluation of data heterogeneity between patient populations of different origin and implications of hospital bias in downstream machine-learning-based data processing: A comparison of 4 critical-care patient datasets. *Front. Big Data* **2022**, *5*, 603429. [CrossRef]
34. He, K.; Zhang, X.; Ren, S.; Sun, J. Deep Residual Learning for Image Recognition. *arXiv* **2015**, arXiv:1512.03385.
35. Luo, G. A review of automatic selection methods for machine learning algorithms and hyper-parameter values. *Netw. Model. Anal. Health Inform. Bioinform.* **2016**, *5*, 1–16. [CrossRef]
36. Liaw, R.; Liang, E.; Nishihara, R.; Moritz, P.; Gonzalez, J.E.; Stoica, I. Tune: A Research Platform for Distributed Model Selection and Training. *arXiv* **2018**, arXiv:1807.05118.
37. Jaderberg, M.; Dalibard, V.; Osindero, S.; Czarnecki, W.M.; Donahue, J.; Razavi, A.; Vinyals, O.; Green, T.; Dunning, I.; Simonyan, K.; et al. Population Based Training of Neural Networks. *arXiv* **2017**, arXiv:1711.09846. [CrossRef]
38. Li, L.; Jamieson, K.; DeSalvo, G.; Rostamizadeh, A.; Talwalkar, A. Hyperband: A Novel Bandit-Based Approach to Hyperparameter Optimization. *J. Mach. Learn. Res.* **2018**, *18*, 1–52.
39. Li, L.; Jamieson, K.; Rostamizadeh, A.; Gonina, E.; Hardt, M.; Recht, B.; Talwalkar, A. A System for Massively Parallel Hyperparameter Tuning. *arXiv* **2018**, arXiv:1810.05934. [CrossRef]

Disclaimer/Publisher's Note: The statements, opinions and data contained in all publications are solely those of the individual author(s) and contributor(s) and not of MDPI and/or the editor(s). MDPI and/or the editor(s) disclaim responsibility for any injury to people or property resulting from any ideas, methods, instructions or products referred to in the content.

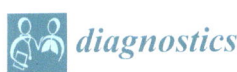

Article

Inter- and Intra-Observer Agreement When Using a Diagnostic Labeling Scheme for Annotating Findings on Chest X-rays—An Early Step in the Development of a Deep Learning-Based Decision Support System

Dana Li [1,2,*], Lea Marie Pehrson [1,3], Lea Tøttrup [4], Marco Fraccaro [4], Rasmus Bonnevie [4], Jakob Thrane [4], Peter Jagd Sørensen [1,2], Alexander Rykkje [1,2], Tobias Thostrup Andersen [1], Henrik Steglich-Arnholm [1], Dorte Marianne Rohde Stærk [1], Lotte Borgwardt [1], Kristoffer Lindskov Hansen [1,2], Sune Darkner [3], Jonathan Frederik Carlsen [1,2] and Michael Bachmann Nielsen [1,2]

1. Department of Diagnostic Radiology, Copenhagen University Hospital, Rigshospitalet, 2100 Copenhagen, Denmark
2. Department of Clinical Medicine, University of Copenhagen, 2100 Copenhagen, Denmark
3. Department of Computer Science, University of Copenhagen, 2100 Copenhagen, Denmark
4. Unumed Aps, 1055 Copenhagen, Denmark
* Correspondence: dana.li@regionh.dk

Citation: Li, D.; Pehrson, L.M.; Tøttrup, L.; Fraccaro, M.; Bonnevie, R.; Thrane, J.; Sørensen, P.J.; Rykkje, A.; Andersen, T.T.; Steglich-Arnholm, H.; et al. Inter- and Intra-Observer Agreement When Using a Diagnostic Labeling Scheme for Annotating Findings on Chest X-rays—An Early Step in the Development of a Deep Learning-Based Decision Support System. *Diagnostics* 2022, *12*, 3112. https://doi.org/10.3390/diagnostics12123112

Academic Editors: Sameer Antani, Zhiyun Xue and Sivaramakrishnan Rajaraman

Received: 19 October 2022
Accepted: 26 November 2022
Published: 9 December 2022

Publisher's Note: MDPI stays neutral with regard to jurisdictional claims in published maps and institutional affiliations.

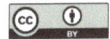

Copyright: © 2022 by the authors. Licensee MDPI, Basel, Switzerland. This article is an open access article distributed under the terms and conditions of the Creative Commons Attribution (CC BY) license (https://creativecommons.org/licenses/by/4.0/).

Abstract: Consistent annotation of data is a prerequisite for the successful training and testing of artificial intelligence-based decision support systems in radiology. This can be obtained by standardizing terminology when annotating diagnostic images. The purpose of this study was to evaluate the annotation consistency among radiologists when using a novel diagnostic labeling scheme for chest X-rays. Six radiologists with experience ranging from one to sixteen years, annotated a set of 100 fully anonymized chest X-rays. The blinded radiologists annotated on two separate occasions. Statistical analyses were done using Randolph's kappa and PABAK, and the proportions of specific agreements were calculated. Fair-to-excellent agreement was found for all labels among the annotators (Randolph's Kappa, 0.40–0.99). The PABAK ranged from 0.12 to 1 for the two-reader inter-rater agreement and 0.26 to 1 for the intra-rater agreement. Descriptive and broad labels achieved the highest proportion of positive agreement in both the inter- and intra-reader analyses. Annotating findings with specific, interpretive labels were found to be difficult for less experienced radiologists. Annotating images with descriptive labels may increase agreement between radiologists with different experience levels compared to annotation with interpretive labels.

Keywords: artificial intelligence; chest X-ray; inter-rater; intra-rater; image annotation; diagnostic scheme; ontology; radiologists

1. Introduction

Plain chest X-rays (CXRs) are the most commonly used diagnostic image modality [1] and the first choice for most diseases of the lung, including pneumonia [2]. Hence, there is a large amount of CXRs every day for radiologists to interpret. With the worldwide shortage of radiologists and the continuing demand for CXRs, artificial intelligence (AI) and deep learning-based decision support systems have emerged as possible solutions to assist radiologists in the backlog of diagnostic images [3]. The large number of CXRs provides diverse information with varying complexity that is beneficial to the development and improvement of AI algorithms [4].

When developing an algorithm for a deep learning-based decision support system in radiology, developers need labeled images for training, validation, and testing [5]. Consistent labeling is a prerequisite for developing an effective algorithm [6]. Previous studies have suggested that variation in interpretation and denomination of CXR findings may be attributed to several factors, including the reader's medical experience, terminology bias, local disease prevalence, and geographic location of the reader's medical background [7,8]. Varying and inconsistent use of terminology, for whatever reason, may decrease the quantity of a given finding and complicate data preparation, which may render the algorithm ineffective.

Consistent labeling can be achieved by creating ontological systems for the annotation of diagnostic images. The importance of creating adequate ontological systems during AI development has previously been highlighted [9]. Several different ontological schemes for annotating CXRs have been developed, ranging from complex schemes with numerous labels to simple schemes consisting of only a handful of labels; PadChest [10] created a complex hierarchical labeling system with >180 unique labels, while Qure.ai [11] and CheXpert [12] had between 10 and 14 labels, respectively, for different chest-specific radiographic findings. Investigations on the construction of ontological schemes contribute to further insights into the challenges of creating suitable annotation labels for AI development [10].

As a step in data preparation for a novel deep learning-based decision support system, a customized diagnostic labeling scheme was developed. Instead of using already existing ontological schemes, customized labels were created to form our diagnostic scheme. The labels were made to be recognizable for Danish radiologists since they would annotate our final training, validation, and test datasets, which would consist of CXR images and text reports of Danish origin.

Our purpose was to collect information on clinicians' behavior when using the diagnostic scheme and receive clinical feedback on the scheme's construction and labels. Thus, this study's main aim was to field test our diagnostic labeling scheme and evaluate the consistency of label use when radiologists of different levels of task experience annotated findings on CXR images. Our results could, in the future, be used to investigate how different deep learning algorithms perform depending on how the labels they used for training were ordered and/or categorized.

2. Materials and Methods

Ethical approval was evaluated and formally waived by the National and Regional Ethics Committee and Knowledge Centre on Data Protection Compliance due to the full anonymity of CXRs.

2.1. Diagnostic Labeling Scheme

The initial structure and labels in the diagnostic labeling scheme were generated with the aid of two radiologists. Labels were chosen based on a combination of the findings' local clinical prevalence, urgency, and potential usefulness for clinicians. The goal of the scheme was that the sum of all labels should cover all the possible findings that are reported in a CXR. Furthermore, each label should be specific enough to be clearly differentiated from other labels and carry individual clinical meaning. Iterations and subsequent corrections were done in cooperation with a team of medical doctors, engineers, and data scientists. The diagnostic labeling scheme was evaluated to match existing collections of CXR ontology schemes or hierarchies, such as the Fleischner criteria and definitions [13], and other machine learning labeling strategies [10–12,14–17]. The annotation labels were represented in hierarchical classes, where a high-level class such as 'Decreased translucency' was divided into lower-level and increasingly more specific classes such as 'Infiltrate', 'Pleural effusion', etc. In this study, we investigated labels in the scheme related to lung tissue findings only (Figure 1).

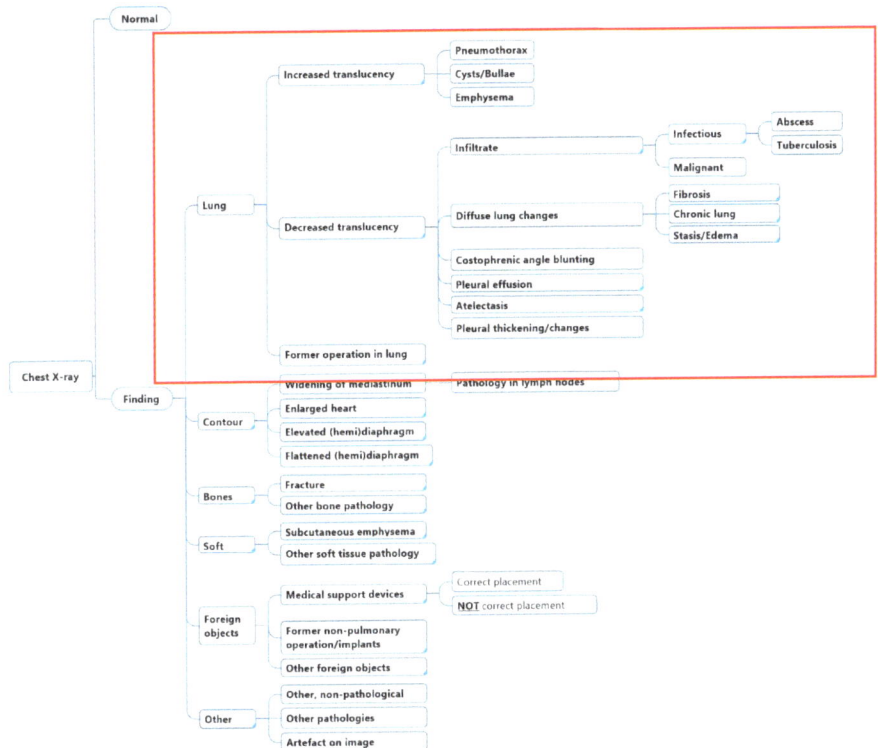

Figure 1. Full diagnostic labeling scheme and annotation labels for lung tissue findings in the diagnostic labeling scheme (red square).

2.2. Dataset and Annotation Software

A selection of 100 fully anonymized CXRs were collected at the Department of Diagnostic Radiology at Rigshospitalet (RH) through the PACS system (AGFA Impax Client 6, Mortsel, Belgium) with the criteria that each label was to be represented in the corresponding text report in at least two cases. CXR images were imported to a proprietary annotation software program (Figure 2a,b) developed by Unumed Aps (Copenhagen, Denmark). Annotators were instructed to mark every single possible finding in both a lateral and frontal projection and select the most suitable annotation label.

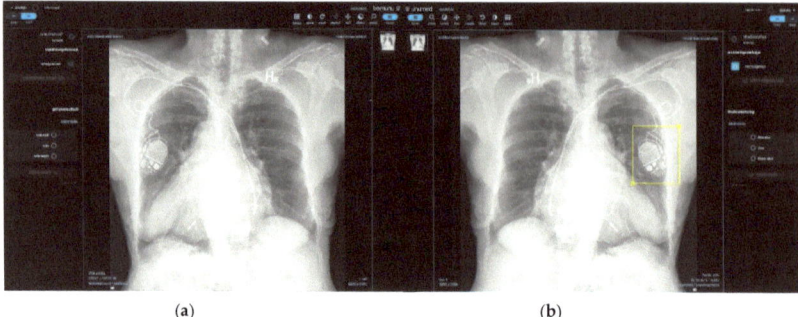

(a) (b)

Figure 2. Image representations of the annotation software interface. (**a**) Front page layout of the annotation software and (**b**) bounding box for annotation of finding in the lower right hemithorax.

2.3. Participants and Image Annotation Process

Six radiologists participated in the study. There were two radiologists at each experience level; novice radiologists with 1–2 years of experience; intermediate radiologists with 3–10 years of experience, and experienced radiologists with >10 years of experience.

Two blinded rounds of annotation were done, and no clinical patient characteristics were given. Rounds were interjected with a wash-out period of a minimum of three weeks from the last day radiologists had access to the CXR cases to the beginning of the second annotation round (Figure 3). Radiologists were allowed to contact the research and data scientist team for technical questions or difficulties. They were not allowed to share or discuss their annotations. No changes to the labels or the composition of the labeling scheme were made while the study ran its course.

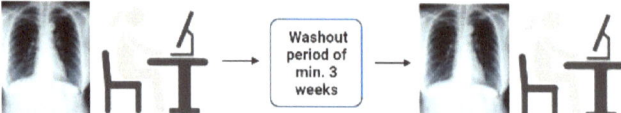

Figure 3. Visualization of the annotation process for each annotator.

2.4. Statistical Analysis

The inter- and intra-reader agreement using annotation labels from the diagnostic scheme on CXR data from Rigshospitalet has not been conducted prior to this study; thus, no formal sample or effect size computation was performed.

For each CXR case, a label would only appear to either have been used or not used for the statistical analysis, despite the label maybe having been used on both posterior–anterior and lateral projections of the same case. Continuous variables were reported in a frequency table.

Inter-reader agreement between all readers and between two readers of the same experience levels was done using data from the first annotation round. Randolph's free-marginal multi-rater Kappa [18] was used to assess the overall degree of agreement between all participants. For two-reader inter-reader agreement between participants of the same level of radiological experience, prevalence-adjusted and bias-adjusted Kappa (PABAK) [19] was used. PABAK was also used to assess intra-reader agreement. Kappa is a commonly used chance-corrected statistic to measure the extent to which readers assign the same score to the same variable. Due to the possible unbalanced distribution of positive and negative labeled cases, we chose to use free-marginal Kappa as opposed to fixed marginal

Kappa measurements. Kappa statistics were interpreted for strength by using the Landis and Koch scale [20].

Additionally, specific agreement, i.e., the proportion of positive agreement (PPA) and proportion of negative agreement (PNA), were calculated [19,21,22]. The PPA describes the shared number of cases in which a label was used out of the total number of cases where the label was used. The PNA describes the shared number of cases in which the label was *not* used out of the total number of cases that did *not* have that label. Analyses were done using RStudio Team (2021). RStudio: Integrated Development Environment for R. RStudio, PBC, Boston, MA URL http://www.rstudio.com (accessed on 2 July 2022), IBM SPSS Statistics for Windows, version 28.0 (IBM Corp. Released 2021, Armonk, NY, USA). Microsoft Excel 365 (2016) and an online kappa calculator were also used [23].

3. Results

Table 1 describes the number of CXR cases in which each label has been used in the first round of annotation. Novices used the broader and less specific label 'Decreased translucency' in 31–51 cases, while experienced radiologists did not use the label at all. However, experienced radiologists used the more specific label 'Infectious infiltrate' in 13–30 cases, while novice radiologists used it in only 0–2 cases. Intermediate radiologists also used the broader label 'Infiltrate' more often (24–33 cases) compared to the more specific label 'Infectious infiltrate' (3–6 cases). The novice and intermediate radiologists used 'Diffuse pulmonary changes' in 6–26 cases, while experienced radiologists only used it in 1 case. The majority of the radiologists marked between 11 and 19 cases as normal, except for one novice and one experienced radiologist, who marked 4 and 23 cases as normal, respectively.

Table 1. Frequency table for each individual participating radiologist. The total number of cases out of 100 CXRs that had been annotated with that specific label by a radiologist. * Does not differentiate between linear and segmental atelectasis, which could explain the difference in frequency of use.

Lung Tissue Findings	Novice 1	Novice 2	Intermediate 1	Intermediate 2	Experienced 1	Experienced 2
Normal	4	11	11	19	11	23
Increased Translucency	7	3	8	0	0	0
Pneumothorax	5	8	11	10	10	9
Cyst/Bullae	0	1	1	0	5	2
Emphysema	0	1	0	3	4	0
Decreased Translucency	51	31	11	0	0	0
Infiltrate	21	12	24	33	24	2
Infection	0	2	3	6	30	13
Abscess	0	0	0	1	0	3
Tuberculosis	0	0	1	0	0	0
Malignant	3	6	1	10	5	3
Diffuse Lung Changes	26	6	7	11	0	1
Fibrosis	1	2	2	2	1	2
Chronic Lung Changes	1	0	1	0	5	2
Stasis/Edema	5	7	9	6	10	9
Costophrenic Angle Blunting	31	21	24	5	3	0
Pleural Effusion	8	22	32	24	38	27
Atelectasis *	14	22	13	9	50	25
Pleural Thickening/Changes	0	7	3	5	3	4
Former Operation in Lung Tissue	0	5	3	5	0	0

3.1. Inter-Reader Agreement

3.1.1. Agreement between Multiple Readers

All readers achieved *fair-to-excellent agreement* on all labels (Randolph's Kappa, 0.40–0.99) (Table 2). 'Atelectasis' had the lowest agreement (Randolph's Kappa, 0.40). Table 1 shows that an experienced radiologist marked 50 cases with 'Atelectasis', whereas the other radiologists marked between 9 and 25 cases. We did not differentiate between linear and segmental atelectasis either in the statistical analysis or in the annotation guidelines, which could explain the difference in frequency of use.

Congregate categories such as 'Decreased translucency including sub-categories' and 'Costophrenic angle blunting AND pleural effusion' reached the highest proportion of positive agreement (PPA) of 0.84 and 0.67, respectively. The congregate category 'Infiltrate incl. sub-categories' reached a PPA of 0.50, which is higher than any of its sub-categories. Otherwise, the only individual labels that reached a PPA above 0.50 were 'Pneumothorax', 'Pleural effusion', and 'Normal'. However, all non-congregate labels reached a minimum of 0.81 in the proportion of negative agreement (PNA) (Table 2).

Table 2. Agreement between all readers measured in Randolph's Kappa, proportion of positive agreement, and proportion of negative agreement. Kappa: <0, poor; 0.01–0.20, slight; 0.21–0.40, fair; 0.41–0.60, moderate; 0.61–0.80, substantial; 0.81–1.00, almost perfect.

All (n = 6)	Randolph's Free-Marginal Multirater Kappa	95% CI for Randolph's Free-Marginal Multirater Kappa	Proportion of Positive Agreement	Proportion of Negative Agreement
Normal	0.79	0.71–0.86	0.59	0.94
Increased Translucency incl. sub-categories	0.73	0.64–0.81	0.47	0.92
Increased Translucency	0.88	0.83–0.93	0	0.97
Pneumothorax	0.83	0.76–0.91	0.53	0.95
Cyst/Bullae	0.98	0.95–1.00	0.1	0.99
Emphysema	0.95	0.91–0.99	0.05	0.99
Decreased Translucency incl. sub-categories	0.55	0.45–0.64	0.84	0.59
Decreased Translucency	0.46	0.38–0.55	0.13	0.84
Infiltrate incl. sub-categories	0.40	0.31–0.48	0.50	0.78
Infiltrate	0.49	0.40–0.58	0.34	0.84
Infection	0.67	0.60–0.75	0.11	0.91
Abscess	0.97	0.95–1.00	0	0.99
Tuberculosis	0.99	0.98–1.00	0	1
Malignant	0.87	0.82–0.93	0.33	0.97
Diffuse Lung Changes incl. sub-categories	0.54	0.45–0.63	0.40	0.85
Diffuse Lung Changes	0.70	0.62–0.78	0.12	0.92
Fibrosis	0.95	0.91–0.99	0.28	0.99
Chronic Lung Changes	0.94	0.90–0.98	0	0.98
Stasis/Edema	0.79	0.71–0.86	0.31	0.94
Costophrenic Angle Blunting	0.58	0.49–0.67	0.25	0.88
Pleural Effusion	0.61	0.51–0.71	0.61	0.87
Costophrenic Angle Blunting AND Pleural Effusion	0.53	0.43–0.62	0.67	0.81
Atelectasis	0.40	0.30–0.50	0.32	0.81
Pleural Thickening/Changes	0.88	0.83–0.94	0.20	0.97
Former Operation in Lung Tissue	0.94	0.90–0.98	0.04	0.98

3.1.2. Agreement between Two Readers with the Same Experience Level

There was *slight-to-excellent* agreement on all labels between radiologists of similar experience levels (Table A1 in Appendix A). The PABAK values ranged from 0.12 to 1.

The wide range in the PABAK values was most noticeable in the label 'Decreased translucency' where novices had the poorest agreement (PABAK 0.12), while experienced radiologists had the best agreement (PABAK 1). Table A2 (Appendix A) shows that the differences in agreement measures were due to the novice radiologists' tendency to use this label more. Despite higher specific agreement on the positive use, it reduced the agreement on its negative use (PPA 0.46, PNA 0.63), while intermediate and experienced radiologists had no use of that label at all, resulting in very high specific agreement on the negative use (PPA 0 and PNA 0.94–1), which lead to the higher overall agreement.

Novice and intermediate radiologists also had a higher agreement on the positive use of the label 'Infiltrate' (PPA 0.48–0.53) (Table A2 in Appendix A), while experienced radiologists did not (PPA 0, PNA 0.84). Experienced radiologists had, however, higher agreement of the positive use of the more specific label 'Infectious infiltrate' compared to novice radiologists (PPA 0.14 vs. 0), despite having a lower overall agreement (PABAK 0.24 vs. 0.96).

Experienced radiologists showed *excellent* agreement on 'Costophrenic angle blunting' (PABAK 0.94), but only due to a high PNA and low PPA (PPA 0, PNA 0.98). However, all levels of radiologists agreed on the positive use of the label 'Pleural effusion' (PPA 0.47–0.86), and all levels of radiologists had a higher positive agreement on this label compared to 'Costophrenic angle blunting' (Table A2 in Appendix A). The congregate category 'Costophrenic angle blunting AND pleural effusion' also achieved a higher PPA compared to 'Costophrenic angle blunting' alone (PPA 0.64–0.72 vs. PPA 0–0.46).

Intermediate radiologists had a positive PPA on a greater number of labels compared to that of both novice and experienced radiologists (Table A2 in Appendix A), suggesting that intermediate radiologists used more labels overall. Despite this, all levels of radiologists had an equally good agreement on 'Normal' (PABAK 0.76–0.80), and intermediate radiologists generally had a comparable number of 'Normal' cases to the other radiologists (Table 1).

While novice radiologists had a higher specific positive agreement on broader and more unspecific labels, intermediate and experienced radiologists had a better specific positive agreement on more detailed and interpretive labels. Figure 4 shows an example of a similar finding on the same CXR case, labeled differently by a novice, intermediate, and experienced radiologist.

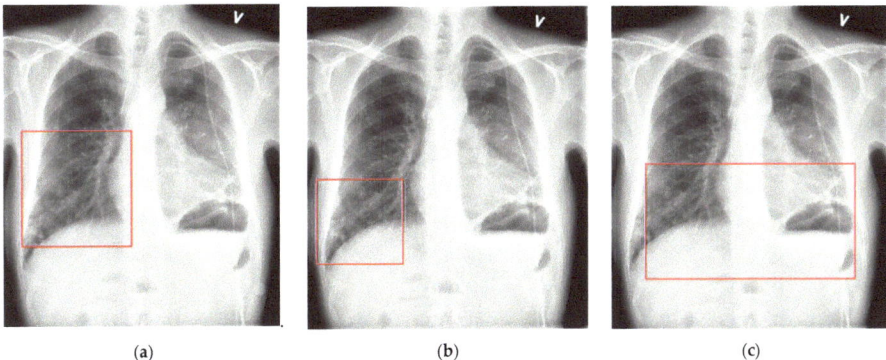

Figure 4. Examples of annotation bounding boxes labeled as (**a**) 'Decreased translucency' by a novice radiologist, (**b**) 'Infiltrate' by an intermediate radiologist, and (**c**) 'Infection' by an experienced radiologist on the same CXR case. Other findings and bounding boxes have also been used in this case but are not represented in this figure.

3.2. Intra-Reader Agreement

All readers reached between 0.26 and 1 in the PABAK (Figure 5a), where 'Decreased translucency', 'Infiltrate incl. sub-categories', and 'Infection' had the lowest intra-reader agreement with PABAK values of 0.28, 0.26, and 0.34, respectively.

On specific agreement, all readers achieved over 0.50 in the PPA on 'Normal', 'Increased translucency incl. sub-categories', 'Pneumothorax', 'Decreased translucency incl. sub-categories', 'Infiltrate incl. sub-categories', 'Pleural effusion', and 'Costophrenic angle blunting AND pleural effusion' (Figure 5b). All readers reached between 0.52 and 1 in the PNA on all labels, with the lowest PNA on the label 'Decreased translucency incl. sub-categories' by one novice reader.

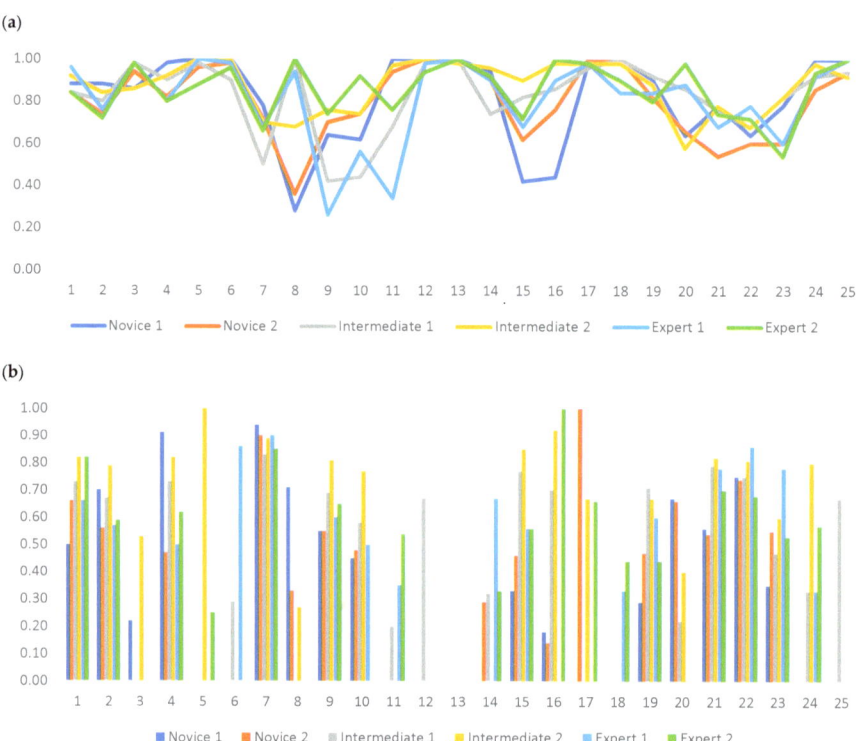

Figure 5. Intra-reader agreement measurements with (**a**) prevalence-adjusted and bias-adjusted Kappa (PABAK) and (**b**) proportion of positive agreement (PPA). 1. Normal, 2. Increased translucency incl. sub-categories, 3. Increased translucency, 4. Pneumothorax, 5. Cysts/bullae, 6. Emphysema, 7. Decreased translucency incl. sub-categories, 8. Decreased translucency, 9. Infiltrate incl. sub-categories, 10. Infiltrate, 11. Infection, 12. Abscess, 13. Tuberculosis, 14. Malignant, 15. Diffuse lung changes incl. sub-categories, 16. Diffuse lung changes, 17. Fibrosis, 18. Chronic pulmonary changes, 19. Stasis/Edema, 20. Costophrenic angle blunting, 21. Pleural effusion, 22. Costophrenic angle blunting AND pleural effusion, 23. Atelectasis, 24. Pleural thickening/changes, 25. Former operation in lung tissue. Kappa: <0, poor; 0.01–0.20, slight; 0.21–0.40, fair; 0.41–0.60, moderate; 0.61–0.80, substantial; 0.81–1.00, almost perfect.

4. Discussion

The main findings of our study were that (1) simple, descriptive, and definitive labels reached greater specific positive agreement among readers with different radiological experience levels, (2) radiologists with less experience more often used and agreed on broader, unspecific labels compared to more experienced radiologists, and (3) the congregation of labels into broader categories increased the agreement for the same radiologists on two separate occasions.

Rudolph et al. [24] found the highest inter-reader agreement on pneumothorax and the lowest agreement on suspicious nodules. This resonated with Christiansen et al. [25], who showed the best performance in detecting pneumothorax and the worst in pneumonic infiltrate amongst a group of junior doctors. In concordance with these studies, our study showed that descriptive and definitive radiological diagnoses, e.g., pneumothorax or pleural effusion, which required nearly no additional patient information, were easier to detect and annotate, resulting in a higher specific positive agreement for all levels of radiologists, compared to interpretive diagnoses, such as infectious infiltrate [26]. Several deep learning solutions have been proposed to assist in the detection of infectious infiltrates [27,28], but due to the lack of consistent image annotation, our study suggests that such solutions must base their training data on multiple sources of information [10]. The integration of multiple sources of information to train an algorithm would be more time-consuming and costly, which could be the reason why several commercially available products have marketed AI-based systems for simple or descriptive findings on CXRs [29–31]. However, further studies are needed to examine the use of such solutions compared to solutions that aid in more interpretive radiological findings.

The strength of our study was the hierarchal layout of our diagnostic scheme. A previous study showed that label extraction following a hierarchical taxonomy increased labeling accuracy and reduced missing annotations [32]. Therefore, even with annotators with different radiological experience levels, there was less risk of missing data due to the option of labeling with a parent label instead of not labeling the finding at all. The hierarchical layout enabled us to analyze the differences in annotation between annotators with different radiological experience levels. Our study showed that experienced radiologists had greater confidence in labeling specific findings, e.g., 'Infectious infiltrate' vs. its parent label 'Infiltrate'. However, novice radiologists were aware of the presence of an infiltrate but did not find confidence in specifying that finding and, therefore, used broader labels such as 'Decreased translucency' or 'Infiltrate'. We showed that novice radiologists had enough training to enable them to recognize a pathological CXR from a normal CXR, but additional clinical training contributes to more confidence and refined recognition skills and detail orientation [33,34].

In terms of AI development, the different annotation behavior due to radiological experience can be used when recruiting data annotators. Our study suggested that the selection of annotators may be dependent on the annotation methodology. If annotations are on simple or broadly defined findings, less experience may be sufficient. However, if annotations on CXR images of complex diagnoses need to be made, our study suggested that more experienced radiologists were needed. It would be optimal to always have an experienced board-certified radiologist as an annotator [34]. Due to difficulties in the recruitment of highly specialized radiologists, AI development projects turn to annotators that are not radiologists [35]. Therefore, every AI development project needs to match the annotation methodology to the annotator's experience to minimize time and cost while preserving accurate and consistent annotation.

Previous studies have shown that readers with less radiological task experience had poorer interpretation skills of diagnostic images compared to more experienced readers [36,37]. In our study, the positive agreement of fewer labels among novice radiologists could, therefore, be due to a lack of radiological experience. Although intermediate radiologists had a positive agreement on a greater number of different labels than the experienced radiologists, it did not result in fewer 'Normal' cases, which suggested that intermediate radiologists tended to over-annotate a single CXR case. This could have been due to either lack of task experience or a fear of missing diagnoses.

A bias in the study was the annotation process itself. The annotation process differs significantly compared to the radiologists' normal free-text reporting, and the choice of annotation labels might be affected. All radiologists were given no clinical information on the cases, which could have been another bias in image interpretation. However, previous studies have not been conclusive in the benefits of additional clinical information on radiologists' interpretive performance of CXRs [38,39].

The study was limited by the number of annotators and included cases. The limited number of cases affected the prevalence and distribution of the labels in the dataset because of natural prevalence patterns in the general population from which the CXR cases were obtained. Kappa statistics are dependent on prevalence. Since Kappa statistics is the agreement compared to chance, studies will inherently return a lower Kappa value if a label is either highly prevalent or highly un-prevalent in a dataset. We have provided the results adjusted for prevalence and bias (Randolph's and PABAK) as a solution to the prevalence problem and as previously recommended [18,19,40]. In addition, deep learning algorithms cannot detect findings that are not there and, therefore, need to train on positively labeled data, which is why we also provided specific agreement measures, such as the proportion of positive agreement. Even though it is still possible for a high PPA when the prevalence is low, the likelihood of achieving a high PPA is low, which is why we reported both specific agreements and chance-adjusted agreements. Another limitation was that we did not test the performance of a deep learning solution that used the proposed labeling scheme as opposed to other labeling tactics. In this study, we, therefore, did not conclude whether our labeling scheme would create better-performing deep learning solutions when compared to deep learning solutions using other labeling schemes. We focused mainly on investigating agreement among radiologists as annotators when using our labeling scheme to annotate CXR image findings.

This is the first study to investigate the inter- and intra-reader agreement when annotating CXR images for the purpose of developing a deep learning-based diagnostic solution. The annotators used bounding boxes when annotating findings to train the deep learning algorithms, but in our study, we did not specifically investigate whether the labeled finding was marked in the same location on the image since it was beyond the scope of this paper. For future perspectives, we suggest revising the diagnostic labeling scheme to include more descriptive labels to potentially increase positive agreement on lower-level labels for radiologists of different levels of task experience (Figure 6). Further studies are needed to investigate inter- and intra-reader agreement when using the suggested revised diagnostic scheme, as proposed in Figure 6.

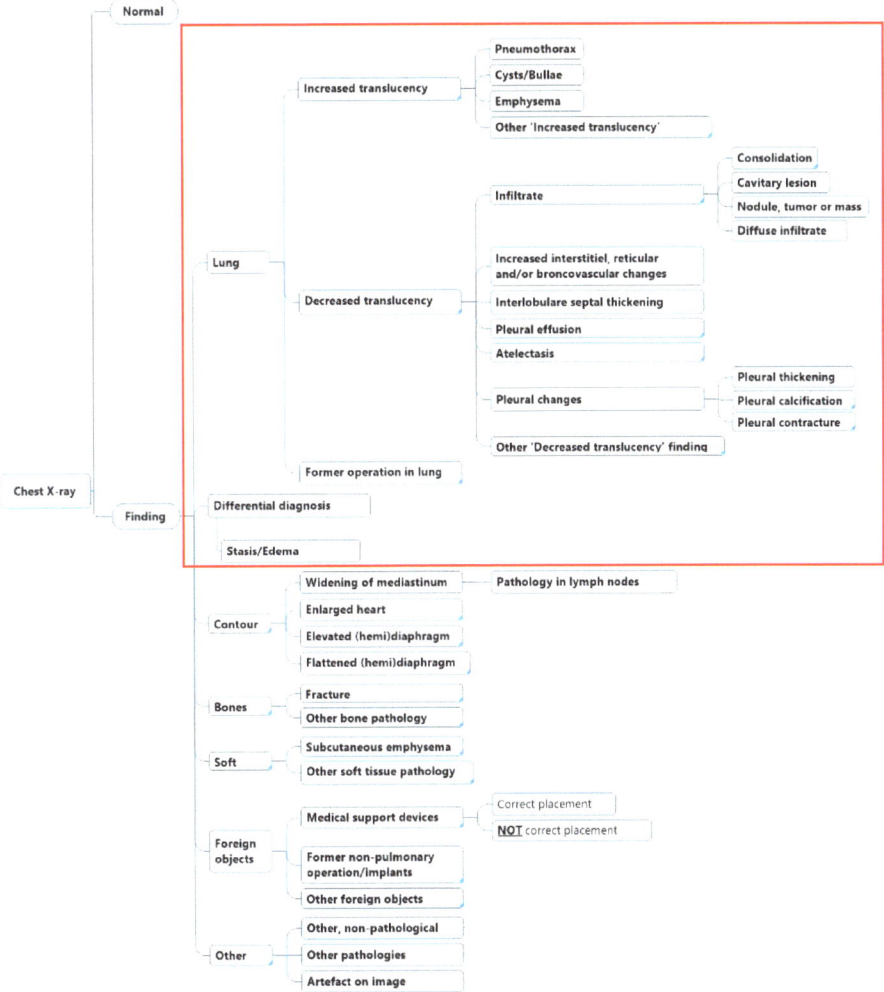

Figure 6. Proposed diagnostic labeling scheme for lung tissue findings (red square) on chest X-ray where interpretive labels have been replaced with more descriptive labels (corresponds to the labels encased with a red square in Figure 1).

5. Conclusions

Readers achieved *fair-to-excellent* agreement on all labels in our diagnostic labeling scheme. Differences in specific agreement showed a tendency to be dependent on radiological experience when distinguishing between using simple, descriptive labels or more complex, interpretive labels. However, further studies are warranted for larger datasets with a higher prevalence of both descriptive and interpretive findings.

Author Contributions: Conceptualization, D.L., J.F.C., L.M.P., L.T., R.B., M.F. and M.B.N.; methodology, D.L., J.F.C., L.T., R.B., M.F. and M.B.N.; formal analysis, D.L., R.B. and J.T.; investigation, D.L., A.R., P.J.S., D.M.R.S., L.B., T.T.A. and H.S.-A.; writing—original draft preparation, D.L.; writing—review and editing, D.L., L.M.P., M.F., R.B., J.T., P.J.S., T.T.A., A.R., D.M.R.S., L.B., H.S.-A., S.D., K.L.H., J.F.C. and M.B.N.; supervision, J.F.C., S.D. and M.B.N.; project administration, D.L.; funding acquisition, S.D. and M.B.N. All authors have read and agreed to the published version of the manuscript.

Funding: This research was funded by Innovation Fund Denmark (IFD) with grant no. 0176-00013B for the AI4Xray project.

Institutional Review Board Statement: Waived due to anonymity. Data storage was applied for and waived by the Knowledge Center of Data Protection Compliance due to full anonymity of images.

Informed Consent Statement: Patient consent was waived due to full anonymity of retrospective chest X-ray images. Informed consent from radiologists were obtained.

Data Availability Statement: Not applicable.

Conflicts of Interest: The funders had no role in the design of the study; in the collection, analyses, or interpretation of data; in the writing of the manuscript; or in the decision to publish the results. Unumed Aps contributed to the design of the study, collection, and analysis of data, but had no role in the outcome of the study or in the decision to publish the results.

Appendix A

Table A1. Prevalence- and bfias-adjusted Kappa (PABAK) for novice, intermediate, and experienced radiologists. Kappa: <0, poor; 0.01–0.20, slight; 0.21–0.40, fair; 0.41–0.60, moderate; 0.61–0.80, substantial; 0.81–1.00, almost perfect.

PABAK	Novice 1 vs. Novice 2	Intermediate 1 vs. Intermediate 2	Experienced 1 vs. Experienced 2
Normal	0.78	0.80	0.76
Increased Translucency incl. sub-categories	0.66	0.80	0.78
Increased Translucency	0.80	0.84	1
Pneumothorax	0.82	0.90	0.82
Cyst/Bullae	0.98	0.98	0.96
Emphysema	0.98	0.94	0.92
Decreased Translucency incl. sub-categories	0.48	0.64	0.50
Decreased Translucency	0.12	0.78	1
Infiltrate incl. sub-categories	0.62	0.56	0.22
Infiltrate	0.66	0.46	0.48
Infection	0.96	0.86	0.24
Abscess	1	0.98	0.94
Tuberculosis	1	0.98	1
Malignant	0.90	0.82	0.88
Diffuse Lung Changes incl. sub-categories	0.28	0.70	0.54
Diffuse Lung Changes	0.36	0.84	0.98
Fibrosis	0.94	0.96	0.94
Chronic Lung Changes	0.98	0.98	0.86
Stasis/Edema	0.84	0.86	0.70
Costophrenic Angle Blunting	0.44	0.54	0.94
Pleural Effusion	0.68	0.84	0.66
Costophrenic Angle Blunting AND Pleural Effusion	0.50	0.56	0.62
Atelectasis	0.44	0.72	0.38
Pleural Changes	0.86	0.88	0.94
Former Operation in Lung Tissue	0.96	0.84	1

Table A2. Specific agreement for novice, intermediate, and experienced radiologists. PPA, Proportion of positive agreement; PNA, Proportion of negative agreement. Kappa: <0, poor; 0.01–0.20, slight; 0.21–0.40, fair; 0.41–0.60, moderate; 0.61–0.80, substantial; 0.81–1.00, almost perfect.

Specific Agreement	Novice 1 vs. Novice 2		Intermediate 1 vs. Intermediate 2		Experienced 1 vs. Experienced 2	
	PPA	PNA	PPA	PNA	PPA	PNA
Normal	0.27	0.94	0.67	0.94	0.65	0.92
Increased Translucency incl. sub-categories	0.19	0.91	0.69	0.94	0.56	0.94
Increased Translucency	0	0.95	0	0.96	—	1
Pneumothorax	0.31	0.96	0.76	0.97	0.52	0.95
Cyst/Bullae	0	0.99	0	0.99	0	0.99
Emphysema	0	0.99	0	0.98	0	0.98
Decreased Translucency incl. sub-categories	0.84	0.32	0.87	0.72	0.81	0.62
Decreased Translucency	0.46	0.63	0	0.94	—	1
Infiltrate incl. sub-categories	0.56	0.88	0.68	0.83	0.43	0.70
Infiltrate	0.48	0.89	0.53	0.81	0	0.85
Infection	0	0.99	0.22	0.96	0.14	0.76
Abscess	—	1	0	0.99	0	0.98
Tuberculosis	—	1	0	0.99	—	1
Malignant	0.44	0.97	0.19	0.95	0.25	0.97
Diffuse Lung Changes incl. sub-categories	0.25	0.76	0.59	0.91	0.21	0.87
Diffuse Lung Changes	0	0.81	0.56	0.96	0	0.99
Fibrosis	0	0.98	0.50	0.98	0	0.98
Chronic Lung Changes	0	0.99	0	0.99	0	0.96
Stasis/Edema	0.33	0.96	0.53	0.96	0.21	0.92
Costophrenic Angle Blunting	0.46	0.81	0.21	0.87	0	0.98
Pleural Effusion	0.47	0.91	0.86	0.94	0.74	0.87
Costophrenic Angle Blunting AND Pleural Effusion	0.64	0.81	0.71	0.82	0.72	0.86
Atelectasis	0.22	0.83	0.36	0.92	0.59	0.75
Pleural Changes	0	0.96	0.25	0.97	0.57	0.98
Former Operation in Lung Tissue	0	0.99	0	0.96	—	1

References

1. Performance Analysis Team, NHS England. *Diagnostic Imaging Dataset Statistical Release*; NHS: London, UK, 2020/2021; Available online: https://www.england.nhs.uk/statistics/statistical-work-areas/diagnostic-imaging-dataset/diagnostic-imaging-dataset-2021-22-data/ (accessed on 15 October 2022).
2. Metlay, J.P.; Kapoor, W.N.; Fine, M.J. Does this patient have community-acquired pneumonia? Diagnosing pneumonia by history and physical examination. *JAMA* **1997**, *278*, 1440–1445. [CrossRef]
3. Kent, C. *Can Tech Solve the UK Radiology Staffing Shortage?* Medical Device Network: London, UK, 2021.
4. Sánchez-Marrè, M. *Intelligent Decision Support Systems*; Springer Nature Swtizerland AG: Cham, Swtizerland, 2022.
5. Li, D.; Mikela Vilmun, B.; Frederik Carlsen, J.; Albrecht-Beste, E.; Ammitzbol Lauridsen, C.; Bachmann Nielsen, M.; Lindskov Hansen, K. The Performance of Deep Learning Algorithms on Automatic Pulmonary Nodule Detection and Classification Tested on Different Datasets That Are Not Derived from LIDC-IDRI: A Systematic Review. *Diagnostics* **2019**, *9*, 207. [CrossRef] [PubMed]
6. Willemink, M.J.; Koszek, W.A.; Hardell, C.; Wu, J.; Fleischmann, D.; Harvey, H.; Folio, L.R.; Summers, R.M.; Rubin, D.L.; Lungren, M.P. Preparing Medical Imaging Data for Machine Learning. *Radiology* **2020**, *295*, 4–15. [CrossRef] [PubMed]
7. Brealey, S.; Westwood, M. Are you reading what we are reading? The effect of who interprets medical images on estimates of diagnostic test accuracy in systematic reviews. *Br. J. Radiol.* **2007**, *80*, 674–677. [CrossRef] [PubMed]
8. Sakurada, S.; Hang, N.T.; Ishizuka, N.; Toyota, E.; le Hung, D.; Chuc, P.T.; Lien, L.T.; Thuong, P.H.; Bich, P.T.; Keicho, N.; et al. Inter-rater agreement in the assessment of abnormal chest X-ray findings for tuberculosis between two Asian countries. *BMC Infect. Dis.* **2012**, *12*, 31. [CrossRef] [PubMed]
9. Lindman, K.; Rose, J.F.; Lindvall, M.; Lundstrom, C.; Treanor, D. Annotations, Ontologies, and Whole Slide Images—Development of an Annotated Ontology-Driven Whole Slide Image Library of Normal and Abnormal Human Tissue. *J. Pathol. Inform.* **2019**, *10*, 22. [CrossRef] [PubMed]
10. Bustos, A.; Pertusa, A.; Salinas, J.-M.; de la Iglesia-Vayá, M. Padchest: A large chest X-ray image dataset with multi-label annotated reports. *Med. Image Anal.* **2020**, *66*, 101797. [CrossRef] [PubMed]

11. Putha, P.; Tadepalli, M.; Reddy, B.; Raj, T.; Chiramal, J.A.; Govil, S.; Sinha, N.; Ks, M.; Reddivari, S.; Jagirdar, A. Can artificial intelligence reliably report chest X-rays? Radiologist validation of an algorithm trained on 2.3 million X-rays. *arXiv* **2018**, arXiv:1807.07455.
12. Irvin, J.; Rajpurkar, P.; Ko, M.; Yu, Y.; Ciurea-Ilcus, S.; Chute, C.; Marklund, H.; Haghgoo, B.; Ball, R.; Shpanskaya, K. Chexpert: A large chest radiograph dataset with uncertainty labels and expert comparison. In Proceedings of the AAAI Conference on Artificial Intelligence, Honolulu, HI, USA, 27 January–1 February 2019; pp. 590–597.
13. Hansell, D.M.; Bankier, A.A.; MacMahon, H.; McLoud, T.C.; Muller, N.L.; Remy, J. Fleischner Society: Glossary of terms for thoracic imaging. *Radiology* **2008**, *246*, 697–722. [CrossRef] [PubMed]
14. Van Leeuwen, K.G.; Schalekamp, S.; Rutten, M.J.; van Ginneken, B.; de Rooij, M. Artificial intelligence in radiology: 100 commercially available products and their scientific evidence. *Eur. Radiol.* **2021**, *31*, 3797–3804. [CrossRef] [PubMed]
15. AI for Radiolgy—Products. Available online: https://grand-challenge.org/aiforradiology/?subspeciality=Chest&modality=X-ray&ce_under=All&ce_class=All&fda_class=All&sort_by=ce%20certification&search= (accessed on 2 February 2022).
16. ChestEye AI Chest X-ray Radiology—Oxipit. Available online: https://oxipit.ai/products/chesteye/ (accessed on 2 February 2022).
17. Annalise.AI—Our Algorithm Can Detect Following Findings. Available online: https://annalise.ai/solutions/annalise-cxr/ (accessed on 2 February 2022).
18. Randolph, J.J. Free-Marginal Multirater Kappa (multirater K[free]): An Alternative to Fleiss' Fixed-Marginal Multirater Kappa. Available online: file:///C:/Users/dana_/Downloads/Free-Marginal_Multirater_Kappa_multirater_kfree_An%20(1).pdf (accessed on 8 December 2022).
19. Byrt, T.; Bishop, J.; Carlin, J.B. Bias, prevalence and kappa. *J. Clin. Epidemiol.* **1993**, *46*, 423–429. [CrossRef] [PubMed]
20. Landis, J.R.; Koch, G.G. The measurement of observer agreement for categorical data. *Biometrics* **1977**, *33*, 159–174. [CrossRef] [PubMed]
21. Cicchetti, D.V.; Feinstein, A.R. High agreement but low kappa: II. Resolving the paradoxes. *J. Clin. Epidemiol.* **1990**, *43*, 551–558. [CrossRef]
22. De Vet, H.C.W.; Dikmans, R.E.; Eekhout, I. Specific agreement on dichotomous outcomes can be calculated for more than two raters. *J. Clin. Epidemiol.* **2017**, *83*, 85–89. [CrossRef]
23. Randolph, J.J. Online Kappa Calculator [Computer Software]. Available online: http://justus.randolph.name/kappa (accessed on 2 July 2022).
24. Rudolph, J.; Fink, N.; Dinkel, J.; Koliogiannis, V.; Schwarze, V.; Goller, S.; Erber, B.; Geyer, T.; Hoppe, B.F.; Fischer, M.; et al. Interpretation of Thoracic Radiography Shows Large Discrepancies Depending on the Qualification of the Physician-Quantitative Evaluation of Interobserver Agreement in a Representative Emergency Department Scenario. *Diagnostics* **2021**, *11*, 1868. [CrossRef] [PubMed]
25. Christiansen, J.M.; Gerke, O.; Karstoft, J.; Andersen, P.E. Poor interpretation of chest X-rays by junior doctors. *Dan. Med. J* **2014**, *61*, A4875. [PubMed]
26. Boersma, W.G.; Daniels, J.M.; Lowenberg, A.; Boeve, W.J.; van de Jagt, E.J. Reliability of radiographic findings and the relation to etiologic agents in community-acquired pneumonia. *Respir. Med.* **2006**, *100*, 926–932. [CrossRef] [PubMed]
27. Salvatore, C.; Interlenghi, M.; Monti, C.B.; Ippolito, D.; Capra, D.; Cozzi, A.; Schiaffino, S.; Polidori, A.; Gandola, D.; Ali, M.; et al. Artificial Intelligence Applied to Chest X-ray for Differential Diagnosis of COVID-19 Pneumonia. *Diagnostics* **2021**, *11*, 530. [CrossRef] [PubMed]
28. Codlin, A.J.; Dao, T.P.; Vo, L.N.Q.; Forse, R.J.; Van Truong, V.; Dang, H.M.; Nguyen, L.H.; Nguyen, H.B.; Nguyen, N.V.; Sidney-Annerstedt, K.; et al. Independent evaluation of 12 artificial intelligence solutions for the detection of tuberculosis. *Sci. Rep.* **2021**, *11*, 23895. [CrossRef]
29. Qure.AI. qXR—Artificial Intelligence for Chest X-ray. Available online: https://www.qure.ai/product/qxr/ (accessed on 6 June 2022).
30. Aidoc. Radiology AI. Available online: https://www.aidoc.com/ (accessed on 8 June 2022).
31. Lunit. Lunit INSIGHT CXR. Available online: https://www.lunit.io/en/products/insight-cxr (accessed on 8 June 2022).
32. Chen, H.; Miao, S.; Xu, D.; Hager, G.D.; Harrison, A.P. Deep hierarchical multi-label classification of chest X-ray images. In Proceedings of the International Conference on Medical Imaging with Deep Learning, London, UK, 8–10 July 2019; pp. 109–120.
33. Miglioretti, D.L.; Gard, C.C.; Carney, P.A.; Onega, T.L.; Buist, D.S.; Sickles, E.A.; Kerlikowske, K.; Rosenberg, R.D.; Yankaskas, B.C.; Geller, B.M.; et al. When radiologists perform best: The learning curve in screening mammogram interpretation. *Radiology* **2009**, *253*, 632–640. [CrossRef]
34. Fabre, C.; Proisy, M.; Chapuis, C.; Jouneau, S.; Lentz, P.A.; Meunier, P.; Mahe, G.; Lederlin, M. Radiology residents' skill level in chest X-ray reading. *Diagn. Interv. Imaging* **2018**, *99*, 361–370. [CrossRef] [PubMed]
35. SimplyJob.com. Medical Student Assistant for Data Annotation—Cerebriu. Available online: https://simplyjob.com/729014/cerebriu/medical-student-assistant-for-data-annotation (accessed on 14 June 2022).
36. Myles-Worsley, M.; Johnston, W.A.; Simons, M.A. The influence of expertise on X-ray image processing. *J. Exp. Psychol. Learn. Mem. Cogn.* **1988**, *14*, 553–557. [CrossRef]
37. Miranda, A.C.G.; Monteiro, C.C.P.; Pires, M.L.C.; Miranda, L.E.C. Radiological imaging interpretation skills of medical interns. *Rev. Bras. Educ. Méd.* **2019**, *43*, 145–154. [CrossRef]

38. Doubilet, P.; Herman, P.G. Interpretation of radiographs: Effect of clinical history. *Am. J. Roentgenol.* **1981**, *137*, 1055–1058. [CrossRef]
39. Test, M.; Shah, S.S.; Monuteaux, M.; Ambroggio, L.; Lee, E.Y.; Markowitz, R.I.; Bixby, S.; Diperna, S.; Servaes, S.; Hellinger, J.C.; et al. Impact of clinical history on chest radiograph interpretation. *J. Hosp. Med.* **2013**, *8*, 359–364. [CrossRef] [PubMed]
40. McHugh, M.L. Interrater reliability: The kappa statistic. *Biochem. Med.* **2012**, *22*, 276–282. [CrossRef]

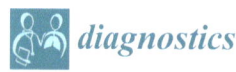

Review

Revolutionizing Cardiology through Artificial Intelligence—Big Data from Proactive Prevention to Precise Diagnostics and Cutting-Edge Treatment—A Comprehensive Review of the Past 5 Years

Elena Stamate [1,2,†], Alin-Ionut Piraianu [2,*], Oana Roxana Ciobotaru [2,3,*], Rodica Crassas [4], Oana Duca [2,4,†], Ana Fulga [2,5,†], Ionica Grigore [2,4], Vlad Vintila [1,6], Iuliu Fulga [2,5,†] and Octavian Catalin Ciobotaru [2,3]

1. Department of Cardiology, Emergency University Hospital of Bucharest, 050098 Bucharest, Romania; elena.stamate94@yahoo.com (E.S.); vladvintila2005@yahoo.com (V.V.)
2. Faculty of Medicine and Pharmacy, University "Dunarea de Jos" of Galati, 35 AI Cuza Street, 800010 Galati, Romania; oanam.duca@gmail.com (O.D.); ana.fulgaa@yahoo.com (A.F.); ionicagrigore2004@yahoo.com (I.G.); fulgaiuliu@yahoo.com (I.F.); coctavian72@gmail.com (O.C.C.)
3. Railway Hospital Galati, 800223 Galati, Romania
4. Emergency County Hospital Braila, 810325 Braila, Romania; rodica.crassas@gmail.com
5. Saint Apostle Andrew Emergency County Clinical Hospital, 177 Brailei Street, 800578 Galati, Romania
6. Clinical Department of Cardio-Thoracic Pathology, University of Medicine and Pharmacy "Carol Davila" Bucharest, 37 Dionisie Lupu Street, 4192910 Bucharest, Romania
* Correspondence: alin.piraianu@gmail.com (A.-I.P.); roxana_hag@yahoo.com (O.R.C.); Tel.: +40-747133397 (A.-I.P.); Tel.: +40-740425597 (O.R.C.)
† These authors contributed equally to this work.

Abstract: Background: Artificial intelligence (AI) can radically change almost every aspect of the human experience. In the medical field, there are numerous applications of AI and subsequently, in a relatively short time, significant progress has been made. Cardiology is not immune to this trend, this fact being supported by the exponential increase in the number of publications in which the algorithms play an important role in data analysis, pattern discovery, identification of anomalies, and therapeutic decision making. Furthermore, with technological development, there have appeared new models of machine learning (ML) and deep learning (DP) that are capable of exploring various applications of AI in cardiology, including areas such as prevention, cardiovascular imaging, electrophysiology, interventional cardiology, and many others. In this sense, the present article aims to provide a general vision of the current state of AI use in cardiology. Results: We identified and included a subset of 200 papers directly relevant to the current research covering a wide range of applications. Thus, this paper presents AI applications in cardiovascular imaging, arithmology, clinical or emergency cardiology, cardiovascular prevention, and interventional procedures in a summarized manner. Recent studies from the highly scientific literature demonstrate the feasibility and advantages of using AI in different branches of cardiology. Conclusions: The integration of AI in cardiology offers promising perspectives for increasing accuracy by decreasing the error rate and increasing efficiency in cardiovascular practice. From predicting the risk of sudden death or the ability to respond to cardiac resynchronization therapy to the diagnosis of pulmonary embolism or the early detection of valvular diseases, AI algorithms have shown their potential to mitigate human error and provide feasible solutions. At the same time, limits imposed by the small samples studied are highlighted alongside the challenges presented by ethical implementation; these relate to legal implications regarding responsibility and decision making processes, ensuring patient confidentiality and data security. All these constitute future research directions that will allow the integration of AI in the progress of cardiology.

Keywords: artificial intelligence; machine learning; deep learning; cardiology; valvular disease; arithmology

Citation: Stamate, E.; Piraianu, A.-I.; Ciobotaru, O.R.; Crassas, R.; Duca, O.; Fulga, A.; Grigore, I.; Vintila, V.; Fulga, I.; Ciobotaru, O.C. Revolutionizing Cardiology through Artificial Intelligence—Big Data from Proactive Prevention to Precise Diagnostics and Cutting-Edge Treatment—A Comprehensive Review of the Past 5 Years. *Diagnostics* **2024**, *14*, 1103. https://doi.org/10.3390/diagnostics14111103

Academic Editor: Michael Henein

Received: 22 April 2024
Revised: 12 May 2024
Accepted: 23 May 2024
Published: 26 May 2024

Copyright: © 2024 by the authors. Licensee MDPI, Basel, Switzerland. This article is an open access article distributed under the terms and conditions of the Creative Commons Attribution (CC BY) license (https://creativecommons.org/licenses/by/4.0/).

1. Introduction

Artificial intelligence (AI) has penetrated all aspects of life and has recently stood out through the development of deep learning models that can generate almost anything with minimal human intervention. However, among all fields of activity, medicine has emerged as a particularly significant one, with great potential for development [1]. Among all specialties wherein AI has found its place through clinical applications, cardiology holds a leading position. According to the World Health Organization, the main cause of death globally, accounting for approximately a third of annual deaths, is cardiovascular disease [2].

When it comes to healthcare, a paradigm shift has been triggered with the integration of AI into various medical disciplines, including cardiology. Therefore, AI could revolutionize cardiology by transforming the way cardiovascular diseases are prevented, diagnosed, and treated. It includes different methods that allow machines to mimic human behaviors such as learning, reasoning, problem solving, perception, and decision making. In cardiology, all of these can lead to providing accurate predictions and personalized information and can even identify patterns [3]. Artificial intelligence techniques have shown their power to enhance progress in the management of atherosclerotic cardiovascular disease, heart failure, atrial fibrillation, pulmonary embolism, hypertension, pulmonary hypertension, valvular heart diseases, cardiomyopathies, congenital heart diseases, and more [4]. However, expertise in pathophysiology and patient clinical knowledge will not be replaced, the human element remaining vital in the medical process, with physicians ultimately deciding where to apply and how to interpret the data provided by AI [5]. The main advantage of AI lies in its ability to analyze a large database in a short time and provide targeted information tailored to each category of patients [6,7]. In addition, deep learning algorithms, which are the most commonly applied AI subcategory in medicine at this moment [8], allow for the partial elimination of human error from the medical process by reducing human involvement, correcting clinician errors, and preventing misdiagnosis, which constitutes another advantage of AI in healthcare [9,10].

In the healthcare field, artificial intelligence has the potential to open up new perspectives through personalized approaches to each patient. Thus, integrating AI into routine medical practice supports medical activity, can increase the success rate in treating cardiovascular diseases, and can improve the quality of medical care whilst recognizing the limits of AI and not minimizing its ethical and legal issues [11]. This summary aims to provide a synthesis of the application of AI in cardiology for easier understanding of AI and to support the use of AI in the daily practice of the cardiologist. The relationship between AI and its subdisciplines—machine learning (ML), deep learning (DL), and cognitive computing—is visually represented in Figure 1. In essence, both machine learning and deep learning fall under the umbrella of artificial intelligence. Machine learning, as an innovative field, enables systems to adapt and improve with minimal human intervention. Deep learning, in turn, is a subset of machine learning that focuses on artificial neural networks to mimic the learning process of the human brain. Deep learning is an evolution of machine learning [12]. Additionally, Table 1 briefly exemplifies the most relevant concepts of AI tools.

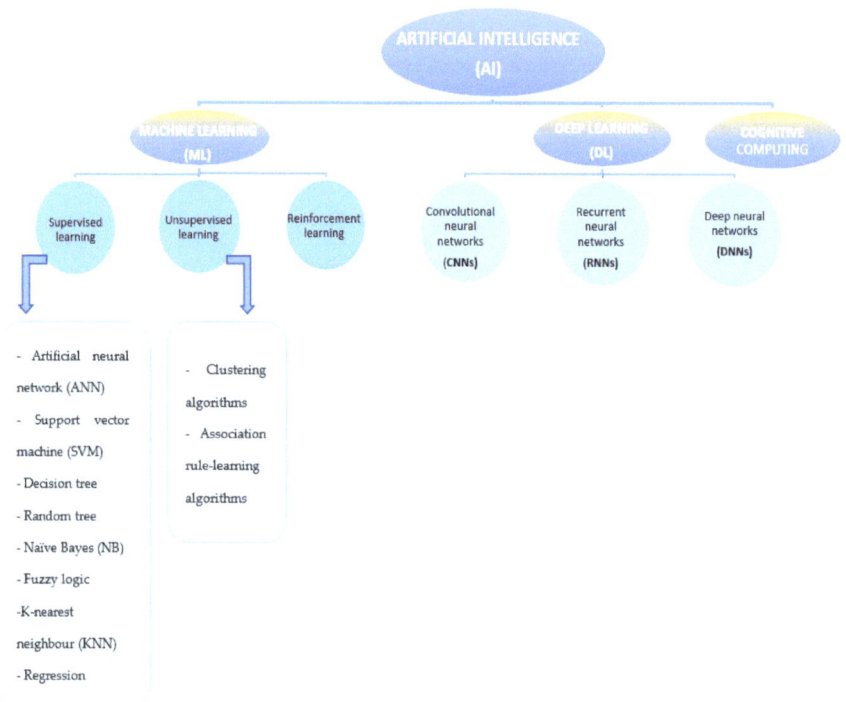

Figure 1. Illustration of the AI subtypes. Created based on information from [4,13].

Table 1. Important AI-related terms and definitions.

Term	Definitions	References
Artificial intelligence (AI)	Artificial intelligence (AI) is a subtype of information technology that through algorithms can analyze (receive, process, and interpret) medical information and perform complex mathematical calculations, simulating artificially what happens in the human mind during learning.	[14]
Machine learning (ML)	Machine learning (ML) is the ability of computer systems to automatically learn from existing data and past experiences to find patterns and make future predictions. ML is a well-known subtype of AI and can be grouped into three categories: supervised learning, unsupervised learning, and reinforcement learning. In medicine, ML can incorporate and manage various data resources (from clinical and biological observations to wearable devices and environmental information) to create models that can predict and diagnose certain diseases. Additionally, ML can personalize disease treatment to improve the healthcare system. In conclusion, ML is one of the fastest, most convenient, and cost-effective ways of detecting disease through artificial intelligence technology.	[15–18]

Table 1. *Cont.*

Term	Definitions	References
Deep learning (DL)	Deep learning (DL) is a subtype of machine learning that can analyze massive amounts of data to provide greater accuracy in creating concepts and accurately predicting pathologies. DL is currently one of the most applied algorithms for medical purposes, alongside support vector machine (SVM) and artificial neural network (ANN).	[4,19]
Cognitive computing	Cognitive computing systems are artificial intelligence systems that are part of machine learning and understand, reason, and enhance human brain capabilities by combining virtual technology and natural language processing.	[20]
Supervised learning	Training the ML algorithm using labeled examples consisting of inputs and outputs provided by an expert is a phenomenon known as supervised learning. Supervised learning encompasses artificial neural networks (ANNs), support vector machine (SVM), decision tree, random forest, fuzzy logic, naive Bayes (NB), K-nearest neighbor (KNN), and regression.	[17,21]
Unsupervised learning	This involves training the ML algorithm to process data and perform classification of samples without category information, thus without human intervention. Unsupervised learning includes clustering algorithms and association rule-learning algorithms.	[21,22]
Reinforcement learning	Reinforcement learning is a subtype of machine learning that can be considered a combination of supervised and unsupervised learning and can facilitate efforts to increase algorithm accuracy. It is a learning strategy for optimal learning regarding a specific criterion in a given situation. This algorithm receives feedback on its performance by comparing rewards obtained during training with the chosen criterion.	[23,24]
Convolutional neural networks (CNNs)	Deep learning (DL), a method primarily used in image processing and understanding or classifying images, involves models similar to those used in the visual cortex for processing images. Convolutional neural networks (CNNs) are neural networks similar to regular neural networks, as they are composed of neurons with weights that can be learned. However, CNNs explicitly assume that inputs have specific structures, such as images.	[21,25,26]
Recurrent neural networks (RNNs)	RNNs are different from CNNs in that the input data are of variable size, which can be processed by the RNN; moreover, the outputs of intermediate-layer neurons are cyclically captured in the original input. When many recurrent neurons exist in a recurrent layer, the sequential data are processed in parallel through different weights, allowing RNNs to generate multiple representations and create effective feature space separation.	[27]
Deep neural networks (DNNs)	A DL architecture with multiple layers between the input and output layers.	[21]
Artificial neural network (ANN)	An ML technique that processes information in an architecture comprising many layers ("neurons"), with each interneuronal connection extracting the desired parameters incrementally from the training data.	[21,28]
Support vector machine (SVM)	A supervised learning model that can efficiently perform linear and nonlinear classifications, implicitly mapping their inputs into high-dimensional feature spaces.	[29]
Decision tree (DT)	This nonparametric supervised learning method is visualized as a graph representing the choices and their outcomes in the form of a tree; each tree consists of branches (values that a node can take) and nodes (attributes in the group to be classified).	[30]
Random tree (RT)	This is an ensemble classification technique that uses "parallel ensembling", fitting several decision tree classifiers in parallel on dataset subsamples.	[30]

Table 1. *Cont.*

Term	Definitions	References
Naïve Bayes (NB)	A classification technique assuming independence among predictors, Naive Bayes is a tool that works with the most basic knowledge of probability. Bayes' rule is a formula that determines the probability that Y will happen with a given X. The Bayes technique makes the naive assumption of independence of all characteristics. It attempts to find probabilities based on known prior probabilities that have been learned from training data.	[29]
Fuzzy logic	Fuzzy logic is part of supervised learning which allows multiple possible truth values to be processed through the same variable.	[30]
K-nearest neighbor (KNN)	This non-generalizing learning algorithm or an "instance-based learning" does not focus on constructing a general internal model but rather stores all instances corresponding to the training data in an n-dimensional space and classifies new data points based on similarity measures.	[30]
Regression	This is an algorithm using a logistic function to estimate probabilities that can overfit high-dimensional datasets, being suitable for datasets that can be linearly separated.	[30]
Clustering algorithms	Data clustering is an essential part of extracting information from databases and is part of unsupervised learning. There are several ways to split the data, the most important of which are horizontal and vertical collaborative clustering.	[31]
Association rule-learning algorithms	Association rule learning and correlation learning methods are used to find and weigh contextual relations between modeled context entities. In the presence of a training dataset, a unique classification strategy is introduced, which can effectively increase classification performance.	[32–34]

2. Literature Review

2.1. Methodology

We conducted a comprehensive review of current literature including original articles that studied various clinical applications of AI in cardiology. We performed extensive searches on PubMed, Google Scholar, ScienceDirect, Elsevier, Scopus, Web of Science, and Cochrane databases to identify relevant manuscripts. We used three sets of keywords to recognize terms from the title, abstract, and keywords of the studies: (i) the first set of keywords included terms associated with artificial intelligence, such as "artificial intelligence", "deep learning", "machine learning", "prediction", "diagnosis", "screening", "treatment", and "prognosis". However, studies using these methodologies are likely to incorporate terms such as "artificial intelligence" or "machine learning" in their abstracts or keywords. (ii) The second set of keywords included domains associated with applicability in clinical practice. Thus, compound searches were performed using the terms "artificial intelligence" combined with a chosen cardiology domain: "arithmology", "cardiac imaging", "ischemic heart disease", "valvular disease", "heart failure", "congenital diseases", "hypertension", and more. We restricted our search to papers published in English in the last 5 years, between 2020 and 2024; additionally, textbooks on AI were consulted, and we found more than 973 relevant manuscripts.

We removed duplicate articles and then conducted a detailed evaluation of abstracts and titles to determine their suitability for inclusion. The selection criteria focused on studies examining the application of artificial intelligence in various branches of cardiology. Subsequently, we systematically applied selection criteria to evaluate the studies. Studies were assessed based on the following criteria: (1) journal, (2) publication date, (3) study design, (4) analysis methods, (5) results, and (6) conclusions. We initially screened abstracts and eliminated studies not written in English. To ensure data quality, we paid close attention to specific aspects regarding the comprehensive evaluation of studies meeting the inclusion criteria, such as justification, method design, results, discussions, conclusions, and any signs of methodological bias or interpretation of data that could have a negative impact on the results of the studies reviewed.

Essentially, the inclusion criteria were as follows:
1. Studies examining the application of artificial intelligence in various branches of cardiology, such as arrhythmology, emergency cardiology, cardiomyopathies, cardiovascular imaging, congenital cardiovascular disease, electrocardiography, heart failure, heart transplantation, hypertension, pulmonary hypertension, infective endocarditis, ischemic heart disease, pericardial disease, peripheral heart disease, thromboembolic disease, and valvular diseases (this is a broad selection criterion focusing on the theme of studies relevant to the proposed review and represents the main topic of the article);
2. Publications in English;
3. Published within the last 5 years, between 2020 and 2024 (this temporal restriction ensures the timeliness and relevance of the information included in the review);
4. Patient batches that included both adults and children (this criterion ensured a larger batch of studies covering cardiology);
5. Studies in the form of an academic journal article.

Exclusion criteria:
1. Articles in languages other than English;
2. Retracted studies (eliminating retracted studies is essential to maintain the integrity and credibility of this review);
3. Applications of artificial intelligence regarding technical functionality data of algorithms (excluding these studies may be justified to focus on the practical and clinical application of artificial intelligence in cardiology, rather than the technical aspects of algorithms);
4. Studies in the form of posters, short papers, or only abstracts;
5. Duplicate studies;
6. Studies with a title and abstract that do not match the review topic.

The limitations of the review process included variations in methodologies among the included studies and potential publication biases. Additionally, the rapidly evolving nature of AI technologies in healthcare may introduce limitations in capturing the latest developments. Additionally, limitations of the study are issues related to ethical implementation and legal issues regarding accountability and decision making; still, in small batches of patients, the susceptibility model is considered a "black box" and standardization of the method. These may be future research directions in AI [34].

2.2. Results

After a thorough review and assessment of the 665 articles, we identified and included a subset of 200 papers that were directly relevant to our research, including 5 on arithmology, 10 on cardiogenic shock, 21 on cardiomyopathies, 18 on cardiac imaging, 6 on congenital heart disease, 11 on electrocardiography, 13 on heart failure, 14 on heart transplant, 14 on hypertension, 25 on pulmonary hypertension, 3 on infective endocarditis, 21 on ischemic heart disease, 5 on pericardial disease, 8 on peripheral artery disease, 12 on thromboembolic disease, and 14 on valvular disease. These areas of application of AI in cardiology are represented in Figure 2. These selected studies provided valuable insights into the use and impact of AI in cardiology, forming the basis of our review.

The 200 scientific articles that analyze the current applications of artificial intelligence in cardiology, as well as future research perspectives, are schematically summarized in Table 2.

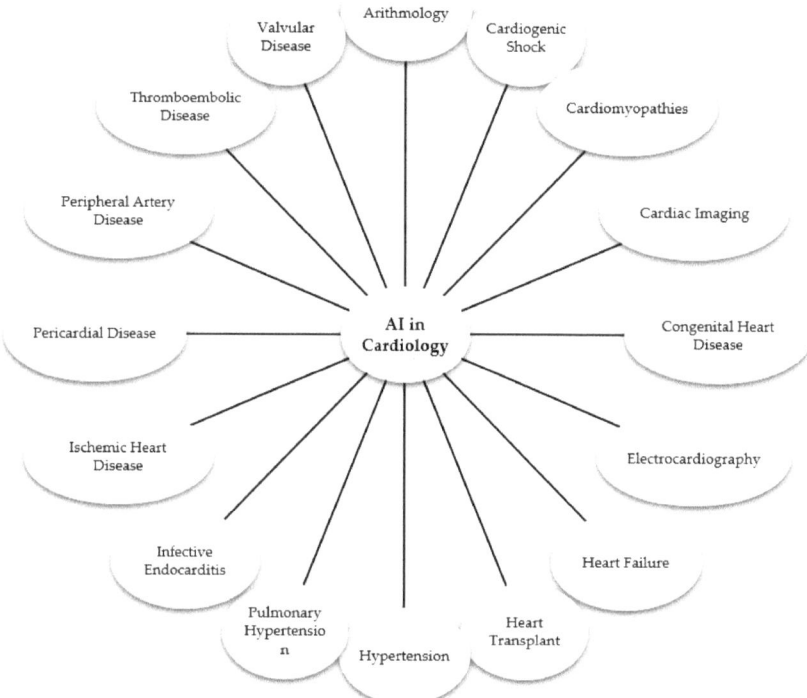

Figure 2. Application areas of AI in cardiology—main points of the review.

Table 2. Scientific articles that analyze the current applications of AI in cardiology as well as future research perspectives.

	Year of Study	Author	Application	Data Source	Machine Learning Method	Future Direction
Arrhythmias	2023	Tran, K.-V. [35]	AF detection	mECG	CNN	Studies to improve the AI algorithm of commercial wearable devices for AF detection
	2023	Baj, G. [36]	Prediction of new-onset AF	ECG	CNN XGB LR	Integration of demographic information (gender, age) or clinical information as predictors in addition to ECG; clinical interpretability is a fundamental step to building predictive tools for clinical usage
	2023	Raghunath, A. [37]	Prediction of AF	mECG	CNN DNN	Differentiating atrial fibrillation from atrial flutter using the availability of information such as clinical indicators, socio-economic status, or racial background
	2023	Jiang, J. [38]	Prediction AF recurrence 12 months after catheter ablation	ECG	CNN	Larger batches of patients are analyzed to improve applicability and accuracy. In addition, a prospective study is needed; other studies assess recurrence after more than 12 months
	2021	Bai, Y. [39]	Prediction of AF recurrence after catheter ablation	ECG	CNN	To generalize the premise, larger batches of patients were analyzed, with more pathologies
Cardiogenic Shock	2022	Rahman, F. [40]	Predicting patients at high risk of developing cardiogenic shock (CS)	Demographic, vital signs, laboratory, medication	DT RF SVM KNN LR	Future studies will assess how early identification of cardiogenic shock and potential effects on prompt treatment may alter patient outcomes
	2021	Bai, Z. [41]	Predictive model of evolution towards CS in patients with STEMI	Demographic, pre-existing diagnoses, ECG, laboratory	LASSO LR SVM DT	Larger groups of patients; blood glucose analysis used as a predictive factor of CS

Table 2. *Cont.*

	Year of Study	Author	Application	Data Source	Machine Learning Method	Future Direction
Cardiogenic Shock	2022	Chang, Y. [42]	CS prediction 2 h before the need for the first intervention	Demographic, vital signs, laboratory	XGB MLP TCN	Future studies to include the integration of HF or AMI specific elements to increase accuracy
	2023	Jaicay, N. [43]	Predicting CS in acute coronary syndrome (ACS) patients	Demographic, vital signs, laboratory, ECG	KNN	Superior computational power would include more models for analysis and allow the imputation analysis of analyzing more datasets
	2022	Jentzer, J. C. [44]	Phenotype CS	Laboratory	HC LCA KMCk	Integration of multi-biomarker/imaging (ECG, echocardiography, angiography) to understand the differences in underlying pathophysiology that separate these clinical subphenotypes could improve phenotyping
	2023	Wang, L. [45]	Clinical phenotypes of CS	Demographic and medical history, vital signs, laboratory, treatment	CA	Association between endpoints within individual SCAI stages and ML-derived phenotypes whose aim is to characterize disease severity as it evolves over the course of a hospital stay
	2022	Bohm, A. [46]	Clinical predictive model of progression to CS in patients with ACS	Demographic, vital signs, laboratory	LR	Validation on an external cohort
	2023	Popat, A. [47]	Early prediction of CS in acute heart failure or MI	Demographic, Laboratory	ML	Conducting studies also outside the USA
	2022	Rong, F. [48]	Predicting the 30-day mortality of elderly patients with CS	Demographic, vital sign, laboratory, comorbidities, Echocardiograpy	Cox model LASSO SAPSII	Larger groups of patients
	2023	Mo, Z. [49]	Assessing the prognosis of ECMO treatment in elderly patients with CS	Demographic, vital sign, laboratory, comorbidities, medications	RF DT	A larger batch of patients followed for more than 6 months

Table 2. Cont.

	Year of Study	Author	Application	Data Source	Machine Learning Method	Future Direction
Cardiomyopathy	2024	Cau, R. [50]	Differential diagnosis of cardiomyopathy phenotypes	Demographic, vital sign, laboratory, ECG	CNN	Randomized trials are crucial
	2023	Haimovich, J. S. [51]	Differential diagnosis between LV hypertrophy: cardiac amyloidosis and hypertrophic cardiomyopathy	Demographic, vital signs, laboratory, medication, ECG	CNN	Studies on cardiomyopathies to include the athletic heart
	2023	Beneyto, M. [52]	Predicting hypertensive origin in left ventricular hypertrophy (LVH)	Clinical, Laboratory, ECG, echocardiograpy	DT RF SVM	Additional studies from non-tertiary centers
	2022	Eckstein, J. [53]	Diagnosis of cardiac amyloidosis (CA)	Demographic, clinical, echocardiogray, CMR	KNN SVM DT	Multicenter evaluation of patients with early stage cardiac amyloidosis
	2021	Siontis, K. C. [54]	Diagnosis of hypertrophic cardiomyopathy (HCM) in children and adolescents	Demographi, ECG,	CNN	Multicenter studies in children under 5 years
	2020	Ko, W.-Y. [55]	Diagnosis of HCM particularly in younger patients	Demographic, ECG	CNN	Further refinement and external validation
	2022	Hwang, I.-C. [56]	Differential diagnosis of LVH	Echocardiography	CNN	Future studies that include rare LVH etiologies: Fabry disease, Danon syndrome, transthyretin amyloidosis
	2023	Zhou, M. [57]	Differentiating ischemic cardiomyopathy from dilated cardiomyopathy	Echocardiography	RF LR CNN XGB	Multicenter external validation on larger patient batches
	2023	Cau, R. [58]	Diagnosis of Takotsubo cardiomyopathy	Demographic, Echocardiography	RT	Longitudinal and prospective studies to assess predictive performance in different cohorts and validate these findings

Table 2. Cont.

	Year of Study	Author	Application	Data Source	Machine Learning Method	Future Direction
Cardiomyopathy	2023	De Filippo, O. [59]	The prediction of prognosis in hospital patients with Takotsubo syndrome	Demographic, ECG, Echocardiography, laboratory, medications	LR CA	Multicenter studies beyond European and Asian ethnicities
	2021	Jefferies, J. L. [60]	Predictive screening model for potential patients with Fabry disease	Demographic, clinical, echocardiography, medications, laboratory	ML	Future clinical implementation studies
	2022	Sotto, J. [61]	The prediction of etiology of LVH	ECG Echocardiography	CNN	Multicenter studies to identify other causes of ventricular hypertrophy, such as Fabry disease or cardiac amyloidosis
	2023	Zhang, Y. [62]	Diagnosis of arrhythmogenic cardiomyopathy (ACM) and dilated cardiomyopathy (DCM)	Echocardiography, Genes	CA RF	Checking for other genes involved in pathogenesis of ACM and DCM
	2022	Papageorgiou, V. E. [63]	Detection of an arrhythmogenic heart disease (ARVD)	ECG	CNN	Checking integration into clinical practice
	2023	Harmon, D.M. [64]	Validation study of cardiac amyloidosis diagnosis	Demographic, ECG	KNN SVM DT CNN	Future multicentric studies to validate the diagnosis in different ethnicities in the presence of left bundle branch block or LVH
	2023	Cotella, J. I. [65]	Measuring ejection fraction and longitudinal strain in cardiac amyloidosis	Echocardiography	LR	Studies on larger batches of patients
	2023	Zhang, X. [66]	Non-invasive diagnostic method for myocardial amyloidosis	Echocardiography	RF SVM LR	Studies on larger, multicentre patient groups

Table 2. Cont.

	Year of Study	Author	Application	Data Source	Machine Learning Method	Future Direction
Cardiomyopathy	2023	Goswami, R. [67]	Predicting death or transplantation of transthyretin amyloid cardiomyopathy (ATTR-CM)	Hemodynamic, clinical, Echocardiograpy	CNN	Larger groups of patients in multicenter studies
	2023	Michalski, A. A. [68]	Diagnosis of Fabry disease	Demographics, clinical, Echocardiograpy, laboratory	NLP	Prospective studies on larger groups of patients with improved NLP
	2023	Jefferies, J. [69]	Predicting the risk of arrhythmias in Fabry disease	Demographics, Clinical data, ECG, Echocardiograpy	ML	Multicentric studies
	2023	Stolpe, G. [70]	The prediction of sudden cardiac death in HCM	Demographic, Clinical data, Echocardiograpy	RF	Definition of sensitivity and specificity
	2022	Zhang, X. [71]	A predictive model for classifying HCM, DCM, and healthy patients	CMR	RF	Multicentric studies
Cardiovascular Imaging	2023	Tatsugami, F. [72]	Prediction of myocardial infarction or cardiac death	CT cardiac	CNN	External validation for cardiac CT on larger datasets
	2022	O'Brien, H. [73]	Diagnosis of myocardial scars	MRI-LGE CT-DE	SVM	Larger studies with larger CT-DE data to establish optimal imaging parameters and characteristics
	2022	Wen, D. [74]	Identification of hemodynamically significant coronary artery stenosis	CCTA FFR	DT	Validation studies on larger groups of patients
	2023	Lara-Hernández, A. [75]	Quantitative myocardial perfusion	CCTA	DL	Extending the method to other dynamic imaging modalities
	2023	Griffin, W.F. [76]	Detection and grading of coronary stenoses	CCTA QCA FFR	ML	Application of the method after the results of the INVICTUS trial

Table 2. Cont.

	Year of Study	Author	Application	Data Source	Machine Learning Method	Future Direction
Cardiovascular Imaging	2022	Bandt, V. [77]	Identify significant CAD pre-TAVR	CCTA	ML	Additional studies on larger batches
	2022	Li, X.-N. [78]	Highlighting the vulnerability of the coronary artery plate	CCTA	ML	Validation studies
	2021	Lyu, T. [79]	Deep learning approach in reducing the radiation dose of CT	CT cardiac	CNN	Additional studies on larger batches
	2023	Zhang, R. [80]	Diagnosis of myocardial perfusion imaging	SPECT-CT	CNN	The larger cohort in the next stage of our study
	2023	Khunte, A. [81]	Detection of left ventricular systolic dysfunction	ECG, Echocardiography	CNN	Use of this algorithm as a screening method for LV systolic dysfunction among individuals with no clinical disease
	2024	Pieszko, K. [82]	Prediction of left atrial appendage thrombus (LAT)	TTE TOE	LR, DT	Studies in different populations to assess the performance and to evaluate performance in specific subgroups based on sex or race
	2023	Liu, Z. [83]	Diagnosis of right ventricular abnormalities	CMR	DNN	Another validation study by comparing with human experts
	2023	Wang, Y. [84]	Improved myocardial strain analysis	CMR	CNN	Larger batches
	2024	Yu, J. [85]	Assessment of LV function	TOE	ML	Larger batches
	2023	Laumer, F. [86]	Differential diagnosis of Takotsubo syndrome (TTS) and acute myocardial infarction (AMI)	TTE	CNN	Future studies on a larger population are to differentiate the two conditions in the acute phase
	2024	Lee, D. [87]	Detecting obstructive CAD	CCTA	DL	Larger batches
	2023	Kapalos, A. [88]	Segmentation of cardiac T1 and T2 mapping images	CMR	DNN	Future work will focus on ensuring the accurate measurement of tissue properties

Table 2. Cont.

	Year of Study	Author	Application	Data Source	Machine Learning Method	Future Direction
Congenital Heart Disease	2023	Ishikita, A. [89]	Prediction of adverse cardiovascular events in adults with repaired tetralogy of Fallot	CMR Clinical data	RF	Follow-up studies including multiple centers with longer follow-up
	2023	De Vries, I.R. [90]	Screening of congenital heart disease (CHD)	ECG	ANN	Future work should aim to improve the signal processing chain to omit or reduce the need for combining multiple heartbeats, potentially further allowing for the additional analysis of arrhythmias and better performance
	2022	Lv, J. [91]	Screening and detecting CHD in children	Heart sounds	CNN	Larger patient cohorts
	2022	Majeed, A. [92]	A greater risk of developing executive function deficits in children with complex CHD	Demographic, medical and surgical history, family social class	RF DT	Larger patient cohorts
	2022	Sakai, A. [93]	Detection of small ventricular septal defects	Fetal cardiac ultrasound	DNN	Multicenter joint research.
	2022	Gearhart, A. [94]	Analysis of pediatric echocardiograms	ETT	CNN	Future work could incorporate transfer learning to reduce the manual workload
	2022	Valente Silva, B. [95]	Diagnosis of pulmonary embolism	ECG	DNN	External samples from other centers
Electrocardiography	2022	Adedinsewo, D. [96]	Detecting moderate-to-severe acute cellular rejection (ACR) among heart transplant (HT) recipients	Demographic, clinical characteristic, ECG, TTE	CNN	Future directions would include evaluating the potential benefit of combining AI-ECG screening with blood testing methods, evaluation of the AI-ECG for detecting ACR and antibody-mediated rejection (AMR) combined
	2023	Shiraishi, Y. [97]	Risk of sudden cardiac death	ECG	CNN RNN	Studies on larger batches of patients; future studies will include batches of patients treated with angiotensin receptor-neprilysin inhibitors and sodium-glucose cotransporter 2 inhibitors

Table 2. Cont.

	Year of Study	Author	Application	Data Source	Machine Learning Method	Future Direction
Electrocardiography	2023	Hirota, N. [98]	The biological age of the patient is associated with cardiovascular events	ECG	CNN	The clinical significance of AgeDiff in patients older than 60 years should be re-evaluated in different cohorts, such as multicenter cohorts or the general population
	2023	Wouters, P. C. [99]	Effects of cardiac resynchronization therapy	ECG	DNN	Prospective studies; the results need to be validated in a patient group that received a CRT-P device
	2023	Raghunath, A. [37]	Onset of atrial fibrillation	ECG	CNN RNN	Future studies with characteristic information for the population (e.g., racial background)
	2023	Liu, C.-W. [100]	Prediction of LVH	ECG	CNN DNN	Analyzing other surrogate end points in cardiovascular diseases (such as left ventricular diastolic dysfunction, new-onset myocardial infarction, or heart failure)
	2023	Zaver, H. [101]	Predicting cardiac events and incident AF in patients who have received a liver transplant	ECG	CNN DNN	Larger patient cohorts
	2023	Naser, J. [102]	Concentration of sex hormones	ECG; Laboratory	CNN	Larger patient cohorts
	2023	Vaid, A. [103]	Valvular diseases	ECG	CNN	Further external validation from another health system
	2023	Jiang, J. [38]	Predicting the risk of recurrence in patients with paroxysmal atrial fibrillation after catheter ablation	ECG	CNN	Further calibration and validation using high-quality prospective studies

Table 2. Cont.

	Year of Study	Author	Application	Data Source	Machine Learning Method	Future Direction
Heart Failure	2023	Khan, M. S. [104]	Early diagnosis of HF, stratifying HF disease severity	Demographic, clinical parameters, ECG, TTE	SVM ANN CNN	More datasets are needed for validation and increased transparency through an understanding of AI models
	2023	Almujally, N. A. [105]	Remote monitoring of patients with acute heart failure	Demographic, clinical, laboratory	CNN RNN	The IoT-based system can be further expanded with different types of wearable medical healthcare devices that can be operated on tablets or smartphones
	2022	Kobayashi, M. [106]	Predicting heart failure incidence in asymptomatic individuals	Demographic, TTE, laboratory, medication, cardiovascular risk factors	CA DT	A further prospective multicenter study is needed to assess the applicability
	2020	Segar, M.W. [107]	Phenomapping of patients with HF with preserved ejection fraction (HFpEF)	TTE, Laboratory,	CA	The use of more comprehensive data, as well as a larger number of patient variables, may have yielded different results
	2024	Bourazana, A. [108]	HF diagnosis, monitoring, and management	Clinical examinations, TTE, laboratory	SVM ANN CNN	Issues that remain unresolved concern diagnosis, classification, and treatment. Future studies will assess heart failure with preserved ejection fraction (HFpEF)
	2022	Bachtiger, P. [109]	Screening for HF with reduced ejection fraction	ECG ETT	CNN	Screening for further priority cardiovascular diseases, such as valvular heart pathology, using AI-enabled phonocardiography
	2021	Harmon, D. M. [110]	Diagnosis of HF with reduced ejection fraction (HFrEF)	ECG	CNN	Prospective evaluation of the AI-ECG for ventricular dysfunction for treatment of HF in the acute setting
	2021	Kwon, J.-M. [111]	Early detection of HFpEF	ECG	DLM	The algorithm used must be further validated in patients with HFrEF in other countries
	2024	Wu, J. [112]	Predicting mortality in patients with undiagnosed HFpEF	Demographic, ETT	NLP	Other observational studies

Table 2. Cont.

	Year of Study	Author	Application	Data Source	Machine Learning Method	Future Direction
Heart Failure	2023	Akerman, A. P. [113]	Detection of HF	ETT ECG	CNN	Future work is required to guide more transparent and patient-level interpretation
	2021	Paná, M.-A. [114]	Predicting HF exacerbation	Patient's voice	SVM ANN KNN	Larger batches of patients
	2024	Cheungpasitporn, W. [115]	Treatment for HF patients with acute kidney disease	Demographic, vital signs, laboratory, medication	ML	External validation
	2023	Kamio, T. [116]	Predicting clinical outcomes in acute heart failure	Demographic, vital signs, laboratory, comorbidities, medication	CNN SVM LSVCe XGB	Further research is required to determine the generalizability of these conclusions to other populations and settings
	2022	Naruka, V. [117]	Predicting graft failure and mortality	Demographic, biomarker, CMR	ANN CNN RF SVM DT	Prospective multicenter studies collecting data on the immunosuppression regime or the causative factors for length of hospital stay were not studied
Heart Transplant	2021	Briasoulis, A. [118]	Predicting survival and acute rejection after HT	Clinical and Laboratory	LR DT SVM KNN	Future studies with analysis of other predictors after heart transplantation
	2023	Seraphin, T. P. [119]	Predicting the degree of cellular rejection from pathology	Pathological archive	CNN	Validation in larger cohorts for clinical-grade AI biomarkers
	2022	Ozcan, I. [120]	Predicting major adverse cardiovascular events (MACE) risk post-HT	Clinical and laboratory, ECG	CNN	Further research is to guide screening and treatment strategies for HT patients using this algorithm
	2023	Sharma, S. [121]	Predicting the susceptibility of HT patients to COVID-19	Demographic, Clinical, Laboratory	CNN MLP	Further research and implementation of these technologies in diagnosis, monitoring, and detection

Table 2. Cont.

	Year of Study	Author	Application	Data Source	Machine Learning Method	Future Direction
	2020	Glass, C. [122]	Identify myocyte damage in HT acute cellular rejection (ACR)	Comorbidities	CNN	Validation in prospective studies with larger cohorts
	2023	Al-Ani, M. A. [123]	Predicting survival rates in intra-aortic balloon pump (IABP) used as a bridge to HT compared to the Impella	Clinical, Laboratory, Related Disease	XGB	External validation
	2021	Peyster, E. G. [124]	Histological grading of cardiac allograft rejection	Endomyocardial biopsy slides	SVM	External validation
Heart Transplant	2022	Lipkova, J. [125]	Assessment of cardiac allograft rejection from	Endomyocardial biopsy slides	CNN	Larger studies
	2023	Gluste, F.O. [126]	Enhancing risk assessment of rare pediatric heart transplant rejection	Heart Biopsy	CNN DNN	Future work will focus on generating additional expert-annotated examples of cellular rejection signs to further improve and validate our model's performance
	2022	Lisboa, P. J. G. [127]	Survival prediction in heart transplantation	Clinical, Demographic	GANN PRN	Prospective studies
	2022	Ruiz Morales, J. [128]	Predicting outcomes after HT	ECG	CNN	Larger studies
	2020	Agasthi, P. [129]	Predicting 5-year mortality and graft failure in patients with HT	Demographic, clinical	GBM	Larger studies
	2021	Ozcan, I. [130]	Predicting MACE after HT	ECG	CNN	Larger studies
Hypertension	2020	Soh, D. C. K. [131]	Diagnosis of hypertension	ECG	KNN	Future studies with larger cohorts and validation studies
	2020	López-Martinez, F. [132]	Predicting hypertension	Demographic, laboratory, vital signs	ANN	Future studies with new risk factors

Table 2. Cont.

	Year of Study	Author	Application	Data Source	Machine Learning Method	Future Direction
Hypertension	2020	Wu, X. [133]	Clinical prediction of hypertension in young patients	Clinical, comorbidities	XGB	Larger studies
	2020	Aziz, F. [134]	Effectiveness of hypertension treatment	Demographic, clinical, treatment	ANN SVR	Studies on larger batches of patients
	2020	Koshimizu, H [135]	Blood pressure variability	Demographic, vital signs	DNN	Longer-term studies
	2023	Hamoud, B. [136]	Estimating blood pressure	Videos of subjects	CNN	Extending the training set with subjects who are older or estimating other vital signs such as heart rate, oxygen saturation, and body temperature
	2023	Cheng, H. [137]	Blood pressure prediction	IPPG	CNN	Larger studies
	2023	Xing, W. [138]	Hypertension screening and disease prevention	Facial videos	DNN	Larger studies
	2023	Visco, V. [139]	Hypertension prediction and management	Clinical, Laboratory, TTE	ANN SVM KNN	Implementation studies
	2022	Maqsood. S. [140]	Blood pressure estimation and measurement	PPG ECG	DNN	Future studies will combat the "Black Box" because they lack the declarative knowledge necessary to explain the outcomes further
	2023	Herzog, L. [141]	Hypertension management	Demograpic, clinical, Comorbidities	DNN	Validation of results with a randomized controlled clinical trial
	2021	Khthir, R. [142]	Predictive factors for hypertension in patients with type 2 diabetes	Demographic, Clinical data, Laboratory	RF	Larger studies
	2023	Aryal, S. [143]	Evidence that blood pressure is closely correlated with the microbiota	Demographic, clinical, laboratory, genetic tests	XGB RF NB	Larger studies and prospective studies

Table 2. Cont.

	Year of Study	Author	Application	Data Source	Machine Learning Method	Future Direction
Hypertension	2023	Lin, Z. [144]	Prediction of hypokalemia in patients with hypertension	Laboratory, comorbidities, antihypertensive medications	RF	Prospective studies
	2020	Kusunose, K. [145]	Confirmation of the need for RHC in patients with suspected pulmonary hypertension (PH)	Clinical Findings CXR ETT PAP	CNN	Further validation is necessary to determine the feasibility of CXR and larger numbers for the differentiation of pre- and post-capillary PH
	2021	Hardacre, C. J. [146]	MRI may allow for reduction of right heart catheterization (RHC)	CMR, laboratory	CNN DT RF	Future studies with AI to diagnose PAH that can be applied to CT
	2022	Ragnarsdottir, H. [147]	Prediction of PH in newborns	ECG	CNN	Larger batches of patients
	2021	Chakravarty, K. [148]	PH therapies for COVID-19 treatment	Clinical, laboratory	RF	Further validation is necessary
Pulmonary Hypertension	2021	Rahaghi, F. N. [149]	Detection of pulmonary arterial disease	Demographic, PAP, CT imaging, ECG, ETT, Laboratory	CNN	Future studies on the multicenter registry; further work is to determine the specificity and sensitivity of such metrics as well as their value for prognostication and monitoring response to therapeutic intervention
	2022	Shi, B. [150]	Prediction of PH	Biomarkers, Hemodynamics, PAP	DT RF RT LR SVM	Prospective studies on human subjects
	2021	Amodeo, I. [151]	Predict PH in newborns with congenital diaphragmatic hernia	CMR images	CNN SVM	Future prospective multicenter cohort study for validation
	2022	Van der Bijl, P. [152]	Diagnosis of PH	ETT CXR	ANN	studies including patients with tricuspid regurgitation

Table 2. Cont.

	Year of Study	Author	Application	Data Source	Machine Learning Method	Future Direction
Pulmonary Hypertension	2021	Swift, A. J. [153]	Diagnosis of PH	CMR PAP, ETT	SVM LR	Larger cohorts
	2022	Charters, P. F. P. [154]	Predicting survival in patients with suspected PH	ETT, CTPA	ML	Larger studies with larger cohorts
	2022	Fortmeier, V. [155]	Predicting PH in patients with severe TR	ETT PAP demographic, laboratory, comorbidities	XGB	Randomized controlled trials to investigate whether specifically patients with elevations of predicted mPAP still benefit from transcatheter interventions
	2022	Liu, C.-M. [156]	Predicting future risk for cardiovascular mortality in patients with PH	ECG ETT	CNN	Further studies on larger cohorts are necessary for validation
	2023	Lu, W. [157]	Diagnostic biomarkers for idiopathic pulmonary hypertension (IPAH)	Gene	RF	Larger studies
	2023	Yu, X. [158]	PH diagnosis	ETT, PAP CT images	KNN	Larger studies
	2023	Hyde, B. [159]	Distinguishing between patients with PAH and those without PAH at 6 months before diagnosis	Demographics, diagnoses, laboratory, medications	RF	External validation
	2023	Zhang, N. [160]	Diagnosis of PH	ETT, CTPA	SVM XGB	Future studies will explore the volumetric information of heart and pulmonary artery morphology as well as the spatial relationship between different intra- and extra-cardiac structures to improve the accuracy of PAP parameter evaluation
	2024	Hirata, Y. [161]	Predicting PH	RHC	LR	Validation and further research to assess clinical utility in PH diagnosis and treatment decision making

174

Table 2. Cont.

	Year of Study	Author	Application	Data Source	Machine Learning Method	Future Direction
	2024	Imai, S. [162]	PAH detection	CXR PAP	CNN	Future studies should include diseases with CXR images similar to PAH, such as cardiac hypertrophy, and collect data from diverse clinical settings
	2024	Ragnarsdottir, H. [163]	Assessing PH in newborns	ETT	CNN	Future studies could be applied to ECHOs from the adult population, with retraining required
	2024	Dwivedi, K. [164]	Improving PH prognosis by detecting pulmonary fibrosis	Demographic, CT pulmonary angiograms, ETT	CNN	Validation study
Pulmonary Hypertension	2023	Griffiths, M. [165]	Risk prediction model for pediatric PH	Demographics, imaging, hemodynamics, laboratory, comorbidities	RF	Future studies could be applied to the adult population
	2023	Mamalakis, M. [166]	Diagnosis of PH	CT images	CNN	Larger studies
	2024	Tchuente Foguem, G. [167]	Prognosis of survival of PH	Demographics, ETT	SVM	Larger studies
	2024	Han, P.-L. [168]	Diagnosis of congenital heart disease and associated PAH	CXR CMR ETT	RF	Larger studies
	2024	Anand, V. [169]	Diagnosis PH	ETT PAP ECG	ML	Larger studies
Infective Endocarditis	2024	Lai, C. K.-C. [170]	Predicting infective endocarditis (IE)	Demographic, clinical, ETT, comorbidities	RF	Multicentric study and prospective studies

Table 2. *Cont.*

	Year of Study	Author	Application	Data Source	Machine Learning Method	Future Direction
Infective Endocarditis	2024	Yi, C. [171]	Common biomarkers in IE and sepsis	Laboratory tests, genes	RF LASSO	Future research will require more extensive datasets and experimental validation. Future studies also demonstrate differences between subtypes of sepsis, including significant variations in the abundance and expression levels of immune cell populations
	2023	Galizzi Fae, I. [172]	Risk stratification of patients hospitalized with IE	Laboratory, imaging, treatment, comorbidities	LR DT	Larger studies
Ischemic Heart Disease	2022	Chen, Z. [173]	Myocardial infarction segmentation	CMR	CNN	Future studies that can differentiate old myocardial scar from acute myocardial infarction
	2021	Rauseo, E. [174]	Diagnosis of chronic ischemic disease	CMR	SVM RF	Further studies to determine whether there is a correlation between the radiomic features and the extent of myocardial scarring
	2021	Liu, W.-C. [175]	Diagnosis of acute myocardial infarction (AMI) at the emergency department (ED)	Clinical, ECG, Laboratory	DL	Future studies on large-scale, multi-institute, prospective, or randomized control studies are necessary to further confirm real-world performance
	2020	Zhao, Y. [176]	Early detection of ST-segment elevated myocardial infarction (STEMI)	ECG	CNN	Future studies should be validated in various ethnics
	2020	Cho, Y. [177]	Diagnosis of AMI	Demographic, ECG, laboratory	CNN	A prospective study specifically designed to confirm the accuracy of data from various wearable or portable ECG devices is warranted to apply the DLA to these devices

Table 2. Cont.

	Year of Study	Author	Application	Data Source	Machine Learning Method	Future Direction
Ischemic Heart Disease	2021	Liu, W.-C. [178]	Detecting AMI	Demographic, ECG, laboratory, angiography	DL LR	Further prospective validation with prehospital and in-hospital ECG tests is needed to confirm the performance of our DLM
	2023	Ciccarelli, M. [11]	Prevention of cardiovascular disease (CAD)	Genetic and epigenetic variables, clinical risk factor	RF	Future studies for the prevention of other pathologies
	2021	Velusamy, D. [179]	Diagnosis and prediction of CAD	Demographic, clinical, laboratory, risk factors	RF SVM KNN	Larger studies
	2021	Muhammad, L. J. [180]	Prediction of CAD	Demographic, clinical, diagnosis	Naive Bayes; SVM RF DT	Future studies on other ethnic groups
	2021	Li, D. [181]	Prediction of CAD	Demographic, clinical, laboratory	ML	Future studies for prediction of other pathologies
	2024	Brendel, J. M. [182]	Assessment of CAD in patients undergoing workup for transcatheter aortic valve replacement (TAVR)	CT angiography, laboratory, ETT, comorbidities	CNN	Multicentric study
	2024	Ihdayhid, A. R. [183]	CAD diagnosis and identification of high-risk plaque	Demographic, CCTA ECG	CNN	Future research is needed to investigate the prognostic impact and value of incorporating deep learning techniques into clinical practice compared to the standard of care
	2024	Uzokov, J. [184]	Diagnosis of ischemic heart disease (IHD)	ECG ETT CCTA	DL	Further management using cloud-based innovative digital technologies and artificial intelligence (AI)

Table 2. Cont.

	Year of Study	Author	Application	Data Source	Machine Learning Method	Future Direction
	2024	Abdelrahman, K. [185]	Coronary artery calcium scoring detection and quantification	ECG, CT imaging	KNN, SVM, CNN, ANN	Future studies to distinguish between non-coronary calcifications such as valvular calcification and other high-density objects (e.g., metal implants) from coronary calcifications
	2024	Park, M. J. [186]	Predicting coronary occlusion in resuscitated out-of-hospital cardiac arrest (OHCA) patients	ECG, Clinical, Biomarkers	DL	Further validation in larger, prospective studies to establish efficacy across diverse clinical settings
	2024	Alkhamis, M. A. [187]	Predicting in-hospital and 30 days adverse events in ACS	Demographic, clinical, ECG, ETT, CCTA	RF, XGB, SVM, LR	Future studies for prediction of 1-year adverse events in ACS
Ischemic Heart Disease	2024	Zhu, X.; Xie, B. [188]	Prediction of death in patients with first AMI	Demographic, Clinical, Laboratory, ECG	LR, RF, XGB, SVM, MLP	Validating studies on other ethnic groups
	2024	Kasim, S. [189]	Predicting outcomes in non-ST-segment elevation myocardial infarction (NSTEMI) or unstable angina (UA)	Demographic, medication	XGB, SVM, NB, RF, GLM	Continuous development, testing, and validation of these ML algorithms hold the promise of enhanced risk stratification, thereby revolutionizing future management strategies and patient outcomes
	2023	Oliveira, M. [190]	AMI mortality prediction	Demographic, laboratory	LR, DT, RF, XGM, SVM	Further studies should be conducted and consider the inclusion of more variables that may be relevant in predicting AMI mortality, such as socioeconomic factors, systolic blood pressure, heart rate, and electrocardiogram results

Table 2. Cont.

	Year of Study	Author	Application	Data Source	Machine Learning Method	Future Direction
Ischemic Heart Disease	2021	Bai, Z. [41]	Prediction for CS risk in patients with STEMI	Demographic ECG laboratory in-hospital events	LR SVM XGB LASSO	Future studies with other risk factor analyses; for example, glycemia is not routinely recorded in our patients and therefore could not be tested as a potential predictor of CS. Further investigations using larger populations are warranted to fully evaluate the applicability of this model
	2024	Azdaki, N. [191]	Predicting CAD in hospital patients	Demographic Clinical comorbidities	ANN	Larger studies on ethnic groups
	2024	Zhan, W. [192]	Prognostic model based on malignant pericardial effusion (PE)	genes	LASSO	Future studies to discover immunotherapy drugs
	2022	Liu, Y.-L. [193]	Diagnosis of acute pericarditis and differentiate it from STEMI in the ED	ECG	XGB	Prospective, multicenter study; large-scale, further external validation
Pericardial Disease	2023	Cheng, C.-Y. [194]	Detecting and measurement of PE	TTE	CNN	Future studies should utilize a multicenter design with greater heterogeneity in the dataset. Further research should evaluate the collapsibility of the cardiac chambers and the presence of tamponade signs
	2022	Wilder-Smith, A. J. [195]	Detection and segmentation of PE	CT images	CNN	Future studies to include CT images of older machines, as this study was performed on state-of-the-art CT
	2022	Piccini, J. P. [196]	Predicting PE after leadless pacemaker implantation	Demographic clinical comorbidities	LASSO LR	A larger number of patients

Table 2. *Cont.*

	Year of Study	Author	Application	Data Source	Machine Learning Method	Future Direction
Peripheral Arterial Disease	2024	McBane, R. D. [197]	Diagnosis patients with peripheral artery disease (PAD) at greatest risk for major adverse events	Demographic Comorbidities Ankle-brachial index	CNN	Future studies to assess the tolerance of such signal acquisition would be important. Further validation studies are required to assess test accuracy and reproducibility in community settings outside of a large-volume academic vascular laboratory
	2024	Rusinovich, Y. [198]	Identifying and classifying the anatomical patterns of PAD	Angiograms	ML	A larger number of patients
	2024	Sasikala, P. [199]	Prediction of PAD and accurate categorization of its severity levels	Demographic clinical angiograms	DT	Future studies for validation
	2024	Li, B. [200]	Prognosis of PAD	Laboratory, Demographic, Comorbidities Treatment	ML	Future validation at other institutions is needed to demonstrate the generalizability of this model
	2024	Masoumi Shahrbabak, S. [201]	Diagnosis of PAD	Arterial pulse waveforms ankle-brachial index BP	DL	External validation.
	2024	McBane, R. D., II [202]	Prediction of major adverse outcomes among patients with diabetes mellitus and PAD	Posterior tibial arterial Doppler waveforms	DNN	Larger studies
	2024	Li, B. [203]	Predict outcomes after infra-inguinal bypass in patients with PAD	Demographic Clinical complications	XGB LR	Larger studies
	2024	Liu, L. [204]	Prediction of PAD in diabetes mellitus (T2DM)	demographic diagnoses, biochemical index test	DT LR RF SVM XGB	Future studies in other regions also need to address the lack of collected and analyzed data on patients' subjective descriptions, such as their duration of diabetes and smoking habits, which have been reported as associated with PVD in T2DM

Table 2. Cont.

	Year of Study	Author	Application	Data Source	Machine Learning Method	Future Direction
Thromboembolic Disease	2024	Nassour, N. [205]	Predicting venous thromboembolism (VTE) in ankle fracture patients	Demographic CXR CT images ultrasonograpy	RF	Studies on larger groups of patients
	2024	Chen, R. [206]	Predicting diagnosis and 1-year risk of VTE	Demographics, laboratory, medications	ML	Future research should focus on refining and validating these models in different healthcare settings as well as informing personalized treatment strategies and exploring their potential utility in predicting VTE recurrence
	2024	Pan, S. [207]	VTE risk prediction for surgical patients	Demographic clinical laboratory comorbidities	ANN LR	Validation studies
	2024	Grdinic, A. G. [208]	Bleeding prediction in patients with cancer-associated thrombosis	Clinical biochemistry diagnosis	LR RF XGB	Validation studies
	2023	Chiasakul, T. [209]	Prediction of VTE	Ultrasonography	LR	Future studies should focus on transparent reporting, external validation, and clinical application of these models
	2023	Wang, X. [210]	Predicting the risk of DVT after knee/hip arthroplasty	Demographic clinical comorbidities	NLP XGB RF SVM RL	In future studies, model accuracy will be further evaluated by performing prospective and real-time predictions of DVT
	2023	Wang, K. Y. [211]	Identification of patients at risk of VTE following posterior lumbar fusion	Demographic, clinical comorbidities	LR XGB	Future studies should seek to externally validate these predictive tools and should examine the potential cost savings provided by predictive analytics models which can accurately identify patients at risk of VTE following spine surgery

Table 2. *Cont.*

	Year of Study	Author	Application	Data Source	Machine Learning Method	Future Direction
Thromboembolic Disease	2023	Muñoz, A. J. [212]	Predicting 6-month VTE recurrence in patients with cancer	Demographic, clinical comorbidities	LR DT RF NLP	Future studies are needed to assess the validity of these results
	2021	Razzaq, M. [213]	Predicting the risk of recurrent VTE by biomarkers	Laboratory	ANN	Further experimental validations for these biomarkers
	2023	Valente Silva, B. [95]	Acute pulmonary embolism (PE) diagnosis	ECG laboratory	DNN	Further application in larger cohorts and external validation of the deep learning model are essential to fully validate its performance. These results should be validated in an external sample from other centers in the future, as well as in high-risk patient subgroups, for example, patients with hemodynamic instability
	2022	Contreras-Luján, E. E [214]	Early diagnosis of DVT	Clinical ultrasonography	KNN DT SVM RF	External validation
	2023	Seo, J. W. [215]	Detecting iliofemoral DVT	CT angiography	CNN	Future studies to extend the detection ranges to the infrapopliteal vein for investigating DVT
Valvular Heart Disease	2023	Alhwiti, T. [216]	Predicting in-hospital mortality post-TAVR	Demographic disease	LR	Future studies looking at long-term mortality post-TAVR
	2023	Strange, G. [217]	Identifying severe aortic stenosis (AS) phenotypes associated with high mortality	TTE	ML	Future studies in other geographic regions/health systems or specific ethnic groups

Table 2. Cont.

	Year of Study	Author	Application	Data Source	Machine Learning Method	Future Direction
Valvular Heart Disease	2023	Ueda, D. [218]	Screening for heart valve disease	CXR TTE	CNN	Further validation with prospectively acquired test datasets from cohorts with various disease prevalences
	2024	Singh, S. [219]	Valvular heart disease screening	TTE	SVM LR CNN	Future studies to validate these data
	2024	Brown, K. [220]	Screening for rheumatic heart disease (RHD) in children	TTE	CNN	Future work needs to be pursued incorporating other features of RHD into our current AI algorithms as well as feasibility testing for field implementation in RHD endemic regions
	2024	Toggweiler, S. [221]	TAVR planning and implantation	Cardiac CT	CNN	Further studies are required to demonstrate if these results can be reproduced by other centers using different scanners and different protocols for image acquisition (external validation)
	2021	Solomun M.D. [222]	Screening of AS	ECG	NLP	Future studies leveraging NLP-derived data to evaluate the association between the severity of AS and clinical outcomes, along with identifying predictors of AS progression
	2022	Aoyama, G. [223]	Diagnosis of AS	Cardiac CT	DNN	In future work, we should compare the intraoperative direct observation and the manual measurements by physicians with the automatic measurements by our proposed method to more concretely verify the clinical effectiveness and risks of the proposed method
	2024	Dasi, A. [224]	Predicting post-transcatheter aortic valve replacement	TTE Cardiac CT	ANN SVR	Future studies can focus on building upon these AI models to account for the nonlinear and complex relationships among postoperative AV pressure gradient, AVA, and patient outcomes

Table 2. Cont.

	Year of Study	Author	Application	Data Source	Machine Learning Method	Future Direction
	2023	Krishna, H. [225]	Assessment of AS	ETT	ANN	Future work will aim to utilize AI to categorize AS severity, incorporating multiple echocardiographic variables
	2024	Xie, L.-F. [226]	Predicting postoperative adverse outcomes following surgical treatment of acute type A aortic dissection	Demographic, clinical	LASSO XGB	Multicenter study; external validation data are needed to test the clinical utility of the model
Valvular Heart Disease	2024	Zhou, M. [227]	Screening of aortic dissection	ECG	CNN	Larger studies; future prospective studies could enhance the efficacy of this AI model
	2023	Irtyuga, O [228]	Screening of AS in patients with and without bicuspid aortic valve	TTE	SVM ANN RF DR	Future research efforts should focus on early diagnostics and strategies to delay the progression of degenerative aortic valve disease
	2023	Kennedy, L. [229]	Prediction of the mechanical function of thoracic aortic aneurysm (TAA) tissue	TTE medical history genetic paneling	SVM GPR	Larger studies and an investigation are needed to compare the accuracy of risk levels assigned by the integrated ML approach compared to that of diameter thresholding using histopathological classification of tissue

2.2.1. AI in Arrhythmias

One of the most common arrhythmias in adults is atrial fibrillation (AF), with an estimated prevalence ranging from 2% to 4% [230]. Because one-third of people with arrhythmia are asymptomatic, diagnosing AF can be challenging. AF often presents intermittently, referred to as paroxysmal atrial fibrillation (AF), which is often undiagnosed, resulting in significant mortality and morbidity. Strategies for detecting AF include serial electrocardiography (ECG), event monitors, long-term outpatient monitoring using wearable continuous ECGs, in-hospital monitoring, or implantable cardiac monitors. However, AF detection rates remain low, between 5% and 20%, despite these measures. Predicting the timing of the onset of AF could improve the treatment of this condition, especially since AF is expected to affect more than 12 million people in the U.S. by 2030. Thus, there is a need to identify innovative and cost-effective techniques, especially in terms of cost, to help clinicians better treat this disease [36,37].

The ECG has been analyzed since the 1970s when ventricular repolarization abnormalities were analyzed by an AI-based model, which finally showed a high correlation with serum potassium levels [231]. In 2023, the way AF prediction and detection are evolving with the availability of new predictive tools was well described in a review carried out by Martínez-Sellés, M. et Marina-Breysse, M [232].

In this review, the authors showed how an AI-enabled ECG acquired during normal sinus rhythm allows point-of-care identification of people with AF. Other authors have explored AF prediction using mobile sinus rhythm electrocardiograms (mECG) and demonstrated that neural networks can predict AF development using mECG data in sinus rhythm. They concluded that mECG data could lower barriers to the implementation of AI-based AF event prediction systems in the modern healthcare environment due to their cost-effectiveness, availability, and scalability [37].

A study of 2530 patients showed that the CNN model had better predictive performance than other current predictive models in effectively predicting the risk of postoperative recurrence in patients with paroxysmal atrial fibrillation by identifying 12-lead ECG characteristics before catheter ablation [38].

In January 2024, a paper was published in JAHA, developing robust deep learning algorithms for automated ECG detection of postoperative AF and its burden using both atrial and surface ECGs. This finding has an important impact on the subsequent management of patients with newly diagnosed AF [233]. Overall, ML models show promise for detecting AF in a stroke population for secondary stroke prevention and for accurately predicting AF in a healthy population for primary prevention.

While previous authors analyze models to predict the risk of FA or to detect FA in at-risk populations, other authors focus on the applicability of these models. Kawamura, Y. concludes in a review that implementation in the real world of AF prediction models requires validation studies and the development of points that would facilitate transparency through reducing potential systemic biases and improving generalizability [234].

However, another review in 2024, which included 14 studies, showed that AI is effective for detecting AF from ECGs. Among DL algorithms, convolutional neural networks (CNNs) demonstrate superior performance in AF detection compared to traditional machine learning (TML) algorithms. Diagnosing AF earlier can integrate ML algorithms that can help wearable devices [235].

2.2.2. AI in Cardiogenic Shock

CS is a pathology represented by low cardiac output causing hypoperfusion of the target organs. CS causes very high short-term mortality of up to 50%. Observational studies have shown that early recognition, protocol management, optimal triage, and risk stratification in hospitals equipped with technology and well-trained staff have led to much better outcomes in the management of CS [236].

In January 2024 Raheem A. et al. published a retrospective study, which looked at 97,333 patients, in which they described a new, much more detailed way to predict

MACE, in-hospital mortality (up to 30 days) from all causes, and cardiac arrest. They used AI and a systemic grid technique in an ANN to robustly analyze the performance of the ANN model compared to RF and LR classifiers and the commonly used Emergency Severity Index (ESI). The authors created a predictive model, based on emergency room presentation criteria, that would make it easier for emergency physicians to triage patients with cardiovascular symptoms. They demonstrated that ANN with systematic grid search predicted MACE, cardiac arrest, and 30-day in-hospital mortality in triaging patients with cardiovascular symptoms with high accuracy, unlike LR and RF models. Their predictive model could therefore help emergency physicians make timely triage choices for patients with cardiovascular symptoms by classifying and prioritizing patients in the early phase based on triage presentation criteria [237]. On the other hand, another study analyzing 2282 STEMI patients demonstrated that for predicting cardiogenic shock in STEMI patients, the linear LASSO model showed superiority over LR, SVM, and XGBoos. In patients with AMI, CS is the most common cause of in-hospital death, accounting for 5–10% of patients [41]. In most of the studies analyzed, the repeatable limitations include retrospective studies conducted on target populations. Future prospective studies are therefore needed, including populations from more than one center [42,47,48].

2.2.3. AI in Cardiomyopathy

Numerous studies have analyzed electrocardiograms using artificial intelligence and have proven their usefulness in detecting cardiomyopathies and more [51,54,55,64]. ECG analysis using AI has shown its usefulness in both adult [51,55] and pediatric hypertrophic cardiomyopathy [54] in the detection of cardiac amyloidosis [64]. Haimovich, J. S. et al. published a study in 2023 that included 93,138 adult patients and concluded that models based on ECG analysis, LVH-NET, and its single-lead versions may be useful in the clinic for screening patients with left ventricular hypertrophy as well as rare diseases such as hypertrophic cardiomyopathy and cardiac amyloidosis [51]. Another previously mentioned study looked at ECGs from 300 children and adolescents under the age of 18 and showed their usefulness in detecting pediatric hypertrophic cardiomyopathy. In 2023, Harmon D.M. et al. studied 676 patients who were evaluated at the Mayo Clinic and diagnosed with AL or ATTR cardiac amyloidosis (CA). The authors demonstrated that AI-ECG achieved very high performance for detecting CA in terms of sex, race, age, and amyloid subtype. On the other hand, the AI-ECG demonstrated lower performance for patients with LBBB [64]. Echocardiography is another tool that with the help of AI can bring closer diagnoses of CA. Cotella J. I et al. studied 51 patients who calculated FEVS and GLS using AI, and they proved that there were no significant differences in manual and automated LVEF and GLS values either pre-CA or at diagnosis. This would allow for a faster evaluation of CA patients [65].

Zhang X. et al. showed in a retrospective analysis of 289 patients that ultrasonic imaging omics and a machine learning model can provide an excellent and non-invasive diagnostic tool for clinical practice for distinguishing CA from non-CA. For left ventricular strain, the machine learning model was slightly better than conventional echocardiography [66]. Another study, which analyzed 128 patients with ATTR-CA using AI, concluded that the ANN model estimated the risk of death or transplantation in patients with ATTR cm with better accuracy compared to traditional risk models [67].

Takotsubo (TTS) cardiomyopathy is another cardiomyopathy in which the application of AI has found a place. Takotsubo cardiomyopathy (transient apical ballooning syndrome or broken heart syndrome) is a form of non-ischemic cardiomyopathy. TTS predominantly affects women and is a regional left ventricular systolic dysfunction; it is transient but occurs without significant coronary artery disease on angiography [238]. Echocardiography, coronary angiography, left ventriculogram, and cardiac magnetic resonance imaging (CMR) are used to diagnose TTS. As a clinical entity of acute transient heart failure, its general management is conventional heart failure therapy if the patient does not show hemodynamic instability or mechanical complications [239].

For patients who are not eligible for gadolinium contrast CMR, the diagnosis of takotsubo cardiomyopathy remains difficult without invasive investigation. One study that analyzed non-contrast CMR images and demographic data of cardiac arrest patients using AI found a model that offers good accuracy in predicting patients with Takotsubo (TTS) cardiomyopathy [58]. Another study, which looked at 3284 patients with TTS, showed that an ML-based approach identified patients at risk of a poor short-term prognosis in the hospital. The Inter-TAK-ML model has shown its usefulness for predicting in-hospital death in patients with TTS [59].

Another rare genetic cardiomyopathy is Fabry disease (FD). It has multisystem involvement and a reported but possibly underestimated annual incidence of 1 in 100,000. Many cases go undiagnosed because there is a large age gap between the age at which the first symptoms appear and the age at which it is diagnosed; this is 13 and 32 for women and 9 and 23 for men [240]. Symptoms of onset include neuropathic pain, recurrent fever, ophthalmic problems, sweating disorders, typical skin changes, gastrointestinal symptoms, heat/cold intolerance, and otolaryngological problems. However, the most serious problems induced by FD include cerebrovascular cardiovascular events and cardiac dysfunction, cardiovascular and cerebrovascular events, and chronic kidney disease, usually with proteinuria. Michalski A.A. et al. evaluated risk factors among patients who may suffer from FD and demonstrated that an NLP tool approach increased diagnostic effectiveness and improved prognosis and quality of life for patients with Fabry disease. The method also recognized its limitations, which consisted of the need for prospective studies, the small sample of patients diagnosed with FD, the analyzed risk factors, and the implemented NLP algorithm which requires further development to improve its accuracy [68]. In patients with FD, cardiac arrhythmias are common, but individual risk varies widely. Among the most common arrhythmias are ventricular tachycardia and atrial fibrillation. Jefferies J. et al. conducted a study on 5904 patients with FD in which AI-machine learning models were applied and demonstrated strong performance in estimating the risk of adverse outcomes. This discovery could be useful in clinical practice where it would be used to reduce patients' adverse outcomes and improve their management [69].

2.2.4. AI in Cardiovascular Imaging

Artificial intelligence (AI) is spreading into every facet of cardiac imaging, from studies to prognostication and personalized risk prediction for each patient. The Food and Drug Administration (FDA) has approved approximately 300 artificial intelligence devices in the combined fields of radiology and cardiovascular, and this number continues to grow. Cardiac magnetic resonance imaging (CMR), echocardiography, and coronary computed tomography angiography (CCTA) derive significant benefits from AI-based solutions. AI has numerous advantages in cardiovascular imaging, from the possibilities of increasing efficiency to reducing inter-observer and intra-observer variability and also reducing human error and reader variability [241].

Artificial intelligence has also found its place in cardiovascular imaging. Using machine learning methods and radiomic features from delayed enhancement CT (CT-DE), myocardial scarring has been identified with good accuracy compared to cardiac magnetic resonance imaging (MRI) with late gadolinium enhancement (LGE) (MRI-LGE), which is the gold standard [73]. Additionally, using CMR radiomic features, other authors in another study created a predictive model to classify patients with hypertrophic cardiomyopathy (HCM) and dilated cardiomyopathy (DCM) [71]. A retrospective study of 303 patients analyzing coronary CT, fractional flow reserve (FFR), and quantitative coronary angiography (QCA) data demonstrated that AI has its place in coronary CT. The authors demonstrated rapid and accurate identification of major stenoses, superimposable with coronary angiography [76]. Zhang R et al. published a retrospective study in which they analyzed 599 patients who underwent myocardial perfusion imaging (MPI). Image analysis was performed using hybrid SPECT-CT systems. The authors aimed to validate and develop an AI (artificial intelligence) aid method applied in myocardial perfusion imaging (MPI) to help clinicians differentiate ischemia in coronary artery disease. They demonstrated the high predictive value and very good efficacy of this system and therefore found a tool to help radiologists in their clinical practice [80]. Another study published in the European Heart Journal of 2827 patients that analyzed echocardiographic images using AI demonstrated increased accuracy in diagnosing left atrial thrombosis (LAT). This finding guides clinicians in the management of patients on oral anticoagulant (OAC) therapy in deciding on transesophageal ultrasound (TOE) [82].

Another large study published in the Jama analyzed transthoracic ultrasounds of 224 patients with Takotsubo and 224 patients with AMI to differentiate between the two diseases. The authors demonstrated that the system created was more accurate than clinical cardiologists in classifying disease based on echocardiography alone, but further studies are needed to put the system into clinical application [86]. High-quality prospective evidence is still needed to show how the benefits of DL cardiovascular imaging systems can outweigh the risks [242].

2.2.5. AI in Congenital Heart Disease

Congenital heart disease (CHD) is a field of application for AI, taking into account the diverse and robust datasets that extend from the management and diagnosis of pathologies to multimodal imaging. It has also increased the cohabitation of patients with CHD due to innovative surgery and new therapies. Thus, the use of AI could improve the quality of patient care, help optimize the treatment of these patients, extend life expectancy, save time for the attending physician, and reduce healthcare costs [243]. Artificial intelligence has found usefulness in current studies in the prediction of cardiovascular events in adults operated on for Fallot tetralogy [89] and the screening of congenital diseases based on ECG [90] based on cardiac auscultation [91] or echocardiography [93,94]. De Vries R.I. et al. conducted a study that developed an ECG-based fetal screening method for CHD. They demonstrated a 63% detection rate for all CHD types and 75% for critical CHD [90]. A study of 386 patients identified predictors of impaired executive function in adolescents after surgical repair of critical congenital heart disease (CHD), which were as follow: social class as the primary predictor and birth weight, neurological events, and number of procedures as other predictors [92].

2.2.6. AI in Electrocardiography

Cardiovascular disease (CVD) crosses geographic, gender, or socioeconomic boundaries. Electrocardiograms (ECGs) are a routine instrument for any complete medical evaluation. ECGs are also used for diagnosis [244].

Artificial intelligence has found its usefulness in ECG for the following purposes: diagnosis of pulmonary thromboembolism [95], prediction of sudden death and cardiovascular events [97,98], prediction of fatal events after cardiac resynchronization [99], prediction of paroxysmal atrial fibrillation [37], detection of ventricular hypertrophy [100], risk prediction in liver transplantation [101], detection of ventricular dysfunction [103], and prediction of recurrence after paroxysmal atrial fibrillation ablation [38].

Valente Silva, B. et al. published a study on a batch of 1014 ECGs from patients presenting to the emergency room with suspected pulmonary embolism (PE). The authors demonstrated and validated a high-specificity pulmonary embolism prediction model for PE diagnosis based on artificial intelligence and ECG [95]. Shiraishi Y. conducted a study enrolling 2559 patients hospitalized for decompensated heart failure. Together with the authors of this study, they demonstrated the prediction of death in cardiac subjects using AI-ECG [97]. Zaver B. H. et al. published a retrospective study in 2023 that enrolled patients from a single center who were evaluated for liver transplantation or who underwent liver transplantation between 2017–2019. During this period, 3202 ECGs were available in the system, of which 1534 were available pre-transplant, 383 on the day of transplant, and 1284 post-transplant. A total of 719 ECGs from a total of 300 patients were analyzed, of which 533 were pre-transplant ECGs and 196 post-transplant ECGs. The study demonstrated AI-ECG performance in patients who were proposed for evaluation for liver transplantation, in addition, it demonstrated performance similar to that in the general population, but which was lower in the presence of an elongated QTc. ECG analysis using AI showed its usefulness in predicting post-transplant de novo AF. AI-based ECG assessment has also shown utility in predicting decreased left ventricular ejection fraction post-transplant. Therefore, AI-ECG can be a useful tool for patients proposed for liver transplantation, as a positive screening for a decreased SV ejection fraction or atrial fibrillation can raise alarm signals for the development of new post-transplant AF or cardiac dysfunction. Therefore, the importance of using a large dataset and artificial intelligence (AI) has increased significantly in medicine [101].

2.2.7. AI in Heart Failure

Heart failure (HF) is increasing in prevalence along with the complexity of its diagnosis and treatment. The management and diagnosis of patients with HF require a huge amount of clinical information, leading to the accumulation of large amounts of data. However, traditional analytical methods are not sufficient to manage large datasets. From HF prediction to HF diagnosis, classification, prevention and management, AI has proven its usefulness [245].

Artificial intelligence has found its place in the prediction of heart failure in asymptomatic patients [106], in the diagnosis and treatment of patients with heart failure with reduced ejection fraction [110], in the diagnosis and treatment of patients with heart failure with low ejection fraction, in the detection of heart failure with preserved ejection fraction [111], and in the prediction of congestive heart failure [114].

Heart failure (HF) with preserved ejection fraction (HFpEF) is common and is associated with a high burden of mortality, morbidity, and high healthcare costs. Currently, compared with low-ejection-fraction HF (HFrEF), few medical therapies have been shown to improve cardiovascular outcomes in studies in patients with HFpEF. A study published by Segar M. et al. on 1767 patients has shown that cl analysis based on machine learning can identify the fenogroups of HFpEF patients with different clinical characteristics and also predict long-term results [107].

Almujalys. N discussed acute heart failure (AHF) monitoring in a study published in 2023. Together with all the study authors, they designed a remote health monitoring system to effectively monitor patients with AHF. This tool also helps both patients and doctors. It concerns Internet of Things (IoT) technology, which has revolutionized data colloquialization and communication by incorporating intelligent sensors that collect data from various sources. In addition, it uses artificial intelligence (AI) approaches to control a huge amount of data, which leads to better storage, management, use, and decision making. The created system monitors the clothing activities of patients, which helps to inform patients about their health status [105].

Kamio T. et al. published a study of 1416 patients who were admitted to the intensive care unit (ICU) for acute heart failure (AHF) and who received furosemide treatment. Using AI, they created a model that predicted in-hospital mortality and mechanical ventilation in patients hospitalized for AHF [116].

2.2.8. AI in Heart Transplant

Regarding heart transplantation, artificial intelligence shows its usefulness in the following situations: in the prediction of post-heart-transplant events [118,128,129], the prediction of rejection after heart transplantation [118,119,122], the prediction of COVID-19 in heart transplantation [121] and pediatric heart transplantation [126], and the prediction of post-transplant survival [127].

One study claims that for patients with end-stage heart failure, heart transplantation remains the only chance of life. Medicine has come a long way, and the number of heart transplants has increased exponentially worldwide, but the number of heart donors is not big enough to meet the high demand. This brings up a particular issue of resource allocation. Artificial intelligence comes to the rescue and allows doctors to quantify the risk of rejection, accurately predict post-transplant prognosis, and determine waiting list mortality [117]. Briasoulis A. et al. published a study on a group of 18,625 patients (mean age 53 ± 13 years, majority male—73%), in which they analyzed the prediction of outcomes after heart transplantation. They concluded that 1 year after heart transplantation, there were 2334 (12.5%) deaths. Additionally, using AI, they demonstrated an ML-based model that proved its effectiveness in predicting post-transplant survival as well as acute rejection after heart transplantation [118]. The prediction of post-heart transplant rejection was also analyzed by Seraphin T.P. et al. in a study published in 2023, which included 1079 histopathology reports of 325 transplant patients in three centers in Germany. The authors detected patterns of cell transplant rejection in routine pathology, even when trained in small cohorts [119]. Since 2021, the rejection of cardiac alograft has been a serious concern in transplant medicine. It is well known that endomyocardial biopsy with histological examination is the gold standard in the diagnosis of rejection, but poor inter-pathology agreement creates important clinical uncertainty. Peyster E.G. et al. published a study that looked at 2472 endomyocardial biopsies, which concluded that the degrees of cellular rejection generated by histological analysis using AI are the same as those provided by expert pathologies [124].

In 2022, Ozcan I. et al. published a study in a cohort of 540 patients in which they looked at the patient's physiological age based on ECG and correlated this information with the risk of post-heart transplantation mortality.

They were able to demonstrate that age-related cardiac aging after transplantation is associated with a higher risk of major cardiovascular events (MACEs), such as mortality, re-transplantation, and hospitalization for heart failure or coronary revascularization. The usefulness of this discovery is that the change in the physiological age of the heart could be an important factor in the risk of post-heart transplant MACE [120]. This study was reinforced by Morales J. R.'s study, which suggested that there may be an association with ECG cardiac age and one-year post-transplant events [128].

2.2.9. AI in Hypertension

Artificial intelligence is increasingly being used in treating hypertension. In the highly scientific literature, numerous machine learning techniques are used to diagnose and detect numerous diseases: hypertension prevention [138], hypertension prediction [132,137,140,142], hypertension prediction in young patients [133], hypertension diagnosis [131,136], hypertension management and treatment [134,139,141], and hypertension variability [135]. Hypertension is found in 1.28 billion adults according to the World Health Organization (WHO). Hypertension has been found in adults aged 30 to 79 worldwide. Of adults with hypertension, about 42% are treatable. WHO data claim that about one in five adults worldwide has achieved optimal blood pressure control through treatment. Hypertension is also the leading cause of death worldwide [246].

Lopez-Martinez F. et al. performed a study that included 24,434 people aged over 20 years in the USA; they developed a neural network model in which they evaluated several factors and their relationship with the prevalence of hypertension. This study focused on using ANN to estimate the association between smoking, sex, age, BMI race, diabetes, and kidney disease in hypertensive patients. The results of this study show a specificity of 87% and sensitivity of 40%, with a precision of 57.8% and a measured AUC of 0.77 (95% CI [75.01–79.01]). The advantage of this study is that the results are more efficient than a previous study by other authors using another statistical model with similar characteristics that showed a lower calculated AUC than the present study (0.73). This model needs validation in other clinical settings, and further studies should include socio-demographic information to increase accuracy and integrate this model with clinical diagnosis [132].

Masked hypertension (MHPT) is ambulatory blood pressure that is not normal but exhibits instant normal blood pressure. Therefore, patients with MHPT are difficult to identify, and they remain untreated. Soh, D. C. K et al. developed a paper in which they analyzed a computational intelligence tool that used electrocardiogram (ECG) signals to detect MHPT. EI demonstrated that the best accuracy for the diagnosis of arthritic hypertension in the ECG signals was KNN, 97.70% [131].

Risk stratification remains an important step in hypertensive patients, especially if they are young patients. Wu X. et al. performed a study on a group of 508 patients, who were followed for an average period of 33 months. Two new ML techniques (RFE and XGBoost) were applied in the study to analyze the future risk of young patients diagnosed with hypertension. Baseline clinical data were analyzed, as well as a composite endpoint including all-cause death, coronary artery revascularization, peripheral artery revascularization, acute myocardial infarction, new-onset stroke, new-onset atrial fibrillation/atrial flutter, new-onset heart failure, sustained ventricular tachycardia/ventricular fibrillation, and end-stage renal disease. These patients were treated in a tertiary hospital. The performance of these models was then compared with that of a traditional statistical model (Cox regression model) and a clinically available model (FRS model). The study showed that the prognostic efficacy of the analyzed ML method was comparable to that of the Cox regression model; moreover, the efficacy of the analyzed ML method was higher than that of the recalibrated FRS model [133].

Herzog L. et al. studied a cohort of 16,917 participants, predicting antihypertensive therapeutic success with the help of AI. With an accuracy of 51.7%, the custom model developed by the authors was based on deep neural networks. The most successful treatment was a combination of an angiotensin-converting enzyme inhibitor and a thiazide (with 44.4% percent), and the angiotensin-converting enzyme inhibitor used alone was the most commonly used treatment (with 39.1%). These results may help with personalized treatment and better management of this pathology [141].

2.2.10. AI in Pulmonary Hypertension

In the last four decades, a considerable number of registries have been published for pulmonary hypertension, which is a rare condition. These data have enabled the management and understanding of this pathology to be improved. However, to increase the understanding of the pathophysiology of pulmonary hypertension, prognostic scales are needed, as well as scales for verifying the transferability of the results from clinical trials in clinical practice. Although there are a huge amount of data from numerous sources, they are not always taken into account by registries. This is why machine learning (ML) provides a great opportunity to manage all these data and subsequently access tools that could help to make an early diagnosis. All of this functions to advance personalized medicine, especially the prognosis of the patient [247].

Many studies have focused on the effects of AI on pulmonary hypertension, from the prediction of this rare pathology in adults [147,150,155,161,162] or children [151,163,165] to the prediction of survival [154,167] or risk in patients with pulmonary hypertension [156], diagnosis of pulmonary hypertension [149,152,153,156–158,160,169], and the treatment of this disease [148].

In 2023, Griffiths M. et al. published a study of 1232 patients in *Circulation*, using data from multicentric registries. The authors developed a predictive model for pulmonary hypertension in children and also with the help of this model discovered a high-risk model for the time of intervention in these children. In the test cohort, the developed model showed very good results, with an AUROC of 87%, sensitivity of 85%, and specificity of 77% [165]. Another study used echocardiographic data to diagnose pulmonary hypertension (PH) in the pediatric population in a cohort of 270 newborns. The results of the study showed an average F1 score of 0.84 for predicting the severity of pulmonary hypertension in newborns, 0.92 for binary detection using a 10-fold cross-validation, 0.63 for predicting severity, and 0.78 for binary detection on the device held by the tests. The authors conclude that the learned model focuses on clinically relevant cardiac structures, motivating its use in clinical practice; at the time, this paper was the first to show automated pH assessment in newborns using echocardiograms [163].

In 2024, Anand V. et al. studied a cohort of 7853 patients who underwent cardiac catheterization and echocardiography and created an ML model for predicting PH using data from echocardiography.

The cohort age was 64 ± 14 years, of which 3467 (44%) were women and 81% (6323/7853) had a diagnosis of PH. The final trained model included 19 measurements and features from the echocardiogram. The model showed high discrimination for diagnosing PH (area under the characteristic operating curve of the receiver, 0.83; 95% CI, 0.80 to 0.85) in the test data. The accuracy, sensitivity, positive predictive value, and negative predictive values of the model were 82% (1267/1554), 88% (1098/1242), 89% (1098/1241), and 54% (169/313), respectively. The authors concluded that the PH could be predicted based on echocardiographic and clinical variables without using the regurgitation rate at tricuspid. Thus, machine learning methods seem to be promising for diagnosing patients with a low pH probability [169].

2.2.11. AI in Infective Endocarditis

Infective endocarditis (IE) is a serious infectious disease that has high morbidity and mortality rates and severe complications. Severe complications include cardiac arrhythmias, embolic events, and valve ruptures leading to acute heart failure. Early risk assessment of patients with IE is crucial to optimize treatment. The prognosis of IE is influenced by many factors, including laboratory tests, clinical factors, cardiovascular and systemic imaging, and a combination of these. In addition, electrocardiographic changes may indicate advanced disease and thus predict high morbidity and mortality [15]. A dynamically modulated heart rate is considered to be a surrogate of the interaction between the parasympathetic and sympathetic nervous systems. This is measured by the variability or fluctuation in the time intervals between normal heartbeats (heart rate variability [HRV]). Inflammation is reflexively inhibited by the vagus, through activation of the hypothalamic–pituitary–adrenal axis, which causes cortisol secretion. Inflammation is also inhibited by the vagus and by vagus-sympathetic innervation of the spleen, where proinflammatory cytokines are no longer released from macrophages, which have in turn been signaled by single T cells. To highlight this mechanism, in 2023, Perek S. et al. published a study on a group of 75 patients with a mean age of 60.3 years from a tertiary center with a diagnosis of infective endocarditis. With the help of logistic regression (LR), it was determined whether laboratory, clinical, and HRV parameters were predictive of severe short-term complications (metastatic infection, cardiac injury, and death) or specific clinical features (staphylococcal infection and type of valve). The authors demonstrated that the standard deviation of normal heartbeat intervals (SDNN) and in particular the root mean square of successive differences (RMSSD), which were derived from very short ECG records, can be used for the prognosis of patients with IE [248].

In 2024, Christopher Koon-Chi Lai et al. discovered a new risk score comparable to existing scores but which is superior to clinical judgment; it applies to patients with *S. aureus* bacteremia (SAB). The authors looked at 15,741 patients with infective endocarditis, 658 of whom had a diagnosis of endocarditis-infective Staphylococcus aureus (SA-IE). The AUCROC was 0.74 (95% CI 0.70–0.76), with a negative predictive value of 0.980 (95% CI 0.977–0.983). Of all the features analyzed, four were the most discriminatory: history of infectious endocarditis, age, community onset, and valvular heart disease [170].

Another study by Galizzi Fae, I. et al. concluded that the most feared complications of infectious endocarditis are cardiovascular and neurological, and they are independently associated with high mortality. In addition to these complications, variables such as older age and elevated CRP levels are also associated with increased mortality. With the help of AI, it has been shown that intra-hospital mortality is determined by cardiovascular complications. Therefore, rapid identification of patients at high risk can prompt more aggressive treatment, which may decrease the mortality rate [172].

2.2.12. AI in Ischemic Heart Disease

When it comes to ischemic heart disease, artificial intelligence can be useful both in the early diagnosis of ischemic heart disease [175–178,184,185] and in the prediction of complications after an acute ischemic event [186–190] and coronary artery disease [179–181,191]; AI can also be used in coronary artery disease prevention [11].

The current guidelines state that natural CAD can be modified by medical therapies, risk stratification, and early detection of CAD. In this way Ciccarelli M. et al. published an article in 2023 in which they mentioned (1) various machine learning algorithms based on single-photon emission computed tomography (SPECT) to facilitate CAD prediction and (2) prediction of major adverse cardiac events (MACE) in patients with the current or prior acute coronary syndrome (ACS) by risk scores such as the SINTAX87 score; however, these tools do not have the expected accuracy. The authors recalled in their study the use of machine learning techniques in identifying patients with increased morbidity and mortality following ACS. To estimate the risk of myocardial infarction, major bleeding, and, death of any cause for a period of 1 year, the PRAISE95 score was used and demonstrated precise discriminatory capabilities [11].

In patients with acute myocardial infarction (AMI), the most common cause of in-hospital death, despite early revascularization, is cardiogenic shock (CS) cauing 5–10% of deaths. Of all cases of CS, about 70% may be due to AMI. Bai Z. et al. published a paper in which five machine learning methods were analyzed to predict in-hospital cardiogenic shock in STEMI patients. These models include least absolute shrinkage and selection operator (LASSO), logistic regression (LR) models, support vector regression (SVM), and the tree-based ensemble machine learning models gradient boosting machine (LightGBM), and extreme gradient boosting (XGBoost). Of all the learning methods, the most successful prediction performance was represented by the LASSO model. The LASSO model in STEMI patients could provide excellent prognostic prediction for the risk of developing CS. The study included a group of 2282 patients with STEMI. The best overall predictive power was shown by linear models constructed using LASSO and LR, with an average accuracy of over 0.93 and an AUC of over 0.82. However, the LASSO nomogram showed adequate calibration and better differentiation, with a C-index of 0.811 [95% confidence interval (CI): 0.769–0.853]. A high C-index value of 0.821 was obtained for the internal validation tests. In terms of the decision curve (DCA) and clinical impact curve (CIC), the LASSO model showed superior clinical relevance compared to previous models that were score-based [41].

In order not to delay acute myocardial infarction (AMI) diagnosis, Liu W. C. et al. published a paper in which they developed a deep learning model (DLM) that analyzed 450 12-lead electrocardiograms (ECGs) for improved diagnosis of AMI. For STEMI detection, in the human–machine comparison, the AUC for DLM was 0.976. This was better than that of the best doctors. DLM also showed sufficient diagnostic capacity for STEMI diagnostics (AUC = 0.997; sensitivity, 98.4%; specificity, 96.9%) independently. Compared to NSTEMI diagnostics, the combined AUC of conventional cardiac troponin I (cTnI) and DLM increased to 0.978, which was superior to that of cTnI (0.950) or DLM (0.877). The authors concluded in their study that DLM can be used as a tool to help clinicians make an objective, timely, and accurate diagnosis for subsequent rapid initiation of reperfusion therapy [178].

Zhao Y. et al. also published a paper in which artificial intelligence (AI) proved able to provide a way to increase the efficiency and accuracy of ECG in STEMI diagnosis. They created an AI-based STEMI self-diagnostic algorithm that used a set of 667 ECG STEMI and 7571 control ECGs. The algorithm proposed in their study reached an area under the receiver operating curve (AUC) of 0.9954 (95% CI, 0.9885 to 1) with sensitivity (recall), specificity, accuracy, and F1 scores of 96.75%, 99.20%, 99.01%, 90.86% and 0.9372, respectively, in the external evaluation. In a comparative test with cardiologists, the algorithm had an AUC of 0.9740 (95% CI, 0.9419 to 1) and sensitivity (recall), specificity, accuracy, and F1 score values of 90%, 98% and 94%, 97.82% and 0.9375, respectively.

Meanwhile, cardiologists had sensitivity (recall), specificity, accuracy, and F1 score values of 71.73%, 89.33%, 80.53%, 87.05%, and 0.8817, respectively [176]. Cho Y. et al. also published a paper in which they concluded that myocardial infarction (MI) could be detected quickly using electrocardiography (ECG) with 6 derivatives, not only ECG with 12 derivatives. The authors developed and validated an algorithm based on deep learning (DLA) for MI diagnostics. The EI analyzed a batch of 412,461 ECGs to create a variational autoencoder (VAE) that reconstructed the precordial ECGs with 6 derivatives [177].

Alkhamis M.A. et al. published a study that developed predictive models for adverse events in the hospital and at 30 days in patients with acute coronary syndrome (ACS). The authors analyzed 1976 patients with ACS and used clinical features and an interpretable multi-algorithm machine learning (ML) approach to match predictive models. EI demonstrated that the RF amplification algorithms and the extreme gradient (XGB) far exceed the traditional logistic regression model (LR) (ASCs = 0.84 and 0.79 for RF and RF, respectively, XGB. The most important predictor of hospital events was the left ventricle ejection fraction. From the point of view of events at 30 days, the most important predictor was the performance of an urgent coronary bypass graft. ML models developed by the authors of this study have elucidated nonlinear relationships that shape the clinical epidemiology of ACS adverse events and have highlighted their risk in individual patients based on their unique characteristics [187].

Kasim. et al. published a paper on 7031 patients in which they developed an ML model that improves mortality prediction accuracy by identifying unique characteristics within individual Asian populations. The performance of the algorithm created by the authors reached an AUC between 0.73 and 0.89. The TIMI risk score was exceeded by the ML algorithm, with superior performance for hospital predictions at 30 days and 1 year (with AUC values of 0.88, 0.88, and 0.81, respectively, all $p < 0.001$), while TIMI scores were much lower, at 0.55, 0.54 and 0.61. This finding shows that the TIMI score seems to underestimate the risk of mortality in patients. Key features identified for both short- and long-term mortality included heart rate, Killip class, age, and low-molecular-weight Heparin (LMWH) administration [189].

2.2.13. AI in Pericardial Disease

AI has proven its usefulness in pericardial diseases; from the diagnosis of liquid pericarditis based on ECG [193] to the measurement of pericardial fluid based on echocardiography [194], automatic detection and classification of pericarditis using CT images of the chest [195], and prediction of fluid pericarditis in patients undergoing cardiac stimulation [196] or in breast cancer patients [192].

Liu Y.L. et al. published a retrospective study, being the first DLM study using a 12-lead electrocardiogram to diagnose acute pericarditis. The strategy developed by the authors is based on discriminating ECGs from acute pericarditis versus ECGs from STEMI in patients presenting with anterior chest pain to the emergency room. This study can be used as a basis for other larger studies and can also be an important support tool for the detection of pericarditis in the on-call room. This method can also be applied remotely and in telemedicine, as well as for portable technologies [193].

Piccini, J. P. et al. published a paper in which they determined predictive factors in which they developed a risk score for pericardial effusion in patients undergoing attempted Micra leadless pacemaker implantation. The authors analyzed a group of 2817 patients and concluded that the overall rate of pericardial effusion following Micra implantation is 1.1%. Using lasso logistic regression, the study authors developed a valid risk score for pericardial effusion composed of 18 preprocedural clinical variables. Using bootstrap resampling, future predictive performance and internal validation were estimated. External validation also benefited the scoring system, using data from the Micra Acute Performance European and Middle East (MAP EMEA) registry. There were 32 patients with pericardial effusion in the study [1.1%, 95% confidence interval (CI) 0.8–1.6%]. The authors demonstrated in the study that the rate of pericardial effusion increased with Micra implantation attempts in patients at medium risk ($p = 0.034$) but also in those at high risk ($p < 0.001$). After the Micra implantation attempt, the risk of developing pericardial effusion can be predicted with reasonable discrimination using preprocedural clinical data [196].

2.2.14. AI in Peripheral Arterial Disease

Patients with a diagnosis of peripheral artery disease (PAD) have a high risk of metabolic events as well as cardiac events but are also at high risk of overall death. To improve outcomes in patients diagnosed with PAD, it is necessary to identify the disease early with prompt initiation of correct risk-managing treatment. McBanell R.D. et al. published a paper in JAHA in which they uncovered an AI algorithm that evaluated the posterior tibial arterial Doppler signal in patients with PAD, with the help of which they determined the patients with the highest risk of death from all causes, MALE, and MACE. A total of 11,384 patients were included in the study, out of which 10,437 underwent ankle–brachial index testing (medium age, 65.8 ± 14.8 years old, 40.6% women). Some 2084 of the patients were followed for 5 years, during which 447 of the patients died, 161 suffered MALE, and 585 suffered MACE events. Adjustments were then made for sex, age and Charlson comorbidity index, and the AI analysis of the posterior tibial artery waveform provided an independent prediction of mortality (hazard ratio [HR], 2.44 [95% CI, 1.78–3.34]), major adverse cardiac events (HR, 1.97 [95% CI, 1.49–2.61]), and major adverse limb events (HR, 11.03 [95% CI, 5.43–22.39]) at 5 years. Their analyses assisted clinicians in detecting peripheral arterial disease (PAD), which can lead to early modification of risk factors and their tailoring to each patient [197].

McBane II R.D. also published a study in which he addressed all major adverse cardiac events (MACEs) and limb events (MALEs), but compared to the previous study, the authors relied only on patients suffering from diabetes mellitus (DM). The authors of this study published in the Journal of Vascular Surgery are developing a tool that can diagnose PAD and predict clinical utility. Like McBanell R.D's study, Doppler arterial waveforms were analyzed to diagnose PAD, but in this study, only patients with a diagnosis of DM were analyzed. This study aimed to identify patients with diabetes who are at highest risk of PAD. Of the 11,384 patients analyzed, only 4211 patients with DM met the study entry criteria (mean age, 68.6 ± 11.9 years; 32.0% female). In the validation set, there was a final subset of testing that included 856 patients. Over 5 years, there were 319 MACEs, 99 MALEs, and 262 patients who died. An independent prediction of death was provided by patients in the upper quartile of prediction based on deep neural network analysis of the posterior tibial artery waveform (hazard ratio [HR], 3.58; 95% confidence interval [CI], 2.31–5.56), MACE (HR, 2.06; 95% CI, 1.49–2.91), and MALE (HR, 13.50; 95% CI, 5.83–31.27).

The authors also concluded that an AI analysis of the arterial Doppler waveform allows the identification of major adverse outcomes, MACEs, and MALEs (including all-cause death) in patients with DM [202].

Masoumi Shahrbabak et al. published a similar paper in which they investigated the feasibility of diagnosing peripheral artery disease (PAD) based on the analysis of non-invasive arterial pulse waveforms. We generated realistic synthetic blood pressure (BP) and pulse volume recording (PVR) waveform signals related to PAD present in the abdominal aorta with a wide range of severity levels using a mathematical model simulating arterial circulation and arterial BP-PVR relationships. We developed a deep learning (DL)-compatible algorithm that can diagnose PAD by analyzing brachial and tibial PVR waveforms and evaluated its effectiveness compared to the same DL-compatible algorithm based on brachial and tibial arterial BP waveforms and the ankle–brachial index (ABI). The results suggested that it is possible to detect PAD based on DL-triggered PVR waveform analysis with adequate accuracy, and its detection efficacy is close to that using blood pressure (positive and negative predictive values in 40% abdominal aortic occlusion: 0.78 vs. 0.89 and 0.85 vs. 0.94; area under the ROC curve (AUC): 0.90 vs. 0.97). The authors concluded that in the diagnosis of PAD, non-invasive arterial pulse wave analysis can be used with the help of DL as it is a non-invasive and accessible means [201].

2.2.15. AI in Thromboembolic Disease

In thromboembolic disease, artificial intelligence has a role, especially in disease prediction [205–207,209–213]. AI is also used in the diagnosis of pulmonary embolism [95] and the diagnosis of deep vein thrombosis [214,215].

Valente Silva B. et al. published a paper in 2023 in which they developed and validated a 12-lead ECG-based deep learning model for the diagnosis of pulmonary embolism. This model shows a high specificity guard in the diagnosis of pulmonary embolism. The authors of the study looked at 1014 ECGs from patients who underwent pulmonary angiography due to suspected pulmonary embolism. Of all these patients, 911 ECGs were used to develop the AI model, and 103 ECGs were used to validate the model. The performance of the AI model used by the authors in this study was compared with the clinical prediction rules recommended by the guidelines in place for EP, such as the Wells and Geneva scores combined with a standard D-dimer threshold of 500 ng/mL and an age-adjusted threshold. The authors concluded that the AI model they developed reached a much higher specificity for diagnosing PE than the commonly used clinical prediction rules. So, the AI model showed 100% specificity (95% confidence interval (CI): 94–100) and 50% sensitivity (IC of 95%: 33–67). Compared to the other models, which had no discriminatory power, the AI model worked much better (area under the curve: 0.75; IC 95% 0.66–0.82; $p < 0.001$). In patients with and without PE, the incidence of typical PE ECG characteristics was similar [95].

Seo J W et al. also addressed the diagnosis of deep vein thrombosis using AI methods and performed a study in which they evaluated the performance of an artificial intelligence algorithm (AI) for the diagnosis of iliofemoral deep vein thrombosis. They used computed tomographic angiography of the lower extremities. The authors concluded that the profuse is an effective method of reporting critical phases of iliofemoral deep vein thrombosis [215]. Contreras-Lujan, E. E. et al. supported previous and public research and used ML methods for more reliable and efficient DVT diagnosis to be incorporated into a high-performance system to develop an intelligent system for the early diagnosis of DVT. The authors concluded that the accuracy of all models trained on PC and Raspberry Pi 4 was greater than 85%, while the area under the curve (AUC) was between 0.81 and 0.86. So, for diagnosing and predicting early DVT, ML models are effective compared to traditional methods [214].

Nassour N. et al. also published a paper in 2024 in which they evaluated new automatic learning techniques to estimate the risk of VTE and the use of prophylaxis after ankle fracture. The authors analyzed using machine learning and conventional statistics 16,421 patients who suffered ankle fractures and were evaluated retrospectively for symptomatic VTE. Of all the patients, 238 patients with VTE confirmed later in the 180 days after the injury either sustained conservative or surgical treatment for ankle fracture. In the control group, there were 937 patients who had no evidence of VTE but who had ankle fractures and had similar treatment. Patients in both groups were divided into those receiving VTE prophylaxis and patients not receiving VTE prophylaxis. More than 110 variables were included. The results of the study were that the higher incidence of VTE was in the group of patients who underwent surgical treatment for ankle fracture, those who had increased hospitalization, and those who were treated with warfarin. The authors concluded that when machine learning was applied to patients with ankle fractures, several predictive factors were successfully found to be related to the appearance or absence of VTE [205].

2.2.16. AI in Valvular Disease

Artificial intelligence seems to be promising in valvular diseases; in this review, we focused our attention mainly on aortic diseases [216,217,222–225,228] and aortic dissection [226,227] as well as aortic aneurysm [229] and rheumatic diseases, focusing on mitral regurgitation [220].

For the treatment of aortic stenosis, transcatheter aortic valve replacement (TAVR) is the procedure increasingly used. Toggweiler, S. et al. have developed automated software to make the necessary measurements for planning TAVR with high reliability and without human help. The authors compared the automatic measurements from 100 CT images with the images from three TAVR expert clinicians. It was noted that the aortic ring measurements generated by AI had very good agreements with those performed manually by doctors, with correlation coefficients of 0.97 for both the perimeter and the area. For the measurement of the ascending aorta at 5 cm above the ring plane, the average difference was 1.4 mm, and the correlation coefficient was 0.95 [221].

Xie, L.-F. et al. published a study in 2024 integrating artificial intelligence to build a predictive model of postoperative adverse events (PAOs) based on clinical data. They wanted to evaluate the incidence of PAO in patients operated with acute aortic dissection type A (AAAD) after total arch repair. The authors included a group of 380 patients with AAAD in the study. They used LASSO regression analysis. After a thorough analysis, the authors concluded that the most optimal model is the extreme gradient growth model (XGBoost) as it showed better performance than other models. Therefore, for patients with AAAD, the prediction model for PAO is based on the XGBoost algorithm, and this model is also interpreted via the SHAP method. This method helps clinicians to identify high-risk AAAD patients at an early stage and choose optimal individualized treatment [226].

Brown, K. et al. published a paper in 2024 in JAHA concluding that artificial intelligence could detect rheumatic heart disease (RHD) in children as well as expert doctors. The authors included 511 ultrasounds from children in their studies, with color Doppler images of the mitral valve. Ultrasound scans were also evaluated by a group of expert doctors. RHD was present in 282 cases out of 511, and 229 were normal. The automatic learning method developed by the authors identified the correct vision of the mitral regurgitation jet and the left atrium, with an average accuracy of 0.99, and the correct systolic frame with an average accuracy of 0.94 (apical) and 0.93 (parallel long axis) [220].

3. Discussion

AI has broad application prospects in cardiovascular disease, and a growing number of scholars are devoted to AI-related research on cardiovascular disease. Cardiovascular imaging techniques (electrocardiography and echocardiography) and the selection of appropriate algorithms (ML or DL) represent the most extensively studied areas, and a considerable boost in these areas is predicted in the coming years.

Strengths: Cardiology leads the way in the artificial intelligence revolution in medicine. AI enables precise prediction of cardiovascular outcomes, non-invasive diagnosis of coronary artery disease, and detection of malignant arrhythmias. Additionally, it facilitates the diagnosis, treatment, and prognosis of heart failure patients. Advances in artificial intelligence and precision medicine will drive future innovations in cardiovascular research.

Limitations: Ethical and data privacy concerns are significant limitations to the widespread adoption of artificial intelligence in cardiology and medicine, requiring careful consideration. Regulations are needed to ensure the safe use of artificial intelligence in cardiology and medicine in the future.

3.1. Perspectives and Directions for the Application of Artificial Intelligence in Cardiology

Artificial intelligence (AI) has been integrated into the healthcare industry as a new technology that uses advanced algorithms to synthesize necessary information from huge databases. Research in the field of AI on cardiology has grown exponentially, as can be seen from the number of articles reviewed above. Arrhythmias, ischemia, diseases of the heart valves, heart failure, myocardial infarction, and problems affecting the peripheral arteries and the aorta are all examples of cardiovascular diseases (CVDs) [249].

A significant number of papers have been published in the field of structural heart disease, especially in the field of cardiomyopathies and ischemic heart disease, but also in pulmonary hypertension. At the opposite end of the spectrum, with a relatively smaller number of articles, is research in the field of AI-based arrhythmia and infective endocarditis. Current research also focuses on machine learning, especially in the use of ECG signals and echocardiograms. As an indispensable tool in cardiology, ECG has become one of the most useful tools for collecting data as input for ML, just like echocardiography. In addition, the role of other instruments that collect data, such as coronary angiography, cardiac MRI, or cardiac CT, should not be minimized. Thus, cardiovascular imaging is one of the main sources of information which is far from being at full capacity. In addition, a tremendous amount of data can come from laboratory data, and hospitals can provide the researcher with data on both patient history and patient profile. These opportunities should be exploited closely, as there is great untapped potential at this time.

Convolutional neural networks, recurrent neural networks, and cross-validation are types of AI much more widely used in publications relevant to this paper, as compared to other machine learning techniques. Deep learning is more widely used in general, compared to unsupervised ML or classical ML models. There are also papers in which predictive values are low, although the negative predictive values are high, which raises the issue of further refinement and further development of these systems. The authors of this article believe that in technology research, close collaboration between AI engineers and clinicians makes effective decision making possible. One potential area of future development is engineering in medical AI and medicine; there will probably be discussion in the future about physicians with exhaustive knowledge of medical AI. For significant technological progress and innovation, close collaborations between healthcare engineering systems and physicians are needed [250].

Finally, through this paper, we also wish to highlight some perspectives for future research, perhaps answering questions about legal and ethical considerations. Who decides whether an AI diagnostic system is safe for the patient, government hospitals, or individual hospitals? Who is directly responsible and who is investigated when a malpractice case is taken up: engineers, technology companies, doctors, or hospitals? What can be done about patients' data privacy and who should be trained to protect it? How can we prevent doctors' judgmental standards from falling due to reliance on AI for diagnosis, which may become a serious problem in a few generations [250]? For correct and complete implementation, this side of AI must be addressed, and for the moment, it is one of the most sensitive issues. Scientific knowledge in the field of artificial intelligence in cardiology is, as we have seen in the analysis carried out, in continuous ascension, and different methods are already being implemented all over the world. We can subdivide these methods into several essential aspects: (1) prevention of cardiovascular diseases; (2) screening; (3) diagnosis of cardiovascular diseases; and (4) treatment, all of which function for the adult population and the pediatric population.

3.1.1. Prevention

Preventive cardiology can be seen today as an understudied specialty within cardiovascular treatments. Preventive cardiology aims to improve the known risk factors for CV disease (CVD). Preventive cardiology has also found a use for AI [11], as AI can introduce new treatment methods and important tools to assist the cardiologist in reducing the risk of CVD. The role of AI has been investigated in weight loss, sleep, nutrition, physical activity, dyslipidemia, blood pressure [138], alcohol, smoking, mental health, and recreational drugs. AI has huge potential to be used for the detection, screening, and monitoring of the mentioned risk factors. However, in terms of preventive cardiology, there is a need for the literature to be complemented by future clinical trials addressing this issue [251].

In cardiovascular disease prevention, artificial intelligence has found its place in several areas; it has an important position in precision cardiovascular disease stratification, integration of multi-omics data, discovery of new therapeutic agents, expanding physician effectiveness and efficiency, remote diagnosis and monitoring, and optimal resource allocation in cardiovascular prevention. The newest applications of artificial intelligence in cardiovascular prevention are addressing the main cardiovascular risk factors, in particular dyslipidemia, hypertension, and diabetes [11].

Diabetes carries twice the risk of coronary heart disease, vascular death, and major stroke subtypes, which is why controlling risk factors, especially diabetes, is crucial from childhood. The age of onset of diabetes is steadily decreasing, with one study noting an age of onset of 6–12 years. The study authors also conclude that glycemic balance in children in particular is increasingly difficult to maintain. This study shows statistically significant differences ($p < 0.05$) in terms of mean systolic SBP values with type I diabetes and type II diabetes, which confirms the importance of controlling cardiovascular risk factors from childhood for the prevention of cardiovascular disease, especially as the study also recommends monitoring lipid profile from childhood and applying therapeutic measures [252].

Japanese researchers used a machine learning approach that looked at more than 18,000 patients, and they developed an algorithm with increased sensitivity for predicting new-onset hypertension that demonstrated greater accuracy than the usual logistic regression model, reaching an AUC close to 0.99 [253]. Another larger study confirmed previous results. It included more than 8,000,000 people from East Asia using an open-source platform with potential large-scale applicability [254].

In dyslipidemia, artificial intelligence has tested applications from diagnosis to the management and prognosis of dyslipidemia. Recent studies have demonstrated the possibility of cardiovascular risk assessment using deep learning, which helps to estimate LDL cholesterol with better accuracy using machine learning [255]. In addition, recent predictive methods for incidental dyslipidemia have been obtained by modeling machine learning on larger datasets considering monogenic or polygenic variants [256,257].

A similar study has pointed out that in screening programs, the use of triglycerides to estimate cardiovascular risk is also recommended from childhood. However, caution should be exercised, as elevated values may be falsely elevated, especially in women with high HDL or in patients with metabolic syndrome or diabetes where low HDL levels may occur frequently. Extrapolating from the above information, future studies may address the analysis of triglyceride values using AI to better control cardiovascular risk factors for optimal cardiovascular disease screening [258].

3.1.2. Screening

A recent article has discussed screening for cardiovascular disease in women using AI [259], this being a subcategory analyzed by the authors within the wide range of areas in which AI has proven effective in screening (e.g., congenital disease screening from both ECG analysis [90] to heart sound analysis [91] and fetal ultrasound [93], screening for reduced fraction heart failure [109], screening for hypertension [138], screening for valvular disease [218–220,222,227,228], and screening for rare diseases such as Fabry disease [60]).

Even though the potential opportunities for AI in CVD screening are enormous, further research is needed to objectively assess whether digital technologies improve patient outcomes [260].

3.1.3. Diagnosis

When it comes to cardiovascular diseases, AI also plays an important role in their diagnosis. From the acute diagnosis of left ventricular hypertrophy using imaging methods such as echocardiography [56], to the diagnosis of amyloidosis also based on TTE [66] or idiopathic pulmonary hypertension [157], artificial intelligence has demonstrated its power to help clinicians.

Echocardiography is an imaging method that detects certain abnormalities in real time and is also one of the few imaging methods that allows real-time imaging. Although artificial intelligence has been around since the 1950s, a major focus in recent years has been on the application of AI to diagnostic imaging. Machine learning and other AI techniques can drive a variety of patterns in imaging modalities, particularly echocardiography [261]. The potential clinical applications of AI in echocardiography have increased exponentially, including the identification of specific disease processes such as coronary heart disease, valvular heart disease, hypertrophic cardiomyopathy, cardiac masses, and cardiac amyloidosis and cardiomyopathies (Figure 3).

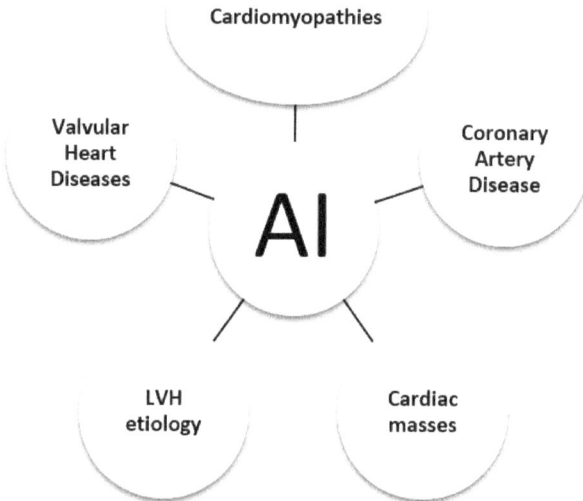

Figure 3. The usefulness of artificial intelligence in echocardiography for diagnosing disease. Created based on information from [261].

In the valvular heart disease subcategory, the focus of AI is on identifying high-risk patients and echocardiographic quantification of the severity of valvular disorders [262]. VHD refers to problems with mitral, aortic, pulmonary, or tricuspid valves. Treatment and identification of cardiovascular diseases could be significantly improved by the application of AI. AI has used various types of echocardiography, ECG, phonocardiography, and ECG to help diagnose valvular diseases.

In this review, we focused our attention on aortic diseases and very little on the mitral valve. Assessment of aortic valve disease's progression can be carried out using AI-based algorithms that integrate the data from the evaluation echocardiography of the aortic valve with additional clinical information [263]. Transcatheter valve replacement decisions, such as the right valve size and selection, can be improved by using AI to automate the measurement of anatomical dimensions derived from imaging data [221].

Recently, a study that included nearly 2000 patients diagnosed with aortic stenosis concluded that AI helped to identify high-risk patients and improved the classification of aortic stenosis severity by integrating echocardiographic measurements. Additionally, identifying subjects at higher risk in this study (patients who had high levels of biomarkers, higher calcium scores of the aortic valve, and higher incidence of negative clinical outcomes) could optimize the timing of aortic valve replacements [264].

Another study, including 1335 test patients and a validated cohort of 311 patients for validation, developed a tool for the automatic screening of echocardiographic videos for aortic and mitral disease. This deep learning algorithm was able to detect the presence of valvular diseases, classify echocardiographic opinions, and quantify the severity of the disease with high accuracy (AOC > 0.88 for all left heart valve diseases) [265]. All of these findings support the effectiveness of a tool to be trained on routine echocardiographic datasets to classify, quantify, and examine the severity of conditions most common in medical practice.

Furthermore, the potential of AI in developing algorithms for CVD diagnosis and prediction will receive major research attention in the coming years. Thus, the application of AI in the field of CVD has gained significant momentum, especially in the diagnosis of coronary heart disease but also in the classification of cardiac arrhythmias, which is a future trend. In addition to echocardiography, other non-invasive imaging techniques such as cardiovascular magnetic resonance imaging (CMRI) possess robust computing power, as well as large datasets and advanced models. In today's world, this is the cornerstone of cardiovascular diagnostics. CMRI is a widely used and accepted tool for assessing cardiovascular risk. It incorporates AI, especially in image recognition and in revolutionizing cardiomyopathy prognostic analyses using late gadolinium enhancement (LGE) [266].

The role of AI extends to minimizing artifacts in CMRI and identifying scar tissues [73,173], thereby increasing diagnostic accuracy and speed [71,153,174]. Studies such as those using RF differentiate hypertrophic from dilated cardiomyopathies and also from healthy patients via CMR analysis [71].

Studies examining ischemic coronary artery disease [11,173–187] use AI both in predicting the disease [180,181,191] and in its diagnosis [179,183,184] or prognosis [41,186–190]. Other studies use machine learning models in patients undergoing coronary artery bypass graft (CABG) surgery to create predictive models of the risk of continuous renal replacement therapy (CRRT) after surgery [267].

A recent study has addressed the topic of CABG patients, who are often frail patients with multiple comorbidities, including chronic obstructive pulmonary disease (COPD), sleep apnea, high blood pressure, and diabetes. COPD is currently one of the most worrying and significant public health problems in many countries. COPD causes an estimated 3.5 million deaths annually and affects over 600 million people worldwide [268]. The most commonly implemented AI algorithms in the diagnosis, prevention, and classification of COPD disease are decision trees and neural networks [269].

In patients with diabetes mellitus, atherosclerotic coronary artery disease is even more common but often more advanced. In these cases, the benefits of percutaneous interventions, which may have a higher risk of in-stent restenosis, have been outweighed by CABG surgery. The authors' perspective thus contributes to a nuanced view of post-CABG outcomes in these patients through appropriate drug treatments but also through post-CABG rehabilitation programs in patients included in their study with/without type 2 diabetes and with/without chronic kidney disease. They demonstrate the clear superior benefit of innovative treatment in cardiology, the SGLT2 inhibitor, which was used during a cardiovascular rehabilitation program and reduced ischemic risk in patients included in their study. This study may represent future research directions in the field of AI in cardiology in patients with ischemic heart disease, especially since the authors mention that their paper is the first in the literature to address this topic (the impact of SGLT2 inhibitors on CABG patients with/without chronic kidney disease and with/without type 2 diabetes mellitus who are undergoing a cardiac rehabilitation program) [270]. There are already studies that have relied on machine learning models that have been designed to perform virtual screening in terms of exploring sodium–glucose cotransporter (SGLT2) inhibitors using AI. The authors have already raised some future research topics, such as identifying new types of drugs as possible next-generation SGLT2 inhibitors and chemotherapy [271].

3.1.4. Treatment

As far as the treatment of cardiovascular disease is concerned, artificial intelligence has found its place even in acute treatment, such as in patients with cardiogenic shock treated with ECMO. When the authors analyzed a group of 258 elderly patients with cardiogenic shock, the mortality rate at 6 months after ECMO treatment was 52 patients (20.16%). Using algorithms, predictive models were constructed to determine the mortality rate and prognosis of the patients in the study. The accuracy, sensitivity, and specificity of the random forest (RF) model were 0.987, 1.000, and 0.929, respectively, which were higher than those of the decision tree model [49]. Additionally, in the treatment of chronic diseases via treatment paradigms for patients with heart failure with acute kidney disease, the authors outlined how AI technologies can be adapted to address major issues among HF patients with acute kidney injury. They identified both personalized interventions and treatment planning using AI without real-time monitoring. In addition, they drew attention to the need for validation and the importance of collaboration between cardiologists and nephrologists [115].

Artificial intelligence has also found its place in the treatment of hypertension [134] and in the treatment of COVID-19 in patients with pulmonary hypertension [148]. The authors discuss patients' adherence to antihypertensive treatment and suggest through this paper that artificial intelligence is an effective alternative to conventional methods for understanding treatment adherence. This finding may be used as a useful tool in educating patients about the importance of medication in the management of hypertension [134].

Artificial intelligence is also involved in the treatment of patients with AMI [175] or acute aortic dissection [226]. The authors created a predictive model based on XGBoost that aims to identify high-risk AAAD patients and develop individualized treatment and diagnostic plans to improve the prognosis of patients diagnosed with AAAD.

To predict the future, we should probably visualize the potential limitations and shortcomings of artificial intelligence at the current stage, as these important elements will have the power to guide us toward new research that will lead to new advances in the years to come. As far as cardiac ultrasound is concerned, AI algorithms are based on datasets that already exist in the real world but which carry the same risks and limits of possible misclassification, the presence of arrhythmias (difficult to handle by artificial intelligence models), and the possibility of sub-optimal image quality (implying limited authenticity or exclusion of some acquisitions, and therefore limited authenticity) when detecting wall motion abnormalities. Additionally, given the frequently inadequate standardization datasets and the limited number and representativeness of datasets, automated software is currently inferior to semi-automatic software in terms of measuring anatomy and morphofunctional structure [272].

3.2. Ethical Considerations of AI in Cardiology

When it comes to artificial intelligence in cardiology, ethical concerns take center stage, especially regarding the privacy of patient data and algorithmic biases. The introduction of AI in cardiology prompts worries about how patient data, often large and sensitive, will be handled to train and test these algorithms. Protecting patient privacy is crucial to maintain trust in the healthcare system. Moreover, there is the issue of algorithmic biases, which can arise from the data used to train AI models. These biases could lead to disparities in healthcare, affecting everything from diagnosis to treatment outcomes. To tackle these ethical challenges, we need transparency in AI development, robust data protection measures, and ongoing efforts to detect and correct algorithmic biases. It is also vital for healthcare professionals, data scientists, ethicists, and policy makers to work together closely to ensure that AI in cardiology is used responsibly and fairly.

3.3. Bias Risk Assessment

A significant concern in the use of AI in cardiology is the risk of bias that can affect outcomes and interpretations. Bias can occur at several stages of the process, including data collection and selection, algorithm construction, and result interpretation. For instance, the input data used for training algorithms may be influenced by population characteristics, collection methods, or human errors. Additionally, the algorithms themselves can be affected by implicit biases embedded in the datasets or in the training process. This can lead to distorted results or incorrect generalizations, compromising the effectiveness and reliability of AI systems in diagnosing and treating cardiac conditions. Therefore, it is crucial to conduct a careful assessment of bias risk in studies utilizing artificial intelligence in cardiology and to apply appropriate methods to minimize and manage this risk.

For a robust design of cardiovascular disease prediction based on machine learning, it is crucial to consider the following aspects: (i) the use of stronger outcomes, such as death, calcium arterial coronary score, or coronary stenosis; (ii) ensuring scientific and clinical validation; (iii) adapting to multi-ethnic groups while practicing unseen AI; and (iv) amalgamating conventional, laboratory, imaging, and pharmacological biomarkers. In the studies we analyzed from the high-quality scientific literature, all these aspects have been assessed and accounted for.

Summary of findings from the papers reviewed:

Common themes: The integration of AI in cardiology has seen substantial growth, particularly in addressing various cardiovascular diseases (CVDs) such as arrhythmias, ischemia, and heart failure. Significant focus on structural heart disease, cardiomyopathies, and ischemic heart disease, alongside emerging areas like pulmonary hypertension, indicates diverse research interests. Utilization of machine learning techniques, especially in analyzing electrocardiogram (ECG) signals and echocardiograms, highlights the importance of AI in data analysis for diagnostic purposes. There is emphasis on the role of cardiovascular imaging techniques, including ECG, echocardiography, coronary angiography, and cardiac MRI, as essential sources of information for AI applications in cardiology.

Challenges: Despite advancements, some AI models exhibit low predictive values, showing the need for further refinement and development. Ethical and legal considerations regarding the safety of AI diagnostic systems, patient data privacy, and potential overreliance on AI for diagnosis pose significant challenges.

Areas of consensus: Collaborative efforts between AI engineers and clinicians are deemed essential for effective technological progress and innovation in medical AI. Future research directions emphasize preventive cardiology, screening, diagnosis, and treatment of cardiovascular diseases using AI, catering to both adult and pediatric populations.

4. Conclusions

The use of artificial intelligence (AI) in the field of cardiovascular diseases represents an emerging paradigm in modern medicine, offering significant advantages in the diagnosis, prognosis, and management of these conditions. From the early identification of thromboembolism and pericarditis to the comprehensive evaluation of valvular and ischemic diseases, AI algorithms provide an essential contribution to improving diagnostic efficiency and clinical decision making.

In the case of thromboembolic diseases, AI algorithms demonstrate an impressive capacity to predict the risk of thromboembolic events and assist in the precise diagnosis of pulmonary embolisms and deep vein thromboses. By identifying subtle patterns in electrocardiographic and medical imaging data, AI enables early detection and prompt intervention, significantly enhancing patient management.

Regarding valvular diseases, AI offers advanced tools for assessment and treatment planning, such as transcatheter aortic valve replacement (TAVR). AI algorithms can make precise and reliable measurements, comparable to those performed manually by physicians, optimizing the decision-making process and ensuring better outcomes for patients.

On the other hand, in pericardial diseases, AI facilitates diagnosis and prognosis, providing a faster and more accurate approach to evaluating ECGs and echocardiographic images. By identifying subtle signs and characteristic patterns, AI algorithms enable early identification of pericarditis and pericardial effusions, contributing to improving patient management.

Last but not least, artificial intelligence holds immense promise in revolutionizing the management of ischemic heart disease, offering enhanced diagnostic accuracy, risk prediction capabilities, and personalized treatment strategies. Its application in cardiovascular care signifies a paradigm shift towards more precise and tailored approaches, ultimately improving patient outcomes and optimizing healthcare delivery.

The use of deep learning algorithms and data processing techniques contributes to optimizing clinical decisions and improving outcomes for patients. However, rigorous implementation and validation are essential to ensure the safety and effectiveness of these technologies in clinical practice.

Author Contributions: Methodology, data curation, writing—original draft preparation, E.S., A.-I.P., O.R.C. and O.C.C.; writing—review and editing, R.C., O.D., A.F., I.G., V.V. and I.F.; supervision, conceptualization and funding, O.R.C. All authors have read and agreed to the published version of the manuscript.

Funding: This research was funded by the "Dunărea de Jos" University of Galati, VAT 27232142, and The APC was paid by the "Dunărea de Jos" University of Galati, VAT 27232142.

Institutional Review Board Statement: Not applicable.

Informed Consent Statement: Not applicable.

Data Availability Statement: Not applicable.

Conflicts of Interest: The authors declare no conflicts of interest.

Abbreviations

ACM	arrhythmogenic cardiomyopathy
ACR	acute cellular rejection
ACS	acute coronary syndrome
AF	atrial fibrillation
AI	artificial intelligence
AI-QCT	artificial intelligence-enabled quantitative coronary computed tomography
AMI	acute myocardial infarction
ARVD	arrhythmogenic heart disease
ATTR-CM	transthyretin amyloid cardiomyopathy
CCTA	coronary computed tomography angiography
CMR	cardiovascular magnetic resonance
CNN	convolutional neural network
DL	deep learning
DCM	dilated cardiomyopathy
DECT	dual-energy computed tomography
ECG	electrocardiogram
FFR	fractional flow reserve
HCA	hierarchical
KMCk	means clustering
IABP	intra-aortic balloon pump
ICA	invasive coronary angiography
IE	infective endocarditis
LA	left atrium
LAAT	left atrial appendage thrombus
LCA	latent class analysis
LV	left ventricle
LVH	left ventricular hypertrophy
MACE	major adverse cardiovascular events
MAPSE	mitral annular plane systolic excursion
MI	myocardial infarction
ML	machine learning
MLP	multiple layer perceptron
MRI	magnetic resonance imagining
PAP	pulmonary artery pressure

PCAT	per coronary adipose tissue
PPG	photoplethysmography
QCA	quantitative coronary angiography
RA	right atrium
RV	right ventricle
STEMI	ST-elevation myocardial infarction
TAVR	transcatheter aortic valve replacement
TTE	transthoracic echocardiography
TOE	transesophageal echocardiography
TCN	temporal convolutional network
XCB	machine learning model based on the xgboost

References

1. Beam, A.L.; Drazen, J.M.; Kohane, I.S.; Leong, T.-Y.; Manrai, A.K.; Rubin, E.J. Artificial Intelligence in Medicine. *N. Engl. J. Med.* **2023**, *388*, 1220–1221. [CrossRef]
2. Lindstrom, M.; DeCleene, N.; Dorsey, H.; Fuster, V.; Johnson, C.O.; LeGrand, K.E.; Mensah, G.A.; Razo, C.; Stark, B.; Turco, J.V.; et al. Global Burden of Cardiovascular Diseases and Risks Collaboration, 1990–2021. *J Am Coll Cardiol.* **2022**, *80*, 2372–2425. [CrossRef]
3. Gala, D.; Behl, H.; Shah, M.; Makaryus, A.N. The Role of Artificial Intelligence in Improving Patient Outcomes and Future of Healthcare Delivery in Cardiology: A Narrative Review of the Literature. *Healthcare* **2024**, *12*, 481. [CrossRef]
4. Sun, X.; Yin, Y.; Yang, Q.; Huo, T. Artificial Intelligence in Cardiovascular Diseases: Diagnostic and Therapeutic Perspectives. *Eur. J. Med. Res.* **2023**, *28*, 242. [CrossRef]
5. Johnson, K.W.; Torres Soto, J.; Glicksberg, B.S.; Shameer, K.; Miotto, R.; Ali, M.; Ashley, E.; Dudley, J.T. Artificial Intelligence in Cardiology. *J. Am. Coll. Cardiol.* **2018**, *71*, 2668–2679. [CrossRef]
6. Shehab, M.; Abualigah, L.; Shambour, Q.; Abu-Hashem, M.A.; Shambour, M.K.Y.; Alsalibi, A.I.; Gandomi, A.H. Machine Learning in Medical Applications: A Review of State-of-the-Art Methods. *Comput. Biol. Med.* **2022**, *145*, 105458. [CrossRef]
7. Yoon, C.H.; Torrance, R.; Scheinerman, N. Machine Learning in Medicine: Should the Pursuit of Enhanced Interpretability Be Abandoned? *J. Med. Ethics* **2022**, *48*, 581–585. [CrossRef]
8. Kahr, M.; Kovács, G.; Loinig, M.; Brückl, H. Condition Monitoring of Ball Bearings Based on Machine Learning with Synthetically Generated Data. *Sensors* **2022**, *22*, 2490. [CrossRef]
9. Mosqueira-Rey, E.; Hernández-Pereira, E.; Alonso-Ríos, D.; Bobes-Bascarán, J.; Fernández-Leal, Á. Human-in-the-Loop Machine Learning: A State of the Art. *Artif. Intell. Rev.* **2023**, *56*, 3005–3054. [CrossRef]
10. Cho, H.; Keenan, G.; Madandola, O.O.; Dos Santos, F.C.; Macieira, T.G.R.; Bjarnadottir, R.I.; Priola, K.J.B.; Dunn Lopez, K. Assessing the Usability of a Clinical Decision Support System: Heuristic Evaluation. *JMIR Hum. Factors* **2022**, *9*, e31758. [CrossRef]
11. Ciccarelli, M.; Giallauria, F.; Carrizzo, A.; Visco, V.; Silverio, A.; Cesaro, A.; Calabrò, P.; De Luca, N.; Mancusi, C.; Masarone, D.; et al. Artificial Intelligence in Cardiovascular Prevention: New Ways Will Open New Doors. *J. Cardiovasc. Med.* **2023**, *24* (Suppl. S2), e106–e115. [CrossRef]
12. Busnatu, Ș.; Niculescu, A.-G.; Bolocan, A.; Petrescu, G.E.D.; Păduraru, D.N.; Năstasă, I.; Lupușoru, M.; Geantă, M.; Andronic, O.; Grumezescu, A.M.; et al. Clinical Applications of Artificial Intelligence—An Updated Overview. *J. Clin. Med.* **2022**, *11*, 2265. [CrossRef]
13. Van den Eynde, J.; Lachmann, M.; Laugwitz, K.-L.; Manlhiot, C.; Kutty, S. Successfully Implemented Artificial Intelligence and Machine Learning Applications in Cardiology: State-of-the-Art Review. *Trends Cardiovasc. Med.* **2023**, *33*, 265–271. [CrossRef]
14. Visco, V.; Ferruzzi, G.J.; Nicastro, F.; Virtuoso, N.; Carrizzo, A.; Galasso, G.; Vecchione, C.; Ciccarelli, M. Artificial Intelligence as a Business Partner in Cardiovascular Precision Medicine: An Emerging Approach for Disease Detection and Treatment Optimization. *Curr. Med. Chem.* **2021**, *28*, 6569–6590. [CrossRef]
15. Soori, M.; Arezoo, B.; Dastres, R. Machine Learning and Artificial Intelligence in CNC Machine Tools, A Review. *Sustain. Manuf. Serv. Econ.* **2023**, *2*, 100009. [CrossRef]
16. Javaid, M.; Haleem, A.; Pratap Singh, R.; Suman, R.; Rab, S. Significance of Machine Learning in Healthcare: Features, Pillars and Applications. *Int. J. Intell. Netw.* **2022**, *3*, 58–73. [CrossRef]
17. Goodswen, S.J.; Barratt, J.L.N.; Kennedy, P.J.; Kaufer, A.; Calarco, L.; Ellis, J.T. Machine Learning and Applications in Microbiology. *FEMS Microbiol. Rev.* **2021**, *45*, fuab015. [CrossRef]
18. Ahmad, A.A.; Polat, H. Prediction of Heart Disease Based on Machine Learning Using Jellyfish Optimization Algorithm. *Diagnostics* **2023**, *13*, 2392. [CrossRef]
19. Alzubaidi, L.; Bai, J.; Al-Sabaawi, A.; Santamaría, J.; Albahri, A.S.; Al-dabba, B.S.N.; Fadhel, M.A.; Manoufali, M.; Zhang, J.; Al-Timemy, A.H.; et al. A Survey on Deep Learning Tools Dealing with Data Scarcity: Definitions, Challenges, Solutions, Tips, and Applications. *J. Big Data* **2023**, *10*, 46. [CrossRef]
20. Srivani, M.; Murugappan, A.; Mala, T. Cognitive Computing Technological Trends and Future Research Directions in Healthcare—A Systematic Literature Review. *Artif. Intell. Med.* **2023**, *138*, 102513. [CrossRef]

21. Vinny, P.W.; Vishnu, V.Y.; Padma Srivastava, M.V. Artificial Intelligence Shaping the Future of Neurology Practice. *Med. J. Armed Forces India* **2021**, *77*, 276–282. [CrossRef] [PubMed]
22. Zhu, R.; Jiang, C.; Wang, X.; Wang, S.; Zheng, H.; Tang, H. Privacy-Preserving Construction of Generalized Linear Mixed Model for Biomedical Computation. *Bioinformatics* **2020**, *36* (Suppl. S1), i128–i135. [CrossRef] [PubMed]
23. Yadav, R.S. Data Analysis of COVID-2019 Epidemic Using Machine Learning Methods: A Case Study of India. *Int. J. Inf. Technol.* **2020**, *12*, 1321–1330. [CrossRef] [PubMed]
24. Hügle, M.; Omoumi, P.; van Laar, J.M.; Boedecker, J.; Hügle, T. Applied Machine Learning and Artificial Intelligence in Rheumatology. *Rheumatol. Adv. Pract.* **2020**, *4*, rkaa005. [CrossRef] [PubMed]
25. Sharma, A.; Pal, T.; Jaiswal, V. Heart Disease Prediction Using Convolutional Neural Network. In *Cardiovascular and Coronary Artery Imaging*; Elsevier: Amsterdam, The Netherlands, 2022; pp. 245–272.
26. Teuwen, J.; Moriakov, N. *Handbook of Medical Image Computing and Computer Assisted Intervention*; Academic Press: Cambridge, MA, USA, 2020.
27. Xiong, Z.; Nash, M.P.; Cheng, E.; Fedorov, V.V.; Stiles, M.K.; Zhao, J. ECG Signal Classification for the Detection of Cardiac Arrhythmias Using a Convolutional Recurrent Neural Network. *Physiol. Meas.* **2018**, *39*, 094006. [CrossRef] [PubMed]
28. Williams, S.; Layard Horsfall, H.; Funnell, J.P.; Hanrahan, J.G.; Khan, D.Z.; Muirhead, W.; Stoyanov, D.; Marcus, H.J. Artificial Intelligence in Brain Tumour Surgery—An Emerging Paradigm. *Cancers* **2021**, *13*, 5010. [CrossRef] [PubMed]
29. Mahesh, B. Machine learning algorithms-a review. *Int. J. Sci. Res.* **2020**, *9*, 381–386.
30. Sarker, I.H. Machine Learning: Algorithms, Real-World Applications and Research Directions. *SN Comput. Sci.* **2021**, *2*, 160. [CrossRef] [PubMed]
31. Al-Sayed, A.; Khayyat, M.M.; Zamzami, N. Predicting Heart Disease Using Collaborative Clustering and Ensemble Learning Techniques. *Appl. Sci.* **2023**, *13*, 13278. [CrossRef]
32. Sahlab, N.; Sonji, I.; Weyrich, M. Graph-Based Association Rule Learning for Context-Based Health Monitoring to Enable User-Centered Assistance. *Artif. Intell. Med.* **2023**, *135*, 102455. [CrossRef]
33. Kumar, K.A.; Gowri, S.; David, J.J.W.; Bevish Jinila, Y. An Efficient Association Rule Mining from Distributed Medical Database for Predicting Heart Disease. In Proceedings of the 2022 6th International Conference on Computing Methodologies and Communication (ICCMC), Erode, India, 29–31 March 2022; IEEE: Piscataway, NJ, USA, 2022; pp. 791–795.
34. Chaudhuri, A.K.; Das, A.; Addy, M. Identifying the Association Rule to Determine the Possibilities of Cardio Vascular Diseases (CVD). In *Advances in Intelligent Systems and Computing*; Springer: Singapore, 2021; pp. 219–229.
35. Tran, K.-V.; Filippaios, A.; Noorishirazi, K.; Ding, E. False Atrial Fibrillation Alerts from Smartwatches Are Associated with Decreased Perceived Physical Well-Being and Confidence in Chronic Symptoms Management. *Cardiol. Cardiovasc. Med.* **2023**, *7*, 97–107. [CrossRef] [PubMed]
36. Baj, G.; Gandin, I.; Scagnetto, A.; Bortolussi, L.; Cappelletto, C.; Di Lenarda, A.; Barbati, G. Comparison of Discrimination and Calibration Performance of ECG-Based Machine Learning Models for Prediction of New-Onset Atrial Fibrillation. *BMC Med. Res. Methodol.* **2023**, *23*, 169. [CrossRef] [PubMed]
37. Raghunath, A.; Nguyen, D.D.; Schram, M.; Albert, D.; Gollakota, S.; Shapiro, L.; Sridhar, A.R. Artificial Intelligence–Enabled Mobile Electrocardiograms for Event Prediction in Paroxysmal Atrial Fibrillation. *Cardiovasc. Digit. Health J.* **2023**, *4*, 21–28. [CrossRef] [PubMed]
38. Jiang, J.; Deng, H.; Liao, H.; Fang, X.; Zhan, X.; Wei, W.; Wu, S.; Xue, Y. An Artificial Intelligence-Enabled ECG Algorithm for Predicting the Risk of Recurrence in Patients with Paroxysmal Atrial Fibrillation after Catheter Ablation. *J. Clin. Med.* **2023**, *12*, 1933. [CrossRef] [PubMed]
39. Bai, Y.; Wang, Z.-Z.; Zhang, G.-G.; Guo, S.-D.; Rivera-Caravaca, J.M.; Wang, Y.-L.; Jin, Y.-Y.; Liu, Y. Validating Scores Predicting Atrial Fibrillation Recurrence Post Catheter Ablation in Patients with Concurrent Atrial Fibrillation and Pulmonary Diseases. *Ann. Palliat. Med.* **2021**, *10*, 4299–4307. [CrossRef] [PubMed]
40. Rahman, F.; Finkelstein, N.; Alyakin, A.; Gilotra, N.A.; Trost, J.; Schulman, S.P.; Saria, S. Using Machine Learning for Early Prediction of Cardiogenic Shock in Patients with Acute Heart Failure. *J. Soc. Cardiovasc. Angiogr. Interv.* **2022**, *1*, 100308. [CrossRef]
41. Bai, Z.; Hu, S.; Wang, Y.; Deng, W.; Gu, N.; Zhao, R.; Zhang, W.; Ma, Y.; Wang, Z.; Liu, Z.; et al. Development of a Machine Learning Model to Predict the Risk of Late Cardiogenic Shock in Patients with ST-Segment Elevation Myocardial Infarction. *Ann. Transl. Med.* **2021**, *9*, 1162. [CrossRef] [PubMed]
42. Chang, Y.; Antonescu, C.; Ravindranath, S.; Dong, J.; Lu, M.; Vicario, F.; Wondrely, L.; Thompson, P.; Swearingen, D.; Acharya, D. Early Prediction of Cardiogenic Shock Using Machine Learning. *Front. Cardiovasc. Med.* **2022**, *9*, 862424. [CrossRef] [PubMed]
43. Jajcay, N.; Bezak, B.; Segev, A.; Matetzky, S.; Jankova, J.; Spartalis, M.; El Tahlawi, M.; Guerra, F.; Friebel, J.; Thevathasan, T.; et al. Data Processing Pipeline for Cardiogenic Shock Prediction Using Machine Learning. *Front. Cardiovasc. Med.* **2023**, *10*, 1132680. [CrossRef]
44. Jentzer, J.C.; Rayfield, C.; Soussi, S.; Berg, D.D.; Kennedy, J.N.; Sinha, S.S.; Baran, D.A.; Brant, E.; Mebazaa, A.; Billia, F.; et al. Machine Learning Approaches for Phenotyping in Cardiogenic Shock and Critical Illness. *JACC Adv.* **2022**, *1*, 100126. [CrossRef]
45. Wang, L.; Zhang, Y.; Yao, R.; Chen, K.; Xu, Q.; Huang, R.; Mao, Z.; Yu, Y. Identification of Distinct Clinical Phenotypes of Cardiogenic Shock Using Machine Learning Consensus Clustering Approach. *BMC Cardiovasc. Disord.* **2023**, *23*, 426. [CrossRef] [PubMed]

46. Bohm, A.; Jajcay, N.; Jankova, J.; Petrikova, K.; Bezak, B. Artificial Intelligence Model for Prediction of Cardiogenic Shock in Patients with Acute Coronary Syndrome. *Eur. Heart J. Acute Cardiovasc. Care* **2022**, *11* (Suppl. S1), zuac041-077. [CrossRef]
47. Popat, A.; Yadav, S.; Patel, S.K.; Baddevolu, S.; Adusumilli, S.; Rao Dasari, N.; Sundarasetty, M.; Anand, S.; Sankar, J.; Jagtap, Y.G. Artificial Intelligence in the Early Prediction of Cardiogenic Shock in Acute Heart Failure or Myocardial Infarction Patients: A Systematic Review and Meta-Analysis. *Cureus* **2023**, *15*, e50395. [CrossRef] [PubMed]
48. Rong, F.; Xiang, H.; Qian, L.; Xue, Y.; Ji, K.; Yin, R. Machine Learning for Prediction of Outcomes in Cardiogenic Shock. *Front. Cardiovasc. Med.* **2022**, *9*, 849688. [CrossRef]
49. Mo, Z.; Lu, Z.; Tang, X.; Lin, X.; Wang, S.; Zhang, Y.; Huang, Z. Construction and Evaluation of Prognostic Models of ECMO in Elderly Patients with Cardiogenic Shock Based on BP Neural Network, Random Forest, and Decision Tree. *Am. J. Transl. Res.* **2023**, *15*, 4639–4648. [PubMed]
50. Cau, R.; Pisu, F.; Suri, J.S.; Montisci, R.; Gatti, M.; Mannelli, L.; Gong, X.; Saba, L. Artificial Intelligence in the Differential Diagnosis of Cardiomyopathy Phenotypes. *Diagnostics* **2024**, *14*, 156. [CrossRef] [PubMed]
51. Haimovich, J.S.; Diamant, N.; Khurshid, S.; Di Achille, P.; Reeder, C.; Friedman, S.; Singh, P.; Spurlock, W.; Ellinor, P.T.; Philippakis, A.; et al. Artificial Intelligence-Enabled Classification of Hypertrophic Heart Diseases Using Electrocardiograms. *Cardiovasc. Digit. Health J.* **2023**, *4*, 48–59. [CrossRef]
52. Beneyto, M.; Ghyaza, G.; Cariou, E.; Amar, J.; Lairez, O. Development and Validation of Machine Learning Algorithms to Predict Posthypertensive Origin in Left Ventricular Hypertrophy. *Arch. Cardiovasc. Dis.* **2023**, *116*, 397–402. [CrossRef] [PubMed]
53. Eckstein, J.; Moghadasi, N.; Körperich, H.; Weise Valdés, E.; Sciacca, V.; Paluszkiewicz, L.; Burchert, W.; Piran, M. A Machine Learning Challenge: Detection of Cardiac Amyloidosis Based on Bi-Atrial and Right Ventricular Strain and Cardiac Function. *Diagnostics* **2022**, *12*, 2693. [CrossRef]
54. Siontis, K.C.; Liu, K.; Bos, J.M.; Attia, Z.I.; Cohen-Shelly, M.; Arruda-Olson, A.M.; Zanjirani Farahani, N.; Friedman, P.A.; Noseworthy, P.A.; Ackerman, M.J. Detection of Hypertrophic Cardiomyopathy by an Artificial Intelligence Electrocardiogram in Children and Adolescents. *Int. J. Cardiol.* **2021**, *340*, 42–47. [CrossRef]
55. Ko, W.-Y.; Siontis, K.C.; Attia, Z.I.; Carter, R.E.; Kapa, S.; Ommen, S.R.; Demuth, S.J.; Ackerman, M.J.; Gersh, B.J.; Arruda-Olson, A.M.; et al. Detection of Hypertrophic Cardiomyopathy Using a Convolutional Neural Network-Enabled Electrocardiogram. *J. Am. Coll. Cardiol.* **2020**, *75*, 722–733. [CrossRef] [PubMed]
56. Hwang, I.-C.; Choi, D.; Choi, Y.-J.; Ju, L.; Kim, M.; Hong, J.-E.; Lee, H.-J.; Yoon, Y.E.; Park, J.-B.; Lee, S.-P.; et al. Differential Diagnosis of Common Etiologies of Left Ventricular Hypertrophy Using a Hybrid CNN-LSTM Model. *Sci. Rep.* **2022**, *12*, 20998. [CrossRef] [PubMed]
57. Zhou, M.; Deng, Y.; Liu, Y.; Su, X.; Zeng, X. Echocardiography-Based Machine Learning Algorithm for Distinguishing Ischemic Cardiomyopathy from Dilated Cardiomyopathy. *BMC Cardiovasc. Disord.* **2023**, *23*, 476. [CrossRef] [PubMed]
58. Cau, R.; Pisu, F.; Porcu, M.; Cademartiri, F.; Montisci, R.; Bassareo, P.; Muscogiuri, G.; Amadu, A.; Sironi, S.; Esposito, A.; et al. Machine Learning Approach in Diagnosing Takotsubo Cardiomyopathy: The Role of the Combined Evaluation of Atrial and Ventricular Strain, and Parametric Mapping. *Int. J. Cardiol.* **2023**, *373*, 124–133. [CrossRef] [PubMed]
59. De Filippo, O.; Cammann, V.L.; Pancotti, C.; Di Vece, D.; Silverio, A.; Schweiger, V.; Niederseer, D.; Szawan, K.A.; Würdinger, M.; Koleva, I.; et al. Machine Learning-based Prediction of In-hospital Death for Patients with Takotsubo Syndrome: The InterTAK-ML Model. *Eur. J. Heart Fail.* **2023**, *25*, 2299–2311. [CrossRef] [PubMed]
60. Jefferies, J.L.; Spencer, A.K.; Lau, H.A.; Nelson, M.W.; Giuliano, J.D.; Zabinski, J.W.; Boussios, C.; Curhan, G.; Gliklich, R.E.; Warnock, D.G. A New Approach to Identifying Patients with Elevated Risk for Fabry Disease Using a Machine Learning Algorithm. *Orphanet J. Rare Dis.* **2021**, *16*, 1–8. [CrossRef] [PubMed]
61. Soto, J.T.; Weston Hughes, J.; Sanchez, P.A.; Perez, M.; Ouyang, D.; Ashley, E.A. Multimodal Deep Learning Enhances Diagnostic Precision in Left Ventricular Hypertrophy. *Eur. Heart J. Digit. Health* **2022**, *3*, 380–389. [CrossRef]
62. Zhang, Y.; Xie, J.; Wu, Y.; Zhang, B.; Zhou, C.; Gao, X.; Xie, X.; Li, X.; Yu, J.; Wang, X.; et al. Novel Algorithm for Diagnosis of Arrhythmogenic Cardiomyopathy and Dilated Cardiomyopathy: Key Gene Expression Profiling Using Machine Learning. *J. Gene Med.* **2023**, *25*, e3468. [CrossRef]
63. Papageorgiou, V.E.; Zegkos, T.; Efthimiadis, G.; Tsaklidis, G. Analysis of Digitalized ECG Signals Based on Artificial Intelligence and Spectral Analysis Methods Specialized in ARVC. *Int. J. Numer. Method. Biomed. Eng.* **2022**, *38*, e3644. [CrossRef]
64. Harmon, D.M.; Mangold, K.; Baez Suarez, A.; Scott, C.G.; Murphree, D.H., Jr.; Malik, A.; Attia, Z.I.; Lopez-Jimenez, F.; Friedman, P.A.; Dispenzieri, A.; et al. Postdevelopment Performance and Validation of the Artificial Intelligence-Enhanced Electrocardiogram for Detection of Cardiac Amyloidosis. *JACC Adv.* **2023**, *2*, 100612. [CrossRef]
65. Cotella, J.I.; Slivnick, J.A.; Sanderson, E.; Singulane, C.; O'Driscoll, J.; Asch, F.M.; Addetia, K.; Woodward, G.; Lang, R.M. Artificial Intelligence Based Left Ventricular Ejection Fraction and Global Longitudinal Strain in Cardiac Amyloidosis. *Echocardiography* **2023**, *40*, 188–195. [CrossRef] [PubMed]
66. Zhang, X.; Liang, Y.; Su, C.; Qin, S.; Li, J.; Zeng, D.; Cai, Y.; Huang, T.; Wu, J. Deep Learn-Based Computer-Assisted Transthoracic Echocardiography: Approach to the Diagnosis of Cardiac Amyloidosis. *Int. J. Cardiovasc. Imaging* **2023**, *39*, 955–965. [CrossRef] [PubMed]
67. Goswami, R.; Jang, J.; Ruiz, J.; Desai, S.; Paghdar, S.; Malkani, S.; Yip, D.; Leoni, J.; Patel, P.; Lyle, M.; et al. (28) Artificial Intelligence to Predict Death or Transplant in ATTR Amyloidosis Cardiomyopathy. *J. Heart Lung Transplant.* **2023**, *42*, S22–S23. [CrossRef]

68. Michalski, A.A.; Lis, K.; Stankiewicz, J.; Kloska, S.M.; Sycz, A.; Dudziński, M.; Muras-Szwedziak, K.; Nowicki, M.; Bazan-Socha, S.; Dabrowski, M.J.; et al. Supporting the Diagnosis of Fabry Disease Using a Natural Language Processing-Based Approach. *J. Clin. Med.* **2023**, *12*, 3599. [CrossRef] [PubMed]
69. Jefferies, J.; Aguiar, P.; Biondetti, G.; Warnock, D.; Kallish, S.; Nelson, M.; Giuliano, J.; Zabinksi, J.; Boussios, C.; Curhan, G.; et al. (751) Estimation of Arrhythmia Risk in Patients with Fabry Disease Using a Machine Learning Model. *J. Heart Lung Transplant* **2023**, *42*, S331. [CrossRef]
70. Stolpe, G.; Didier, R.; Martel, H.; Claire, L.; Michel, N.; Sellami, S.; Essayagh, B.; Réant, P.; Donal, E.; Habib, G. Contribution of Artificial Intelligence and Left Atrial Strain in the Prediction of Sudden Cardiac Death in Hypertrophic Cardiomyopathy. Results of a Multicentric Cohort. *Arch. Cardiovasc. Dis. Suppl.* **2023**, *15*, 237. [CrossRef]
71. Zhang, X.; Cui, C.; Zhao, S.; Xie, L.; Tian, Y. Cardiac Magnetic Resonance Radiomics for Disease Classification. *Eur. Radiol.* **2022**, *33*, 2312–2323. [CrossRef] [PubMed]
72. Tatsugami, F.; Nakaura, T.; Yanagawa, M.; Fujita, S.; Kamagata, K.; Ito, R.; Kawamura, M.; Fushimi, Y.; Ueda, D.; Matsui, Y.; et al. Recent Advances in Artificial Intelligence for Cardiac CT: Enhancing Diagnosis and Prognosis Prediction. *Diagn. Interv. Imaging* **2023**, *104*, 521–528. [CrossRef]
73. O'Brien, H.; Williams, M.C.; Rajani, R.; Niederer, S. Radiomics and Machine Learning for Detecting Scar Tissue on CT Delayed Enhancement Imaging. *Front. Cardiovasc. Med.* **2022**, *9*, 847825. [CrossRef]
74. Wen, D.; Xu, Z.; An, R.; Ren, J.; Jia, Y.; Li, J.; Zheng, M. Predicting Haemodynamic Significance of Coronary Stenosis with Radiomics-Based Pericoronary Adipose Tissue Characteristics. *Clin. Radiol.* **2022**, *77*, e154–e161. [CrossRef]
75. Lara-Hernández, A.; Rienmüller, T.; Juárez, I.; Pérez, M.; Reyna, F.; Baumgartner, D.; Makarenko, V.N.; Bockeria, O.L.; Maksudov, M.; Rienmüller, R.; et al. Deep Learning-Based Image Registration in Dynamic Myocardial Perfusion CT Imaging. *IEEE Trans. Med. Imaging* **2023**, *42*, 684–696. [CrossRef]
76. Griffin, W.F.; Choi, A.D.; Riess, J.S.; Marques, H.; Chang, H.-J.; Choi, J.H.; Doh, J.-H.; Her, A.-Y.; Koo, B.-K.; Nam, C.-W.; et al. AI Evaluation of Stenosis on Coronary CTA, Comparison with Quantitative Coronary Angiography and Fractional Flow Reserve. *JACC Cardiovasc. Imaging* **2023**, *16*, 193–205. [CrossRef]
77. Brandt, V.; Schoepf, U.J.; Aquino, G.J.; Bekeredjian, R.; Varga-Szemes, A.; Emrich, T.; Bayer, R.R., II; Schwarz, F.; Kroencke, T.J.; Tesche, C.; et al. Impact of Machine-Learning-Based Coronary Computed Tomography Angiography–Derived Fractional Flow Reserve on Decision-Making in Patients with Severe Aortic Stenosis Undergoing Transcatheter Aortic Valve Replacement. *Eur. Radiol.* **2022**, *32*, 6008–6016. [CrossRef]
78. Li, X.-N.; Yin, W.-H.; Sun, Y.; Kang, H.; Luo, J.; Chen, K.; Hou, Z.-H.; Gao, Y.; Ren, X.-S.; Yu, Y.-T.; et al. Identification of Pathology-Confirmed Vulnerable Atherosclerotic Lesions by Coronary Computed Tomography Angiography Using Radiomics Analysis. *Eur. Radiol.* **2022**, *32*, 4003–4013. [CrossRef]
79. Lyu, T.; Zhao, W.; Zhu, Y.; Wu, Z.; Zhang, Y.; Chen, Y.; Luo, L.; Li, S.; Xing, L. Estimating Dual-Energy CT Imaging from Single-Energy CT Data with Material Decomposition Convolutional Neural Network. *Med. Image Anal.* **2021**, *70*, 102001. [CrossRef] [PubMed]
80. Zhang, R.; Wang, P.; Bian, Y.; Fan, Y.; Li, J.; Liu, X.; Shen, J.; Hu, Y.; Liao, X.; Wang, H.; et al. Establishment and Validation of an AI-Aid Method in the Diagnosis of Myocardial Perfusion Imaging. *BMC Med. Imaging* **2023**, *23*, 84. [CrossRef] [PubMed]
81. Khunte, A.; Sangha, V.; Oikonomou, E.K.; Dhingra, L.S.; Aminorroaya, A.; Mortazavi, B.J.; Coppi, A.; Brandt, C.A.; Krumholz, H.M.; Khera, R. Detection of Left Ventricular Systolic Dysfunction from Single-Lead Electrocardiography Adapted for Portable and Wearable Devices. *NPJ Digit. Med.* **2023**, *6*, 1–10. [CrossRef] [PubMed]
82. Pieszko, K.; Hiczkiewicz, J.; Łojewska, K.; Uziębło-Życzkowska, B.; Krzesiński, P.; Gawałko, M.; Budnik, M.; Starzyk, K.; Wożakowska-Kapłon, B.; Daniłowicz-Szymanowicz, L.; et al. Artificial Intelligence in Detecting Left Atrial Appendage Thrombus by Transthoracic Echocardiography and Clinical Features: The Left Atrial Thrombus on Transoesophageal Echocardiography (LATTEE) Registry. *Eur. Heart J.* **2024**, *45*, 32–41. [CrossRef] [PubMed]
83. Liu, Z.; Li, H.; Li, W.; Zhang, F.; Ouyang, W.; Wang, S.; Zhi, A.; Pan, X. Development of an Expert-Level Right Ventricular Abnormality Detection Algorithm Based on Deep Learning. *Interdiscip. Sci.* **2023**, *15*, 653–662. [CrossRef]
84. Wang, Y.; Sun, C.; Ghadimi, S.; Auger, D.C.; Croisille, P.; Viallon, M.; Mangion, K.; Berry, C.; Haggerty, C.M.; Jing, L.; et al. StrainNet: Improved Myocardial Strain Analysis of Cine MRI by Deep Learning from DENSE. *Radiol. Cardiothorac. Imaging* **2023**, *5*, e220196. [CrossRef]
85. Yu, J.; Taskén, A.A.; Flade, H.M.; Skogvoll, E.; Berg, E.A.R.; Grenne, B.; Rimehaug, A.; Kirkeby-Garstad, I.; Kiss, G.; Aakhus, S. Automatic Assessment of Left Ventricular Function for Hemodynamic Monitoring Using Artificial Intelligence and Transesophageal Echocardiography. *J. Clin. Monit. Comput.* **2024**, *38*, 281–291. [CrossRef]
86. Laumer, F.; Di Vece, D.; Cammann, V.L.; Würdinger, M.; Petkova, V.; Schönberger, M.; Schönberger, A.; Mercier, J.C.; Niederseer, D.; Seifert, B.; et al. Assessment of Artificial Intelligence in Echocardiography Diagnostics in Differentiating Takotsubo Syndrome from Myocardial Infarction. *JAMA Cardiol.* **2022**, *7*, 494. [CrossRef] [PubMed]
87. Lee, D.-Y.; Chang, C.-C.; Ko, C.-F.; Lee, Y.-H.; Tsai, Y.-L.; Chou, R.-H.; Chang, T.-Y.; Guo, S.-M.; Huang, P.-H. Artificial Intelligence Evaluation of Coronary Computed Tomography Angiography for Coronary Stenosis Classification and Diagnosis. *Eur. J. Clin. Investig.* **2024**, *54*, e14089. [CrossRef] [PubMed]

88. Kalapos, A.; Szabó, L.; Dohy, Z.; Kiss, M.; Merkely, B.; Gyires-Tóth, B.; Vágó, H. Automated T1 and T2 Mapping Segmentation on Cardiovascular Magnetic Resonance Imaging Using Deep Learning. *Front. Cardiovasc. Med.* **2023**, *10*, 1147581. [CrossRef] [PubMed]
89. Ishikita, A.; McIntosh, C.; Hanneman, K.; Lee, M.M.; Liang, T.; Karur, G.R.; Roche, S.L.; Hickey, E.; Geva, T.; Barron, D.J.; et al. Machine Learning for Prediction of Adverse Cardiovascular Events in Adults with Repaired Tetralogy of Fallot Using Clinical and Cardiovascular Magnetic Resonance Imaging Variables. *Circ. Cardiovasc. Imaging* **2023**, *16*, e015205. [CrossRef] [PubMed]
90. De Vries, I.R.; van Laar, J.O.E.H.; van der Hout-van der Jagt, M.B.; Clur, S.-A.B.; Vullings, R. Fetal Electrocardiography and Artificial Intelligence for Prenatal Detection of Congenital Heart Disease. *Acta Obstet. Gynecol. Scand.* **2023**, *102*, 1511–1520. [CrossRef] [PubMed]
91. Lv, J.; Dong, B.; Lei, H.; Shi, G.; Wang, H.; Zhu, F.; Wen, C.; Zhang, Q.; Fu, L.; Gu, X.; et al. Artificial Intelligence-Assisted Auscultation in Detecting Congenital Heart Disease. *Eur. Heart J. Digit. Health* **2021**, *2*, 119–124. [CrossRef] [PubMed]
92. Majeed, A.; Rofeberg, V.; Bellinger, D.C.; Wypij, D.; Newburger, J.W. Machine Learning to Predict Executive Function in Adolescents with Repaired D-Transposition of the Great Arteries, Tetralogy of Fallot, and Fontan Palliation. *J. Pediatr.* **2022**, *246*, 145–153. [CrossRef] [PubMed]
93. Sakai, A.; Komatsu, M.; Komatsu, R.; Matsuoka, R.; Yasutomi, S.; Dozen, A.; Shozu, K.; Arakaki, T.; Machino, H.; Asada, K.; et al. Medical Professional Enhancement Using Explainable Artificial Intelligence in Fetal Cardiac Ultrasound Screening. *Biomedicines* **2022**, *10*, 551. [CrossRef]
94. Gearhart, A.; Goto, S.; Deo, R.C.; Powell, A.J. An Automated View Classification Model for Pediatric Echocardiography Using Artificial Intelligence. *J. Am. Soc. Echocardiogr.* **2022**, *35*, 1238–1246. [CrossRef]
95. Valente Silva, B.; Marques, J.; Nobre Menezes, M.; Oliveira, A.L.; Pinto, F.J. Artificial Intelligence-Based Diagnosis of Acute Pulmonary Embolism: Development of a Machine Learning Model Using 12-Lead Electrocardiogram. *Rev. Port. Cardiol.* **2023**, *42*, 643–651. [CrossRef] [PubMed]
96. Adedinsewo, D.; Hardway, H.D.; Morales-Lara, A.C.; Wieczorek, M.A.; Johnson, P.W.; Douglass, E.J.; Dangott, B.J.; Nakhleh, R.E.; Narula, T.; Patel, P.C.; et al. Non-Invasive Detection of Cardiac Allograft Rejection among Heart Transplant Recipients Using an Electrocardiogram Based Deep Learning Model. *Eur. Heart J. Digit. Health* **2023**, *4*, 71–80. [CrossRef] [PubMed]
97. Shiraishi, Y.; Goto, S.; Niimi, N.; Katsumata, Y.; Goda, A.; Takei, M.; Saji, M.; Sano, M.; Fukuda, K.; Kohno, T.; et al. Improved Prediction of Sudden Cardiac Death in Patients with Heart Failure through Digital Processing of Electrocardiography. *Europace* **2023**, *25*, 922–930. [CrossRef] [PubMed]
98. Hirota, N.; Suzuki, S.; Motogi, J.; Nakai, H.; Matsuzawa, W.; Takayanagi, T.; Umemoto, T.; Hyodo, A.; Satoh, K.; Arita, T.; et al. Cardiovascular Events and Artificial Intelligence-Predicted Age Using 12-Lead Electrocardiograms. *Int. J. Cardiol. Heart Vasc.* **2023**, *44*, 101172. [CrossRef] [PubMed]
99. Wouters, P.C.; van de Leur, R.R.; Vessies, M.B.; van Stipdonk, A.M.W.; Ghossein, M.A.; Hassink, R.J.; Doevendans, P.A.; van der Harst, P.; Maass, A.H.; Prinzen, F.W.; et al. Electrocardiogram-Based Deep Learning Improves Outcome Prediction Following Cardiac Resynchronization Therapy. *Eur. Heart J.* **2023**, *44*, 680–692. [CrossRef] [PubMed]
100. Liu, C.-W.; Wu, F.-H.; Hu, Y.-L.; Pan, R.-H.; Lin, C.-H.; Chen, Y.-F.; Tseng, G.-S.; Chan, Y.-K.; Wang, C.-L. Left Ventricular Hypertrophy Detection Using Electrocardiographic Signal. *Sci. Rep.* **2023**, *13*, 2556. [CrossRef] [PubMed]
101. Zaver, H.B.; Mzaik, O.; Thomas, J.; Roopkumar, J.; Adedinsewo, D.; Keaveny, A.P.; Patel, T. Utility of an Artificial Intelligence Enabled Electrocardiogram for Risk Assessment in Liver Transplant Candidates. *Dig. Dis. Sci.* **2023**, *68*, 2379–2388. [CrossRef] [PubMed]
102. Naser, J.A.; Lopez-Jimenez, F.; Chang, A.Y.; Baez-Suarez, A.; Attia, Z.I.; Pislaru, S.V.; Pellikka, P.A.; Lin, G.; Kapa, S.; Friedman, P.A.; et al. Artificial Intelligence-Augmented Electrocardiogram in Determining Sex. *Mayo Clin. Proc.* **2023**, *98*, 541–548. [CrossRef] [PubMed]
103. Vaid, A.; Argulian, E.; Lerakis, S.; Beaulieu-Jones, B.K.; Krittanawong, C.; Klang, E.; Lampert, J.; Reddy, V.Y.; Narula, J.; Nadkarni, G.N.; et al. Multi-Center Retrospective Cohort Study Applying Deep Learning to Electrocardiograms to Identify Left Heart Valvular Dysfunction. *Commun. Med.* **2023**, *3*, 24. [CrossRef]
104. Khan, M.S.; Arshad, M.S.; Greene, S.J.; Van Spall, H.G.C.; Pandey, A.; Vemulapalli, S.; Perakslis, E.; Butler, J. Artificial Intelligence and Heart Failure: A State-of-the-art Review. *Eur. J. Heart Fail.* **2023**, *25*, 1507–1525. [CrossRef]
105. Almujally, N.A.; Aljrees, T.; Saidani, O.; Umer, M.; Faheem, Z.B.; Abuzinadah, N.; Alnowaiser, K.; Ashraf, I. Monitoring Acute Heart Failure Patients Using Internet-of-Things-Based Smart Monitoring System. *Sensors* **2023**, *23*, 4580. [CrossRef] [PubMed]
106. Kobayashi, M.; Huttin, O.; Magnusson, M.; Ferreira, J.P.; Bozec, E.; Huby, A.-C.; Preud'homme, G.; Duarte, K.; Lamiral, Z.; Dalleau, K.; et al. Machine Learning-Derived Echocardiographic Phenotypes Predict Heart Failure Incidence in Asymptomatic Individuals. *JACC Cardiovasc. Imaging* **2022**, *15*, 193–208. [CrossRef] [PubMed]
107. Segar, M.W.; Patel, K.V.; Ayers, C.; Basit, M.; Tang, W.H.W.; Willett, D.; Berry, J.; Grodin, J.L.; Pandey, A. Phenomapping of Patients with Heart Failure with Preserved Ejection Fraction Using Machine Learning-based Unsupervised Cluster Analysis. *Eur. J. Heart Fail.* **2020**, *22*, 148–158. [CrossRef]
108. Bourazana, A.; Xanthopoulos, A.; Briasoulis, A.; Magouliotis, D.; Spiliopoulos, K.; Athanasiou, T.; Vassilopoulos, G.; Skoularigis, J.; Triposkiadis, F. Artificial Intelligence in Heart Failure: Friend or Foe? *Life* **2024**, *14*, 145. [CrossRef] [PubMed]

109. Bachtiger, P.; Petri, C.F.; Scott, F.E.; Ri Park, S.; Kelshiker, M.A.; Sahemey, H.K.; Dumea, B.; Alquero, R.; Padam, P.S.; Hatrick, I.R.; et al. Point-of-Care Screening for Heart Failure with Reduced Ejection Fraction Using Artificial Intelligence during ECG-Enabled Stethoscope Examination in London, UK: A Prospective, Observational, Multicentre Study. *Lancet Digit. Health* **2022**, *4*, e117–e125. [CrossRef] [PubMed]
110. Harmon, D.M.; Witt, D.R.; Friedman, P.A.; Attia, Z.I. Diagnosis and Treatment of New Heart Failure with Reduced Ejection Fraction by the Artificial Intelligence–Enhanced Electrocardiogram. *Cardiovasc. Digit. Health J.* **2021**, *2*, 282–284. [CrossRef] [PubMed]
111. Kwon, J.-M.; Kim, K.-H.; Eisen, H.J.; Cho, Y.; Jeon, K.-H.; Lee, S.Y.; Park, J.; Oh, B.-H. Artificial Intelligence Assessment for Early Detection of Heart Failure with Preserved Ejection Fraction Based on Electrocardiographic Features. *Eur. Heart J. Digit. Health* **2021**, *2*, 106–116. [CrossRef] [PubMed]
112. Wu, J.; Biswas, D.; Ryan, M.; Bernstein, B.S.; Rizvi, M.; Fairhurst, N.; Kaye, G.; Baral, R.; Searle, T.; Melikian, N.; et al. Artificial Intelligence Methods for Improved Detection of Undiagnosed Heart Failure with Preserved Ejection Fraction. *Eur. J. Heart Fail.* **2024**, *11*, 11728. [CrossRef] [PubMed]
113. Akerman, A.P.; Porumb, M.; Scott, C.G.; Beqiri, A.; Chartsias, A.; Ryu, A.J.; Hawkes, W.; Huntley, G.D.; Arystan, A.Z.; Kane, G.C.; et al. Automated Echocardiographic Detection of Heart Failure with Preserved Ejection Fraction Using Artificial Intelligence. *JACC Adv.* **2023**, *2*, 100452. [CrossRef]
114. Pană, M.-A.; Busnatu Ștefan, S.; Serbanoiu, L.-I.; Vasilescu, E.; Popescu, N.; Andrei, C.; Sinescu, C.-J. Reducing the Heart Failure Burden in Romania by Predicting Congestive Heart Failure Using Artificial Intelligence: Proof of Concept. *Appl. Sci.* **2021**, *11*, 11728. [CrossRef]
115. Cheungpasitporn, W.; Thongprayoon, C.; Kashani, K.B. Artificial Intelligence in Heart Failure and Acute Kidney Injury: Emerging Concepts and Controversial Dimensions. *Cardiorenal Med.* **2024**, *14*, 147–159. [CrossRef] [PubMed]
116. Kamio, T.; Ikegami, M.; Machida, Y.; Uemura, T.; Chino, N.; Iwagami, M. Machine Learning-Based Prognostic Modeling of Patients with Acute Heart Failure Receiving Furosemide in Intensive Care Units. *Digit. Health* **2023**, *9*, 20552076231194933. [CrossRef] [PubMed]
117. Naruka, V.; Arjomandi Rad, A.; Subbiah Ponniah, H.; Francis, J.; Vardanyan, R.; Tasoudis, P.; Magouliotis, D.E.; Lazopoulos, G.L.; Salmasi, M.Y.; Athanasiou, T. Machine Learning and Artificial Intelligence in Cardiac Transplantation: A Systematic Review. *Artif. Organs* **2022**, *46*, 1741–1753. [CrossRef] [PubMed]
118. Briasoulis, A.; Moustakidis, S.; Tzani, A.; Doulamis, I.; Kampaktsis, P. Prediction of Outcomes after Heart Transplantation by Machine Learning Models. *Eur. Heart J.* **2021**, *42* (Suppl. S1), ehab724.0957. [CrossRef]
119. Seraphin, T.P.; Luedde, M.; Roderburg, C.; van Treeck, M.; Scheider, P.; Buelow, R.D.; Boor, P.; Loosen, S.H.; Provaznik, Z.; Mendelsohn, D.; et al. Prediction of Heart Transplant Rejection from Routine Pathology Slides with Self-Supervised Deep Learning. *Eur. Heart J. Digit. Health* **2023**, *4*, 265–274. [CrossRef] [PubMed]
120. Ozcan, I.; Toya, T.; Cohen-Shelly, M.; Park, H.W.; Ahmad, A.; Ozcan, A.; Noseworthy, P.A.; Kapa, S.; Lerman, L.O.; Attia, Z.I.; et al. Artificial Intelligence–Derived Cardiac Ageing Is Associated with Cardiac Events Post-Heart Transplantation. *Eur. Heart J. Digit. Health* **2022**, *3*, 516–524. [CrossRef] [PubMed]
121. Sharma, S.; Menon, N.; Ruiz, J.; Luce, C.; Brumble, L.; Bhattacharya, A.; Goswami, R. Developing a Risk Prediction Model for COVID-19 Infection in Heart Transplant Recipients Using Artificial Intelligence. *Future Virol.* **2023**, *18*, 1123–1136. [CrossRef]
122. Glass, C.; Davis, R.; Xiong, B.; Dov, D.; Glass, M. The Use of Artificial Intelligence (AI) Machine Learning to Determine Myocyte Damage in Cardiac Transplant Acute Cellular Rejection. *J. Heart Lung Transplant.* **2020**, *39*, S59. [CrossRef]
123. Al-Ani, M.A.; Bai, C.; Shickel, B.; Bledsoe, M.; Ahmed, M.M.; Vilaro, J.; Parker, A.; Aranda, J.; Jeng, E.; Bleiweis, M.; et al. (750) Determinants of Successful Bridging to Heart Transplantation on Temporary Percutaneous Left Ventricular Support—An Insight Using Artificial Intelligence. *J. Heart Lung Transplant.* **2023**, *42*, S331. [CrossRef]
124. Peyster, E.G.; Arabyarmohammadi, S.; Janowczyk, A.; Azarianpour-Esfahani, S.; Sekulic, M.; Cassol, C.; Blower, L.; Parwani, A.; Lal, P.; Feldman, M.D.; et al. An Automated Computational Image Analysis Pipeline for Histological Grading of Cardiac Allograft Rejection. *Eur. Heart J.* **2021**, *42*, 2356–2369. [CrossRef]
125. Lipkova, J.; Chen, T.Y.; Lu, M.Y.; Chen, R.J.; Shady, M.; Williams, M.; Wang, J.; Noor, Z.; Mitchell, R.N.; Turan, M.; et al. Deep Learning-Enabled Assessment of Cardiac Allograft Rejection from Endomyocardial Biopsies. *Nat. Med.* **2022**, *28*, 575–582. [CrossRef] [PubMed]
126. Giuste, F.O.; Sequeira, R.; Keerthipati, V.; Lais, P.; Mirzazadeh, A.; Mohseni, F.; Zhu, Y.; Shi, W.; Marteau, B.; Zhong, Y.; et al. Explainable Synthetic Image Generation to Improve Risk Assessment of Rare Pediatric Heart Transplant Rejection. *J. Biomed. Inform.* **2023**, *139*, 104303. [CrossRef] [PubMed]
127. Lisboa, P.J.G.; Jayabalan, M.; Ortega-Martorell, S.; Olier, I.; Medved, D.; Nilsson, J. Enhanced Survival Prediction Using Explainable Artificial Intelligence in Heart Transplantation. *Sci. Rep.* **2022**, *12*, 19525. [CrossRef] [PubMed]
128. Ruiz Morales, J.; Nativi-Nicolau, J.; Jang, J.; Patel, P.; Yip, D.; Leoni-Moreno, J.; Goswami, R. Artificial Intelligence 12 Lead ECG Based Heart Age Estimation and 1-Year Outcomes after Heart Transplantation. *J. Heart Lung Transplant.* **2022**, *41*, S213. [CrossRef]
129. Agasthi, P.; Smith, S.D.; Murphy, K.M.; Buras, M.R.; Golafshar, M.; Herner, M.; Anand, S.; Pujari, S.; Allam, M.N.; Mookadam, F.; et al. Artificial Intelligence Helps Predict 5-Year Mortality and Graft Failure in Patients Undergoing Orthotopic Heart Transplantation. *J. Heart Lung Transplant.* **2020**, *39*, S142. [CrossRef]

130. Ozcan, I.; Toya, T.; Cohen-Shelly, M.; Ahmad, A.; Corban, M.T.; Noseworthy, P.A.; Kapa, S.; Lerman, L.O.; Attia, Z.I.; Friedman, P.A.; et al. Artificial Intelligence Derived Age Algorithm after Heart Transplantation. *Eur. Heart J.* **2021**, *42* (Suppl. S1), ehab724.2272. [CrossRef]
131. Soh, D.C.K.; Ng, E.Y.K.; Jahmunah, V.; Oh, S.L.; San, T.R.; Acharya, U.R. A Computational Intelligence Tool for the Detection of Hypertension Using Empirical Mode Decomposition. *Comput. Biol. Med.* **2020**, *118*, 103630. [CrossRef] [PubMed]
132. López-Martínez, F.; Núñez-Valdez, E.R.; Crespo, R.G.; García-Díaz, V. An Artificial Neural Network Approach for Predicting Hypertension Using NHANES Data. *Sci. Rep.* **2020**, *10*, 10620. [CrossRef] [PubMed]
133. Wu, X.; Yuan, X.; Wang, W.; Liu, K.; Qin, Y.; Sun, X.; Ma, W.; Zou, Y.; Zhang, H.; Zhou, X.; et al. Value of a Machine Learning Approach for Predicting Clinical Outcomes in Young Patients with Hypertension. *Hypertension* **2020**, *75*, 1271–1278. [CrossRef] [PubMed]
134. Aziz, F.; Malek, S.; Mhd Ali, A.; Wong, M.S.; Mosleh, M.; Milow, P. Determining Hypertensive Patients' Beliefs towards Medication and Associations with Medication Adherence Using Machine Learning Methods. *PeerJ* **2020**, *8*, e8286. [CrossRef]
135. Koshimizu, H.; Kojima, R.; Kario, K.; Okuno, Y. Prediction of Blood Pressure Variability Using Deep Neural Networks. *Int. J. Med. Inform.* **2020**, *136*, 104067. [CrossRef]
136. Hamoud, B.; Kashevnik, A.; Othman, W.; Shilov, N. Neural Network Model Combination for Video-Based Blood Pressure Estimation: New Approach and Evaluation. *Sensors* **2023**, *23*, 1753. [CrossRef]
137. Cheng, H.; Xiong, J.; Chen, Z.; Chen, J. Deep Learning-Based Non-Contact IPPG Signal Blood Pressure Measurement Research. *Sensors* **2023**, *23*, 5528. [CrossRef]
138. Xing, W.; Shi, Y.; Wu, C.; Wang, Y.; Wang, X. Predicting Blood Pressure from Face Videos Using Face Diagnosis Theory and Deep Neural Networks Technique. *Comput. Biol. Med.* **2023**, *164*, 107112. [CrossRef] [PubMed]
139. Visco, V.; Izzo, C.; Mancusi, C.; Rispoli, A.; Tedeschi, M.; Virtuoso, N.; Giano, A.; Gioia, R.; Melfi, A.; Serio, B.; et al. Artificial Intelligence in Hypertension Management: An Ace up Your Sleeve. *J. Cardiovasc. Dev. Dis.* **2023**, *10*, 74. [CrossRef] [PubMed]
140. Maqsood, S.; Xu, S.; Tran, S.; Garg, S.; Springer, M.; Karunanithi, M.; Mohawesh, R. A Survey: From Shallow to Deep Machine Learning Approaches for Blood Pressure Estimation Using Biosensors. *Expert Syst. Appl.* **2022**, *197*, 116788. [CrossRef]
141. Herzog, L.; Ilan Ber, R.; Horowitz-Kugler, Z.; Rabi, Y.; Brufman, I.; Paz, Y.E.; Lopez-Jimenez, F. Causal Deep Neural Network-Based Model for First-Line Hypertension Management. *Mayo Clin. Proc. Digit. Health* **2023**, *1*, 632–640. [CrossRef]
142. Khthir, R.; Santhanam, P. Artificial Intelligence (AI) Approach to Identifying Factors That Determine Systolic Blood Pressure in Type 2 Diabetes (Study from the LOOK AHEAD Cohort). *Diabetes Metab. Syndr.* **2021**, *15*, 102278. [CrossRef]
143. Aryal, S.; Manandhar, I.; Mei, X.; Yeoh, B.S.; Tummala, R.; Saha, P.; Osman, I.; Zubcevic, J.; Durgan, D.J.; Vijay-Kumar, M.; et al. Combating Hypertension beyond GWAS: Microbiome and Artificial Intelligence as Opportunities for Precision Medicine. *Camb. Prisms Precis. Med.* **2023**, *1*, e26. [CrossRef] [PubMed]
144. Lin, Z.; Cheng, Y.T.; Cheung, B.M.Y. Machine Learning Algorithms Identify Hypokalaemia Risk in People with Hypertension in the United States National Health and Nutrition Examination Survey 1999–2018. *Ann. Med.* **2023**, *55*, 2209336. [CrossRef]
145. Kusunose, K.; Hirata, Y.; Tsuji, T.; Kotoku, J.; Sata, M. Deep Learning to Predict Elevated Pulmonary Artery Pressure in Patients with Suspected Pulmonary Hypertension Using Standard Chest X ray. *Sci. Rep.* **2020**, *10*, 19311. [CrossRef]
146. Hardacre, C.J.; Robertshaw, J.A.; Barratt, S.L.; Adams, H.L.; MacKenzie Ross, R.V.; Robinson, G.R.E.; Suntharalingam, J.; Pauling, J.D.; Rodrigues, J.C.L. Diagnostic Test Accuracy of Artificial Intelligence Analysis of Cross-Sectional Imaging in Pulmonary Hypertension: A Systematic Literature Review. *Br. J. Radiol.* **2021**, *94*, 19311. [CrossRef] [PubMed]
147. Ragnarsdottir, H.; Manduchi, L.; Michel, H.; Laumer, F.; Wellmann, S.; Ozkan, E.; Vogt, J.E. Interpretable Prediction of Pulmonary Hypertension in Newborns Using Echocardiograms. In *Lecture Notes in Computer Science*; Springer International Publishing: Cham, Switzerland, 2022; pp. 529–542.
148. Chakravarty, K.; Antontsev, V.G.; Khotimchenko, M.; Gupta, N.; Jagarapu, A.; Bundey, Y.; Hou, H.; Maharao, N.; Varshney, J. Accelerated Repurposing and Drug Development of Pulmonary and Systemic Hypertension Therapies for COVID-19 Treatment Using an AI-Integrated Biosimulation Platform. *Molecules* **2021**, *26*, 1912. [CrossRef]
149. Rahaghi, F.N.; Nardelli, P.; Harder, E.; Singh, I.; Sánchez-Ferrero, G.V.; Ross, J.C.; San José Estépar, R.; Ash, S.Y.; Hunsaker, A.R.; Maron, B.A.; et al. Quantification of Arterial and Venous Morphologic Markers in Pulmonary Arterial Hypertension Using CT Imaging. *Chest* **2021**, *160*, 2220–2231. [CrossRef]
150. Shi, B.; Zhou, T.; Lv, S.; Wang, M.; Chen, S.; Heidari, A.A.; Huang, X.; Chen, H.; Wang, L.; Wu, P. An Evolutionary Machine Learning for Pulmonary Hypertension Animal Model from Arterial Blood Gas Analysis. *Comput. Biol. Med.* **2022**, *146*, 105529. [CrossRef]
151. Amodeo, I.; De Nunzio, G.; Raffaeli, G.; Borzani, I.; Griggio, A.; Conte, L.; Macchini, F.; Condò, V.; Persico, N.; Fabietti, I.; et al. A maChine and Deep Learning Approach to Predict pulmoNary hypertNsIon in newbornS with Congenital Diaphragmatic Hernia (CLANNISH): Protocol for a Retrospective Study. *PLoS ONE* **2021**, *16*, e0259724. [CrossRef] [PubMed]
152. Van der Bijl, P.; Bax, J.J. Using Deep Learning to Diagnose Pulmonary Hypertension. *Eur. Heart J. Cardiovasc. Imaging* **2022**, *23*, 1457–1458. [CrossRef] [PubMed]
153. Swift, A.J.; Lu, H.; Uthoff, J.; Garg, P.; Cogliano, M.; Taylor, J.; Metherall, P.; Zhou, S.; Johns, C.S.; Alabed, S.; et al. A Machine Learning Cardiac Magnetic Resonance Approach to Extract Disease Features and Automate Pulmonary Arterial Hypertension Diagnosis. *Eur. Heart J. Cardiovasc. Imaging* **2021**, *22*, 236–245. [CrossRef]

154. Charters, P.F.P.; Rossdale, J.; Brown, W.; Burnett, T.A.; Komber, H.M.E.I.; Thompson, C.; Robinson, G.; MacKenzie Ross, R.; Suntharalingam, J.; Rodrigues, J.C.L. Diagnostic Accuracy of an Automated Artificial Intelligence Derived Right Ventricular to Left Ventricular Diameter Ratio Tool on CT Pulmonary Angiography to Predict Pulmonary Hypertension at Right Heart Catheterisation. *Clin. Radiol.* **2022**, *77*, e500–e508. [CrossRef] [PubMed]
155. Fortmeier, V.; Lachmann, M.; Körber, M.I.; Unterhuber, M.; von Scheidt, M.; Rippen, E.; Harmsen, G.; Gerçek, M.; Friedrichs, K.P.; Roder, F.; et al. Solving the Pulmonary Hypertension Paradox in Patients with Severe Tricuspid Regurgitation by Employing Artificial Intelligence. *JACC Cardiovasc. Interv.* **2022**, *15*, 381–394. [CrossRef]
156. Liu, C.-M.; Shih, E.S.C.; Chen, J.-Y.; Huang, C.-H.; Wu, I.-C.; Chen, P.-F.; Higa, S.; Yagi, N.; Hu, Y.-F.; Hwang, M.-J.; et al. Artificial Intelligence-Enabled Electrocardiogram Improves the Diagnosis and Prediction of Mortality in Patients with Pulmonary Hypertension. *JACC Asia* **2022**, *2*, 258–270. [CrossRef]
157. Lu, W.; Huang, J.; Shen, Q.; Sun, F.; Li, J. Identification of Diagnostic Biomarkers for Idiopathic Pulmonary Hypertension with Metabolic Syndrome by Bioinformatics and Machine Learning. *Sci. Rep.* **2023**, *13*, 615. [CrossRef] [PubMed]
158. Yu, X.; Qin, W.; Lin, X.; Shan, Z.; Huang, L.; Shao, Q.; Wang, L.; Chen, M. Synergizing the Enhanced RIME with Fuzzy K-Nearest Neighbor for Diagnose of Pulmonary Hypertension. *Comput. Biol. Med.* **2023**, *165*, 107408. [CrossRef] [PubMed]
159. Hyde, B.; Paoli, C.J.; Panjabi, S.; Bettencourt, K.C.; Bell Lynum, K.S.; Selej, M. A Claims-based, Machine-learning Algorithm to Identify Patients with Pulmonary Arterial Hypertension. *Pulm. Circ.* **2023**, *13*, e12237. [CrossRef] [PubMed]
160. Zhang, N.; Zhao, X.; Li, J.; Huang, L.; Li, H.; Feng, H.; Garcia, M.A.; Cao, Y.; Sun, Z.; Chai, S. Machine Learning Based on Computed Tomography Pulmonary Angiography in Evaluating Pulmonary Artery Pressure in Patients with Pulmonary Hypertension. *J. Clin. Med.* **2023**, *12*, 1297. [CrossRef] [PubMed]
161. Hirata, Y.; Tsuji, T.; Kotoku, J.; Sata, M.; Kusunose, K. Echocardiographic Artificial Intelligence for Pulmonary Hypertension Classification. *Heart* **2024**, *110*, heartjnl-2023-323320. [CrossRef] [PubMed]
162. Imai, S.; Sakao, S.; Nagata, J.; Naito, A.; Sekine, A.; Sugiura, T.; Shigeta, A.; Nishiyama, A.; Yokota, H.; Shimizu, N.; et al. Artificial Intelligence-Based Model for Predicting Pulmonary Arterial Hypertension on Chest X-ray Images. *BMC Pulm. Med.* **2024**, *24*, 101. [CrossRef] [PubMed]
163. Ragnarsdottir, H.; Ozkan, E.; Michel, H.; Chin-Cheong, K.; Manduchi, L.; Wellmann, S.; Vogt, J.E. Deep Learning Based Prediction of Pulmonary Hypertension in Newborns Using Echocardiograms. *Int. J. Comput. Vis.* **2024**, 1–18. [CrossRef]
164. Dwivedi, K.; Sharkey, M.; Delaney, L.; Alabed, S.; Rajaram, S.; Hill, C.; Johns, C.; Rothman, A.; Mamalakis, M.; Thompson, A.A.R.; et al. Improving Prognostication in Pulmonary Hypertension Using AI-Quantified Fibrosis and Radiologic Severity Scoring at Baseline CT. *Radiology* **2024**, *310*, e231718. [CrossRef]
165. Griffiths, M.; Manlhiot, C.; Chinni, B.K.; Sleeper, L.A.; Abman, S.; Rosenzweig, E.; Romer, L.H.; Mullen, M.P.; Lin, S.; Benza, R.; et al. Abstract 15889: An Artificial Intelligence-Derived Pediatric Pulmonary Hypertension Risk Prediction Model from the Pediatric Pulmonary Hypertension Network (PPHNet) Registry. *Circulation* **2023**, *148* (Suppl. S1), A15889. [CrossRef]
166. Mamalakis, M.; Dwivedi, K.; Sharkey, M.; Alabed, S.; Kiely, D.; Swift, A.J. A Transparent Artificial Intelligence Framework to Assess Lung Disease in Pulmonary Hypertension. *Sci. Rep.* **2023**, *13*, 3812. [CrossRef]
167. Tchuente Foguem, G.; Coulibaly, L.; Diamoutene, A. Combined Learning Models for Survival Analysis of Patients with Pulmonary Hypertension. *Intell. Syst. Appl.* **2024**, *21*, 200321. [CrossRef]
168. Han, P.-L.; Jiang, L.; Cheng, J.-L.; Shi, K.; Huang, S.; Jiang, Y.; Jiang, L.; Xia, Q.; Li, Y.-Y.; Zhu, M.; et al. Artificial Intelligence-Assisted Diagnosis of Congenital Heart Disease and Associated Pulmonary Arterial Hypertension from Chest Radiographs: A Multi-Reader Multi-Case Study. *Eur. J. Radiol.* **2024**, *171*, 111277. [CrossRef] [PubMed]
169. Anand, V.; Weston, A.D.; Scott, C.G.; Kane, G.C.; Pellikka, P.A.; Carter, R.E. Machine Learning for Diagnosis of Pulmonary Hypertension by Echocardiography. *Mayo Clin. Proc.* **2024**, *99*, 260–270. [CrossRef] [PubMed]
170. Lai, C.K.-C.; Leung, E.; He, Y.; Cheung, C.-C.; Oliver, M.O.Y.; Yu, Q.; Li, T.C.-M.; Lee, A.L.-H.; Yu, L.; Lui, G.C.-Y. A Machine Learning-Based Risk Score for Prediction of Infective Endocarditis among Patients with *Staphylococcus Aureus* Bacteraemia—The SABIER Score. *J. Infect. Dis.* **2024**, jiae080. [CrossRef] [PubMed]
171. Yi, C.; Zhang, H.; Yang, J.; Chen, D.; Jiang, S. Elucidating Common Pathogenic Transcriptional Networks in Infective Endocarditis and Sepsis: Integrated Insights from Biomarker Discovery and Single-Cell RNA Sequencing. *Front. Immunol.* **2024**, *14*, 1298041. [CrossRef] [PubMed]
172. Galizzi Fae, I.; Murta Pinto, P.H.O.; De Oliveira, G.B.; Taconeli, C.A.; De Andrade, A.B.; De Padua, L.B.; Diamante, L.C.; Ferrari, T.C.A.; Nunes, M.C.P. Cardiac Complications as a Major Predictor of In-Hospital Death in Infective Endocarditis Using Machine-Learning Algorithm Analysis. *Eur. Heart J.* **2023**, *44* (Suppl. S2), ehad655.1773. [CrossRef]
173. Chen, Z.; Lalande, A.; Salomon, M.; Decourselle, T.; Pommier, T.; Qayyum, A.; Shi, J.; Perrot, G.; Couturier, R. Automatic Deep Learning-Based Myocardial Infarction Segmentation from Delayed Enhancement MRI. *Comput. Med. Imaging Graph.* **2022**, *95*, 102014. [CrossRef] [PubMed]
174. Rauseo, E.; Izquierdo Morcillo, C.; Raisi-Estabragh, Z.; Gkontra, P.; Aung, N.; Lekadir, K.; Petersen, S.E. New Imaging Signatures of Cardiac Alterations in Ischaemic Heart Disease and Cerebrovascular Disease Using CMR Radiomics. *Front. Cardiovasc. Med.* **2021**, *8*, 716577. [CrossRef] [PubMed]
175. Liu, W.-C.; Lin, C.; Lin, C.-S.; Tsai, M.-C.; Chen, S.-J.; Tsai, S.-H.; Lin, W.-S.; Lee, C.-C.; Tsao, T.-P.; Cheng, C.-C. An Artificial Intelligence-Based Alarm Strategy Facilitates Management of Acute Myocardial Infarction. *J. Pers. Med.* **2021**, *11*, 1149. [CrossRef]

176. Zhao, Y.; Xiong, J.; Hou, Y.; Zhu, M.; Lu, Y.; Xu, Y.; Teliewubai, J.; Liu, W.; Xu, X.; Li, X.; et al. Early Detection of ST-Segment Elevated Myocardial Infarction by Artificial Intelligence with 12-Lead Electrocardiogram. *Int. J. Cardiol.* **2020**, *317*, 223–230. [CrossRef]
177. Cho, Y.; Kwon, J.-M.; Kim, K.-H.; Medina-Inojosa, J.R.; Jeon, K.-H.; Cho, S.; Lee, S.Y.; Park, J.; Oh, B.-H. Artificial Intelligence Algorithm for Detecting Myocardial Infarction Using Six-Lead Electrocardiography. *Sci. Rep.* **2020**, *10*, 20495. [CrossRef] [PubMed]
178. Liu, W.-C.; Lin, C.-S.; Tsai, C.-S.; Tsao, T.-P.; Cheng, C.-C.; Liou, J.-T.; Lin, W.-S.; Cheng, S.-M.; Lou, Y.-S.; Lee, C.-C.; et al. A Deep Learning Algorithm for Detecting Acute Myocardial Infarction. *EuroIntervention* **2021**, *17*, 765–773. [CrossRef]
179. Velusamy, D.; Ramasamy, K. Ensemble of Heterogeneous Classifiers for Diagnosis and Prediction of Coronary Artery Disease with Reduced Feature Subset. *Comput. Methods Programs Biomed.* **2021**, *198*, 105770. [CrossRef] [PubMed]
180. Muhammad, L.J.; Al-Shourbaji, I.; Haruna, A.A.; Mohammed, I.A.; Ahmad, A.; Jibrin, M.B. Machine Learning Predictive Models for Coronary Artery Disease. *SN Comput. Sci.* **2021**, *2*, 350. [CrossRef]
181. Li, D.; Xiong, G.; Zeng, H.; Zhou, Q.; Jiang, J.; Guo, X. Machine Learning-Aided Risk Stratification System for the Prediction of Coronary Artery Disease. *Int. J. Cardiol.* **2021**, *326*, 30–34. [CrossRef] [PubMed]
182. Brendel, J.M.; Walterspiel, J.; Hagen, F.; Kübler, J.; Paul, J.-F.; Nikolaou, K.; Gawaz, M.; Greulich, S.; Krumm, P.; Winkelmann, M. Coronary Artery Disease Evaluation during Transcatheter Aortic Valve Replacement Work-up Using Photon-Counting CT and Artificial Intelligence. *Diagn. Interv. Imaging* **2024**. [CrossRef]
183. Ihdayhid, A.R.; Sehly, A.; He, A.; Joyner, J.; Flack, J.; Konstantopoulos, J.; Newby, D.E.; Williams, M.C.; Ko, B.S.; Chow, B.J.W.; et al. Coronary Artery Stenosis and High-Risk Plaque Assessed with an Unsupervised Fully Automated Deep Learning Technique. *JACC Adv.* **2024**, *2024*, 100861. [CrossRef]
184. Uzokov, J.; Alyavi, A.; Alyavi, B.; Abdullaev, A. How Artificial Intelligence Can Assist with Ischaemic Heart Disease. *Eur. Heart J.* **2024**, ehae030. [CrossRef] [PubMed]
185. Abdelrahman, K.; Shiyovich, A.; Huck, D.; Berman, A.; Weber, B.; Gupta, S.; Cardoso, R.; Blankstein, R. Artificial Intelligence in Coronary Artery Calcium Scoring Detection and Quantification. *Diagnostics* **2024**, *14*, 125. [CrossRef]
186. Park, M.J.; Choi, Y.J.; Shim, M.; Cho, Y.; Park, J.; Choi, J.; Kim, J.; Lee, E.; Kim, S.-Y. Performance of ECG-Derived Digital Biomarker for Screening Coronary Occlusion in Resuscitated out-of-Hospital Cardiac Arrest Patients: A Comparative Study between Artificial Intelligence and a Group of Experts. *J. Clin. Med.* **2024**, *13*, 1354. [CrossRef]
187. Alkhamis, M.A.; Al Jarallah, M.; Attur, S.; Zubaid, M. Interpretable Machine Learning Models for Predicting In-Hospital and 30 Days Adverse Events in Acute Coronary Syndrome Patients in Kuwait. *Sci. Rep.* **2024**, *14*, 1243. [CrossRef] [PubMed]
188. Zhu, X.; Xie, B.; Chen, Y.; Zeng, H.; Hu, J. Machine Learning in the Prediction of In-Hospital Mortality in Patients with First Acute Myocardial Infarction. *Clin. Chim. Acta* **2024**, *554*, 117776. [CrossRef]
189. Kasim, S.; Amir Rudin, P.N.F.; Malek, S.; Aziz, F.; Wan Ahmad, W.A.; Ibrahim, K.S.; Muhmad Hamidi, M.H.; Raja Shariff, R.E.; Fong, A.Y.Y.; Song, C. Data Analytics Approach for Short- and Long-Term Mortality Prediction Following Acute Non-ST-Elevation Myocardial Infarction (NSTEMI) and Unstable Angina (UA) in Asians. *PLoS ONE* **2024**, *19*, e0298036. [CrossRef] [PubMed]
190. Oliveira, M.; Seringa, J.; Pinto, F.J.; Henriques, R.; Magalhães, T. Machine Learning Prediction of Mortality in Acute Myocardial Infarction. *BMC Med. Inform. Decis. Mak.* **2023**, *23*, 70. [CrossRef] [PubMed]
191. Azdaki, N.; Salmani, F.; Kazemi, T.; Partovi, N.; Bizhaem, S.K.; Moghadam, M.N.; Moniri, Y.; Zarepur, E.; Mohammadifard, N.; Alikhasi, H.; et al. Which Risk Factor Best Predicts Coronary Artery Disease Using Artificial Neural Network Method? *BMC Med. Inform. Decis. Mak.* **2024**, *24*, 52. [CrossRef] [PubMed]
192. Zhan, W.; Hu, H.; Hao, B.; Zhu, H.; Yan, T.; Zhang, J.; Wang, S.; Liu, S.; Zhang, T. Development of Machine Learning-Based Malignant Pericardial Effusion-Related Model in Breast Cancer: Implications for Clinical Significance, Tumor Immune and Drug-Therapy. *Heliyon* **2024**, *10*, e27507. [CrossRef]
193. Liu, Y.-L.; Cheng, C.-C.; Lin, C. A Deep Learning Algorithm for Detecting Acute Pericarditis by Electrocardiogram. *J. Pers. Med.* **2022**, *12*, 1150. [CrossRef] [PubMed]
194. Cheng, C.-Y.; Wu, C.-C.; Chen, H.-C.; Hung, C.-H.; Chen, T.-Y.; Lin, C.-H.R.; Chiu, I.-M. Development and Validation of a Deep Learning Pipeline to Measure Pericardial Effusion in Echocardiography. *Front. Cardiovasc. Med.* **2023**, *10*, 1195235. [CrossRef]
195. Wilder-Smith, A.J.; Yang, S.; Weikert, T.; Bremerich, J.; Haaf, P.; Segeroth, M.; Ebert, L.C.; Sauter, A.; Sexauer, R. Automated Detection, Segmentation, and Classification of Pericardial Effusions on Chest CT Using a Deep Convolutional Neural Network. *Diagnostics* **2022**, *12*, 1045. [CrossRef]
196. Piccini, J.P.; Cunnane, R.; Steffel, J.; El-Chami, M.F.; Reynolds, D.; Roberts, P.R.; Soejima, K.; Steinwender, C.; Garweg, C.; Chinitz, L.; et al. Development and Validation of a Risk Score for Predicting Pericardial Effusion in Patients Undergoing Leadless Pacemaker Implantation: Experience with the Micra Transcatheter Pacemaker. *Europace* **2022**, *24*, 1119–1126. [CrossRef]
197. McBane, R.D., II; Murphree, D.H.; Liedl, D.; Lopez-Jimenez, F.; Attia, I.Z.; Arruda-Olson, A.M.; Scott, C.G.; Prodduturi, N.; Nowakowski, S.E.; Rooke, T.W.; et al. Artificial Intelligence of Arterial Doppler Waveforms to Predict Major Adverse Outcomes among Patients Evaluated for Peripheral Artery Disease. *J. Am. Heart Assoc.* **2024**, *13*, e031880. [CrossRef]
198. Rusinovich, Y.; Rusinovich, V.; Buhayenka, A.; Liashko, V.; Sabanov, A.; Holstein, D.J.F.; Aldmour, S.; Doss, M.; Branzan, D. Classification of Anatomic Patterns of Peripheral Artery Disease with Automated Machine Learning (AutoML). *Vascular* **2024**, 17085381241236571. [CrossRef] [PubMed]

199. Sasikala, P.; Mohanarathinam, A. A Powerful Peripheral Arterial Disease Detection Using Machine Learning-Based Severity Level Classification Model and Hyper Parameter Optimization Methods. *Biomed. Signal Process. Control* **2024**, *90*, 105842. [CrossRef]
200. Li, B.; Shaikh, F.; Zamzam, A.; Syed, M.H.; Abdin, R.; Qadura, M. A Machine Learning Algorithm for Peripheral Artery Disease Prognosis Using Biomarker Data. *iScience* **2024**, *27*, 109081. [CrossRef]
201. Masoumi Shahrbabak, S.; Kim, S.; Youn, B.D.; Cheng, H.-M.; Chen, C.-H.; Mukkamala, R.; Hahn, J.-O. Peripheral Artery Disease Diagnosis Based on Deep Learning-Enabled Analysis of Non-Invasive Arterial Pulse Waveforms. *Comput. Biol. Med.* **2024**, *168*, 107813. [CrossRef]
202. McBane, R.D., II; Murphree, D.H.; Liedl, D.; Lopez-Jimenez, F.; Arruda-Olson, A.; Scott, C.G.; Prodduturi, N.; Nowakowski, S.E.; Rooke, T.W.; Casanegra, A.I.; et al. Artificial Intelligence of Arterial Doppler Waveforms to Predict Major Adverse Outcomes among Patients with Diabetes Mellitus. *J. Vasc. Surg.* **2024**. [CrossRef] [PubMed]
203. Li, B.; Eisenberg, N.; Beaton, D.; Lee, D.S.; Aljabri, B.; Verma, R.; Wijeysundera, D.N.; Rotstein, O.D.; de Mestral, C.; Mamdani, M.; et al. Using Machine Learning (XGBoost) to Predict Outcomes after Infrainguinal Bypass for Peripheral Artery Disease. *Ann. Surg.* **2024**, *279*, 705–713. [CrossRef]
204. Liu, L.; Bi, B.; Cao, L.; Gui, M.; Ju, F. Predictive Model, and Risk Analysis for Peripheral Vascular Disease in Type 2 Diabetes Mellitus Patients Using Machine Learning and Shapley Additive Explanation. *Front. Endocrinol.* **2024**, *15*, 1320335. [CrossRef]
205. Nassour, N.; Akhbari, B.; Ranganathan, N.; Shin, D.; Ghaednia, H.; Ashkani-Esfahani, S.; DiGiovanni, C.W.; Guss, D. Using Machine Learning in the Prediction of Symptomatic Venous Thromboembolism Following Ankle Fracture. *Foot Ankle Surg.* **2024**, *30*, 110–116. [CrossRef]
206. Chen, R.; Petrazzini, B.O.; Malick, W.A.; Rosenson, R.S.; Do, R. Prediction of Venous Thromboembolism in Diverse Populations Using Machine Learning and Structured Electronic Health Records. *Arterioscler. Thromb. Vasc. Biol.* **2024**, *44*, 491–504. [CrossRef]
207. Pan, S.; Bian, L.; Luo, H.; Conway, A.; Qiao, W.; Win, T.; Wang, W. Risk Factor Analysis and Prediction Model Construction for Surgical Patients with Venous Thromboembolism: A Prospective Study. *Interdiscip. Nurs. Res.* **2024**. [CrossRef]
208. Grdinic, A.G.; Radovanovic, S.; Gleditsch, J.; Jørgensen, C.T.; Asady, E.; Pettersen, H.H.; Delibasic, B.; Ghanima, W. Developing a Machine Learning Model for Bleeding Prediction in Patients with Cancer-Associated Thrombosis Receiving Anticoagulation Therapy. *J. Thromb. Haemost.* **2024**. [CrossRef] [PubMed]
209. Chiasakul, T.; Lam, B.D.; McNichol, M.; Robertson, W.; Rosovsky, R.P.; Lake, L.; Vlachos, I.S.; Adamski, A.; Reyes, N.; Abe, K.; et al. Artificial Intelligence in the Prediction of Venous Thromboembolism: A Systematic Review and Pooled Analysis. *Eur. J. Haematol.* **2023**, *111*, 951–962. [CrossRef] [PubMed]
210. Wang, X.; Xi, H.; Geng, X.; Li, Y.; Zhao, M.; Li, F.; Li, Z.; Ji, H.; Tian, H. Artificial Intelligence-Based Prediction of Lower Extremity Deep Vein Thrombosis Risk after Knee/Hip Arthroplasty. *Clin. Appl. Thromb. Hemost.* **2023**, *29*, 107602962211392. [CrossRef]
211. Wang, K.Y.; Ikwuezunma, I.; Puvanesarajah, V.; Babu, J.; Margalit, A.; Raad, M.; Jain, A. Using Predictive Modeling and Supervised Machine Learning to Identify Patients at Risk for Venous Thromboembolism Following Posterior Lumbar Fusion. *Glob. Spine J.* **2023**, *13*, 1097–1103. [CrossRef] [PubMed]
212. Muñoz, A.J.; Souto, J.C.; Lecumberri, R.; Obispo, B.; Sanchez, A.; Aparicio, J.; Aguayo, C.; Gutierrez, D.; Palomo, A.G.; Fanjul, V.; et al. Development of a Predictive Model of Venous Thromboembolism Recurrence in Anticoagulated Cancer Patients Using Machine Learning. *Thromb. Res.* **2023**, *228*, 181–188. [CrossRef] [PubMed]
213. Razzaq, M.; Goumidi, L.; Iglesias, M.-J.; Munsch, G.; Bruzelius, M.; Ibrahim-Kosta, M.; Butler, L.; Odeberg, J.; Morange, P.-E.; Tregouet, D.A. Explainable Artificial Neural Network for Recurrent Venous Thromboembolism Based on Plasma Proteomics. In *Computational Methods in Systems Biology*; Springer International Publishing: Cham, Switzerland, 2021; pp. 108–121.
214. Contreras-Luján, E.E.; García-Guerrero, E.E.; López-Bonilla, O.R.; Tlelo-Cuautle, E.; López-Mancilla, D.; Inzunza-González, E. Evaluation of Machine Learning Algorithms for Early Diagnosis of Deep Venous Thrombosis. *Math. Comput. Appl.* **2022**, *27*, 24. [CrossRef]
215. Seo, J.W.; Park, S.; Kim, Y.J.; Hwang, J.H.; Yu, S.H.; Kim, J.H.; Kim, K.G. Artificial Intelligence-Based Iliofemoral Deep Venous Thrombosis Detection Using a Clinical Approach. *Sci. Rep.* **2023**, *13*, 967. [CrossRef]
216. Alhwiti, T.; Aldrugh, S.; Megahed, F.M. Predicting In-Hospital Mortality after Transcatheter Aortic Valve Replacement Using Administrative Data and Machine Learning. *Sci. Rep.* **2023**, *13*, 10252. [CrossRef]
217. Strange, G.; Stewart, S.; Watts, A.; Playford, D. Enhanced Detection of Severe Aortic Stenosis via Artificial Intelligence: A Clinical Cohort Study. *Open Heart* **2023**, *10*, e002265. [CrossRef]
218. Ueda, D.; Matsumoto, T.; Ehara, S.; Yamamoto, A.; Walston, S.L.; Ito, A.; Shimono, T.; Shiba, M.; Takeshita, T.; Fukuda, D.; et al. Artificial Intelligence-Based Model to Classify Cardiac Functions from Chest Radiographs: A Multi-Institutional, Retrospective Model Development and Validation Study. *Lancet Digit. Health* **2023**, *5*, e525–e533. [CrossRef] [PubMed]
219. Singh, Y.; Chaudhary, R.; Bliden, K.P.; Tantry, U.S.; Gurbel, P.A.; Visweswaran, S.; Harinstein, M.E. Meta-Analysis of the Performance of AI-Driven ECG Interpretation in the Diagnosis of Valvular Heart Diseases. *Am. J. Cardiol.* **2024**, *213*, 126–131. [CrossRef] [PubMed]
220. Brown, K.; Roshanitabrizi, P.; Rwebembera, J.; Okello, E.; Beaton, A.; Linguraru, M.G.; Sable, C.A. Using Artificial Intelligence for Rheumatic Heart Disease Detection by Echocardiography: Focus on Mitral Regurgitation. *J. Am. Heart Assoc.* **2024**, *13*, e031257. [CrossRef] [PubMed]

221. Toggweiler, S.; Wyler von Ballmoos, M.C.; Moccetti, F.; Douverny, A.; Wolfrum, M.; Imamoglu, Z.; Mohler, A.; Gülan, U.; Kim, W.-K. A Fully Automated Artificial Intelligence-Driven Software for Planning of Transcatheter Aortic Valve Replacement. *Cardiovasc. Revasc. Med.* **2024**. [CrossRef] [PubMed]
222. Solomon, M.D.; Tabada, G.; Allen, A.; Sung, S.H.; Go, A.S. Large-Scale Identification of Aortic Stenosis and Its Severity Using Natural Language Processing on Electronic Health Records. *Cardiovasc. Digit. Health J.* **2021**, *2*, 156–163. [CrossRef] [PubMed]
223. Aoyama, G.; Zhao, L.; Zhao, S.; Xue, X.; Zhong, Y.; Yamauchi, H.; Tsukihara, H.; Maeda, E.; Ino, K.; Tomii, N.; et al. Automatic Aortic Valve Cusps Segmentation from CT Images Based on the Cascading Multiple Deep Neural Networks. *J. Imaging* **2022**, *8*, 11. [CrossRef] [PubMed]
224. Dasi, A.; Lee, B.; Polsani, V.; Yadav, P.; Dasi, L.P.; Thourani, V.H. Predicting Pressure Gradient Using Artificial Intelligence for Transcatheter Aortic Valve Replacement. *JTCVS Technol.* **2024**, *23*, 5–17. [CrossRef] [PubMed]
225. Krishna, H.; Desai, K.; Slostad, B.; Bhayani, S.; Arnold, J.H.; Ouwerkerk, W.; Hummel, Y.; Lam, C.S.P.; Ezekowitz, J.; Frost, M.; et al. Fully Automated Artificial Intelligence Assessment of Aortic Stenosis by Echocardiography. *J. Am. Soc. Echocardiogr.* **2023**, *36*, 769–777. [CrossRef] [PubMed]
226. Xie, L.-F.; Xie, Y.-L.; Wu, Q.-S.; He, J.; Lin, X.-F.; Qiu, Z.-H.; Chen, L.-W. A Predictive Model for Postoperative Adverse Outcomes Following Surgical Treatment of Acute Type A Aortic Dissection Based on Machine Learning. *J. Clin. Hypertens.* **2024**, *26*, 251–261. [CrossRef]
227. Zhou, M.; Lei, L.; Chen, W.; Luo, Q.; Li, J.; Zhou, F.; Yang, X.; Pan, Y. Deep Learning-Based Diagnosis of Aortic Dissection Using an Electrocardiogram: Development, Validation, and Clinical Implications of the AADE Score. *Kardiol. Pol.* **2024**, *82*, 63–71. [CrossRef]
228. Irtyuga, O.; Babakekhyan, M.; Kostareva, A.; Uspensky, V.; Gordeev, M.; Faggian, G.; Malashicheva, A.; Metsker, O.; Shlyakhto, E.; Kopanitsa, G. Analysis of Prevalence and Clinical Features of Aortic Stenosis in Patients with and without Bicuspid Aortic Valve Using Machine Learning Methods. *J. Pers. Med.* **2023**, *13*, 1588. [CrossRef] [PubMed]
229. Kennedy, L.; Bates, K.; Therrien, J.; Grossman, Y.; Kodaira, M.; Pressacco, J.; Rosati, A.; Dagenais, F.; Leask, R.L.; Lachapelle, K. Thoracic Aortic Aneurysm Risk Assessment. *JACC Adv.* **2023**, *2*, 100637. [CrossRef]
230. Benjamin, E.J.; Muntner, P.; Alonso, A.; Bittencourt, M.S.; Callaway, C.W.; Carson, A.P.; Chamberlain, A.M.; Chang, A.R.; Cheng, S.; Das, S.R.; et al. Heart Disease and Stroke Statistics—2019 Update: A Report from the American Heart Association. *Circulation* **2019**, *139*, e56–e528. [CrossRef]
231. Frohnert, P.P.; Gluliani, E.R.; Friedberg, M.; Johnson, W.J.; Tauxe, W.N. Statistical Investigation of Correlations between Serum Potassium Levels and Electrocardiographic Findings in Patients on Intermittent Hemodialysis Therapy. *Circulation* **1970**, *41*, 667–676. [CrossRef] [PubMed]
232. Martínez-Sellés, M.; Marina-Breysse, M. Current and Future Use of Artificial Intelligence in Electrocardiography. *J. Cardiovasc. Dev. Dis.* **2023**, *10*, 175. [CrossRef] [PubMed]
233. Zhang, Y.; Xu, J.; Xing, W.; Chen, Q.; Liu, X.; Pu, Y.; Xin, F.; Jiang, H.; Yin, Z.; Tao, D.; et al. Robust Artificial Intelligence Tool for Atrial Fibrillation Diagnosis: Novel Development Approach Incorporating Both Atrial Electrograms and Surface ECG and Evaluation by Head-to-head Comparison with Hospital-based Physician ECG Readers. *J. Am. Heart Assoc.* **2024**, *13*, e032100. [CrossRef] [PubMed]
234. Kawamura, Y.; Vafaei Sadr, A.; Abedi, V.; Zand, R. Many Models, Little Adoption—What Accounts for Low Uptake of Machine Learning Models for Atrial Fibrillation Prediction and Detection? *J. Clin. Med.* **2024**, *13*, 1313. [CrossRef] [PubMed]
235. Xie, C.; Wang, Z.; Yang, C.; Liu, J.; Liang, H. Machine Learning for Detecting Atrial Fibrillation from ECGs: Systematic Review and Meta-Analysis. *Rev. Cardiovasc. Med.* **2024**, *25*, 8. [CrossRef]
236. Tehrani, B.N.; Truesdell, A.G.; Psotka, M.A.; Rosner, C.; Singh, R.; Sinha, S.S.; Damluji, A.A.; Batchelor, W.B. A Standardized and Comprehensive Approach to the Management of Cardiogenic Shock. *JACC Heart Fail.* **2020**, *8*, 879–891. [CrossRef]
237. Raheem, A.; Waheed, S.; Karim, M.; Khan, N.U.; Jawed, R. Prediction of Major Adverse Cardiac Events in the Emergency Department Using an Artificial Neural Network with a Systematic Grid Search. *Int. J. Emerg. Med.* **2024**, *17*, 4. [CrossRef]
238. Abusnina, W.; Elhouderi, E.; Walters, R.W.; Al-Abdouh, A.; Mostafa, M.R.; Liu, J.L.; Mazozy, R.; Mhanna, M.; Ben-Dor, I.; Dufani, J.; et al. Sex Differences in the Clinical Outcomes of Patients with Takotsubo Stress Cardiomyopathy: A Meta-Analysis of Observational Studies. *Am. J. Cardiol.* **2024**, *211*, 316–325. [CrossRef] [PubMed]
239. Matta, A.; Delmas, C.; Campelo-Parada, F.; Lhermusier, T.; Bouisset, F.; Elbaz, M.; Nader, V.; Blanco, S.; Roncalli, J.; Carrié, D. Takotsubo Cardiomyopathy. *Rev. Cardiovasc. Med.* **2022**, *23*, 1. [CrossRef] [PubMed]
240. Moynihan, D.; Monaco, S.; Ting, T.W.; Narasimhalu, K.; Hsieh, J.; Kam, S.; Lim, J.Y.; Lim, W.K.; Davila, S.; Bylstra, Y.; et al. Cluster Analysis and Visualisation of Electronic Health Records Data to Identify Undiagnosed Patients with Rare Genetic Diseases. *Sci. Rep.* **2024**, *14*, 5056. [CrossRef] [PubMed]
241. van Assen, M.; Razavi, A.C.; Whelton, S.P.; De Cecco, C.N. Artificial Intelligence in Cardiac Imaging: Where We Are and What We Want. *Eur. Heart J.* **2023**, *44*, 541–543. [CrossRef] [PubMed]
242. Wehbe, R.M.; Katsaggelos, A.K.; Hammond, K.J.; Hong, H.; Ahmad, F.S.; Ouyang, D.; Shah, S.J.; McCarthy, P.M.; Thomas, J.D. Deep Learning for Cardiovascular Imaging: A Review. *JAMA Cardiol.* **2023**, *8*, 1089. [CrossRef] [PubMed]
243. Jone, P.-N.; Gearhart, A.; Lei, H.; Xing, F.; Nahar, J.; Lopez-Jimenez, F.; Diller, G.-P.; Marelli, A.; Wilson, L.; Saidi, A.; et al. Artificial Intelligence in Congenital Heart Disease. *JACC Adv.* **2022**, *1*, 100153. [CrossRef]

244. Dahiya, E.S.; Kalra, A.M.; Lowe, A.; Anand, G. Wearable Technology for Monitoring Electrocardiograms (ECGs) in Adults: A Scoping Review. *Sensors* **2024**, *24*, 1318. [CrossRef] [PubMed]
245. Yoon, M.; Park, J.J.; Hur, T.; Hua, C.-H.; Hussain, M.; Lee, S.; Choi, D.-J. Application and Potential of Artificial Intelligence in Heart Failure: Past, Present, and Future. *Int. J. Heart Fail.* **2024**, *6*, 11. [CrossRef]
246. Dogan, S.; Barua, P.D.; Tuncer, T.; Acharya, U.R. An Accurate Hypertension Detection Model Based on a New Odd-Even Pattern Using Ballistocardiograph Signals. *Eng. Appl. Artif. Intell.* **2024**, *133*, 108306. [CrossRef]
247. Becerra-Muñoz, V.M.; Gómez Sáenz, J.T.; Escribano Subías, P. La importancia de los datos en la hipertensión arterial pulmonar: De los registros internacionales al machine learning. *Med. Clin.* **2024**. [CrossRef]
248. Perek, S.; Nussinovitch, U.; Sagi, N.; Gidron, Y.; Raz-Pasteur, A. Prognostic Implications of Ultra-Short Heart Rate Variability Indices in Hospitalized Patients with Infective Endocarditis. *PLoS ONE* **2023**, *18*, e0287607. [CrossRef] [PubMed]
249. Virani, S.S.; Alonso, A.; Benjamin, E.J.; Bittencourt, M.S.; Callaway, C.W.; Carson, A.P.; Chamberlain, A.M.; Chang, A.R.; Cheng, S.; Delling, F.N.; et al. Heart Disease and Stroke Statistics—2020 Update: A Report from the American Heart Association. *Circulation* **2020**, *141*, e139–e596. [CrossRef] [PubMed]
250. Uzun Ozsahin, D.; Ozgocmen, C.; Balcioglu, O.; Ozsahin, I.; Uzun, B. Diagnostic AI and Cardiac Diseases. *Diagnostics* **2022**, *12*, 2901. [CrossRef] [PubMed]
251. El Sherbini, A.; Rosenson, R.S.; Al Rifai, M.; Virk, H.U.H.; Wang, Z.; Virani, S.; Glicksberg, B.S.; Lavie, C.J.; Krittanawong, C. Artificial Intelligence in Preventive Cardiology. *Prog. Cardiovasc. Dis.* **2024**. [CrossRef] [PubMed]
252. Bușilă, C.; Stuparu-Crețu, M.; Nechita, A.; Grigore, C.A.; Balan, G. Good Glycemic Control for a Low Cardiovascular Risk in Children Suffering from Diabetes. *Rev. De Chim.* **2017**, *68*, 358–361. [CrossRef]
253. Kanegae, H.; Suzuki, K.; Fukatani, K.; Ito, T.; Harada, N.; Kario, K. Highly Precise Risk Prediction Model for New-onset Hypertension Using Artificial Intelligence Techniques. *J. Clin. Hypertens.* **2020**, *22*, 445–450. [CrossRef] [PubMed]
254. Islam, S.M.S.; Talukder, A.; Awal, M.A.; Siddiqui, M.M.U.; Ahamad, M.M.; Ahammed, B.; Rawal, L.B.; Alizadehsani, R.; Abawajy, J.; Laranjo, L.; et al. Machine Learning Approaches for Predicting Hypertension and Its Associated Factors Using Population-Level Data from Three South Asian Countries. *Front. Cardiovasc. Med.* **2022**, *9*, 839379. [CrossRef]
255. Oh, G.C.; Ko, T.; Kim, J.-H.; Lee, M.H.; Choi, S.W.; Bae, Y.S.; Kim, K.H.; Lee, H.-Y. Estimation of Low-Density Lipoprotein Cholesterol Levels Using Machine Learning. *Int. J. Cardiol.* **2022**, *352*, 144–149. [CrossRef] [PubMed]
256. Wu, J.; Qin, S.; Wang, J.; Li, J.; Wang, H.; Li, H.; Chen, Z.; Li, C.; Wang, J.; Yuan, J. Develop and Evaluate a New and Effective Approach for Predicting Dyslipidemia in Steel Workers. *Front. Bioeng. Biotechnol.* **2020**, *8*, 839. [CrossRef]
257. Correia, M.; Kagenaar, E.; van Schalkwijk, D.B.; Bourbon, M.; Gama-Carvalho, M. Machine Learning Modelling of Blood Lipid Biomarkers in Familial Hypercholesterolaemia versus Polygenic/EnvironmentalDyslipidaemia. *Sci. Rep.* **2021**, *11*, 3801. [CrossRef]
258. Bușilă, C.; Stuparu-Crețu, M.; Barna, O.; Balan, G. Dyslipidemia in Children as a Risk Factor for Cardiovascular Diseases. *Biotechnol. Biotechnol. Equip.* **2017**, *31*, 1192–1197. [CrossRef]
259. Adedinsewo, D.A.; Pollak, A.W.; Phillips, S.D.; Smith, T.L.; Svatikova, A.; Hayes, S.N.; Mulvagh, S.L.; Norris, C.; Roger, V.L.; Noseworthy, P.A.; et al. Cardiovascular Disease Screening in Women: Leveraging Artificial Intelligence and Digital Tools. *Circ. Res.* **2022**, *130*, 673–690. [CrossRef] [PubMed]
260. Tseng, A.S.; Thao, V.; Borah, B.J.; Attia, I.Z.; Medina Inojosa, J.; Kapa, S.; Carter, R.E.; Friedman, P.A.; Lopez-Jimenez, F.; Yao, X.; et al. Cost Effectiveness of an Electrocardiographic Deep Learning Algorithm to Detect Asymptomatic Left Ventricular Dysfunction. *Mayo Clin. Proc.* **2021**, *96*, 1835–1844. [CrossRef] [PubMed]
261. Barry, T.; Farina, J.M.; Chao, C.-J.; Ayoub, C.; Jeong, J.; Patel, B.N.; Banerjee, I.; Arsanjani, R. The Role of Artificial Intelligence in Echocardiography. *J. Imaging* **2023**, *9*, 50. [CrossRef] [PubMed]
262. Nedadur, R.; Wang, B.; Tsang, W. Artificial Intelligence for the Echocardiographic Assessment of Valvular Heart Disease. *Heart* **2022**, *108*, 1592–1599. [CrossRef]
263. Almansouri, N.E.; Awe, M.; Rajavelu, S.; Jahnavi, K.; Shastry, R.; Hasan, A.; Hasan, H.; Lakkimsetti, M.; AlAbbasi, R.K.; Gutiérrez, B.C.; et al. Early Diagnosis of Cardiovascular Diseases in the Era of Artificial Intelligence: An in-Depth Review. *Cureus* **2024**, *16*, e55869. [CrossRef] [PubMed]
264. Sengupta, P.P.; Shrestha, S.; Kagiyama, N.; Hamirani, Y.; Kulkarni, H.; Yanamala, N.; Bing, R.; Chin, C.W.L.; Pawade, T.A.; Messika-Zeitoun, D.; et al. A Machine-Learning Framework to Identify Distinct Phenotypes of Aortic Stenosis Severity. *JACC Cardiovasc. Imaging* **2021**, *14*, 1707–1720. [CrossRef] [PubMed]
265. Yang, F.; Chen, X.; Lin, X.; Chen, X.; Wang, W.; Liu, B.; Li, Y.; Pu, H.; Zhang, L.; Huang, D.; et al. Automated Analysis of Doppler Echocardiographic Videos as a Screening Tool for Valvular Heart Diseases. *JACC Cardiovasc. Imaging* **2022**, *15*, 551–563. [CrossRef] [PubMed]
266. Zhang, J.; Zhang, J.; Jin, J.; Jiang, X.; Yang, L.; Fan, S.; Zhang, Q.; Chi, M. Artificial Intelligence Applied in Cardiovascular Disease: A Bibliometric and Visual Analysis. *Front. Cardiovasc. Med.* **2024**, *11*, 1323918. [CrossRef]
267. Zhang, Q.; Zheng, P.; Hong, Z.; Li, L.; Liu, N.; Bian, Z.; Chen, X.; Wu, H.; Zhao, S. Machine Learning in Risk Prediction of Continuous Renal Replacement Therapy after Coronary Artery Bypass Grafting Surgery in Patients. *Clin. Exp. Nephrol.* **2024**, 1–11. [CrossRef]
268. Bivolaru, S.; Constantin, A.; Vlase, C.M.; Gutu, C. COPD Patients' Behaviour When Involved in the Choice of Inhaler Device. *Healthcare* **2023**, *11*, 1606. [CrossRef] [PubMed]

269. De Ramón Fernández, A.; Ruiz Fernández, D.; Gilart Iglesias, V.; Marcos Jorquera, D. Analyzing the Use of Artificial Intelligence for the Management of Chronic Obstructive Pulmonary Disease (COPD). *Int. J. Med. Inform.* **2022**, *158*, 104640. [CrossRef] [PubMed]
270. Al Namat, R.; Duceac, L.D.; Chelaru, L.; Dabija, M.G.; Guțu, C.; Marcu, C.; Popa, M.V.; Popa, F.; Bogdan Goroftei, E.R.; Tarcă, E. Post-Coronary Artery Bypass Grafting Outcomes of Patients with/without Type-2 Diabetes Mellitus and Chronic Kidney Disease Treated with SGLT2 Inhibitor Dapagliflozin: A Single-Center Experience Analysis. *Diagnostics* **2023**, *14*, 16. [CrossRef] [PubMed]
271. Moinul, M.; Amin, S.A.; Kumar, P.; Patil, U.K.; Gajbhiye, A.; Jha, T.; Gayen, S. Exploring Sodium Glucose Cotransporter (SGLT2) Inhibitors with Machine Learning Approach: A Novel Hope in Anti-Diabetes Drug Discovery. *J. Mol. Graph. Model.* **2022**, *111*, 108106. [CrossRef]
272. Vidal-Perez, R.; Grapsa, J.; Bouzas-Mosquera, A.; Fontes-Carvalho, R.; Vazquez-Rodriguez, J.M. Current Role and Future Perspectives of Artificial Intelligence in Echocardiography. *World J. Cardiol.* **2023**, *15*, 284–292. [CrossRef]

Disclaimer/Publisher's Note: The statements, opinions and data contained in all publications are solely those of the individual author(s) and contributor(s) and not of MDPI and/or the editor(s). MDPI and/or the editor(s) disclaim responsibility for any injury to people or property resulting from any ideas, methods, instructions or products referred to in the content.

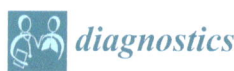

Review

Diagnostic AI and Cardiac Diseases

Dilber Uzun Ozsahin [1,2,*], Cemre Ozgocmen [3,*], Ozlem Balcioglu [2,4], Ilker Ozsahin [2,5] and Berna Uzun [2,6,7]

1. Medical Diagnostic Imaging Department, College of Health Sciences, University of Sharjah, Sharjah 27272, United Arab Emirates
2. Operational Research Center in Healthcare, Near East University, TRNC Mersin 10, 99138 Nicosia, Turkey
3. Department of Biomedical Engineering, Faculty of Engineering, Near East University, TRNC Mersin 10, 99138 Nicosia, Turkey
4. Department of Cardiovascular Surgery, Faculty of Medicine, Near East University, TRNC Mersin 10, 99138 Nicosia, Turkey
5. Brain Health Imaging Institute, Department of Radiology, Weill Cornell Medicine, New York, NY 10025, USA
6. Department of Statistics, Carlos III University of Madrid, 28903 Madrid, Spain
7. Department of Mathematics, Faculty of Sciences and Letters, Near East University, TRNC Mersin 10, 99138 Nicosia, Turkey
* Correspondence: dozsahin@sharjah.ac.ae (D.U.O.); cemreozgocmen@hotmail.com (C.O.)

Abstract: (1) Background: The purpose of this study is to review and highlight recent advances in diagnostic uses of artificial intelligence (AI) for cardiac diseases, in order to emphasize expected benefits to both patients and healthcare specialists; (2) Methods: We focused on four key search terms (Cardiac Disease, diagnosis, artificial intelligence, machine learning) across three different databases (Pubmed, European Heart Journal, Science Direct) between 2017–2022 in order to reach relatively more recent developments in the field. Our review was structured in order to clearly differentiate publications according to the disease they aim to diagnose (coronary artery disease, electrophysiological and structural heart diseases); (3) Results: Each study had different levels of success, where declared sensitivity, specificity, precision, accuracy, area under curve and F1 scores were reported for every article reviewed; (4) Conclusions: the number and quality of AI-assisted cardiac disease diagnosis publications will continue to increase through each year. We believe AI-based diagnosis should only be viewed as an additional tool assisting doctors' own judgement, where the end goal is to provide better quality of healthcare and to make getting medical help more affordable and more accessible, for everyone, everywhere.

Keywords: artificial intelligence; machine learning; cardiac disease; diagnosis

1. Introduction

As it is with other parts of our body, there are many things that can go wrong with our heart. Structural heart defects at birth, lesions in blood vessels, heart valve calcification over time, heart muscle inefficiency for various reasons and electrical signal conduction abnormalities are all examples of cardiac diseases anyone can experience throughout their lifetime.

The Centers for Disease Control and Prevention (CDC) statistics show that 20% of deaths in U.S.A. were caused by cardiac diseases in 2020. This amounts to 696,962 people and it is the leading cause of death in the country [1]. Although cardiac diseases are much more prevalent with elderly patients, it is statistically relevant for all age groups, depending on risk factors present in a patient's life. Therefore, it is easy to understand the amount of research that goes into understanding, diagnosing and treating cardiac diseases. By extension, it is also inevitable that artificial intelligence (AI) research also crosses its path with cardiac disease diagnosis, where earlier and non-invasive diagnosis of as many patients as possible can be seen as the ultimate goal, saving many lives in the process.

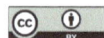

Artificial intelligence (AI), first elaborated by Alan Turing in 1950 [2], is the concept of creating a digital mind that can learn, adapt, react and "think" in a similar manner as a human being. Machine learning (ML) is a process that is closely linked to the concept of AI, where a computer model is enabled to learn new skills and information, and as a result, it can provide useful feedback and perform tasks where classical algorithm-based computer programming falls short. In theory, it is possible for an AI to perform any task imaginable as long as the ML process is sufficiently advanced and robust [3,4].

There are two main approaches to machine learning with many more under each archetype. First is "supervised machine learning", where a dataset is introduced to the model with each case labelled with a class. Computer model then finds commonalities between each case that belongs to the same class and thus "learns" to identify any new unlabelled case as belonging to one of those classes. Supervised ML is especially useful if the task at hand requires the input data to be sorted into predetermined classes or making predictions. However, labelling the dataset for training requires expert knowledge and is time consuming [5,6].

The second approach of "unsupervised machine learning" involves giving the computer model all the data without telling the model which cases belong to which class, and letting it make connections itself where it will sort cases into different classes according to the connections it made while learning. Unsupervised ML can be extremely useful in gaining new understanding about complex systems with many variables as it will make clustering decisions and feature associations by itself, sometimes surprising the experts of the field. However, database size required by an unsupervised ML model is comparatively much larger, where sometimes building the database itself becomes an issue on its own [5,6]. Figure 1 shows the diagram of the AI and machine learning relationship.

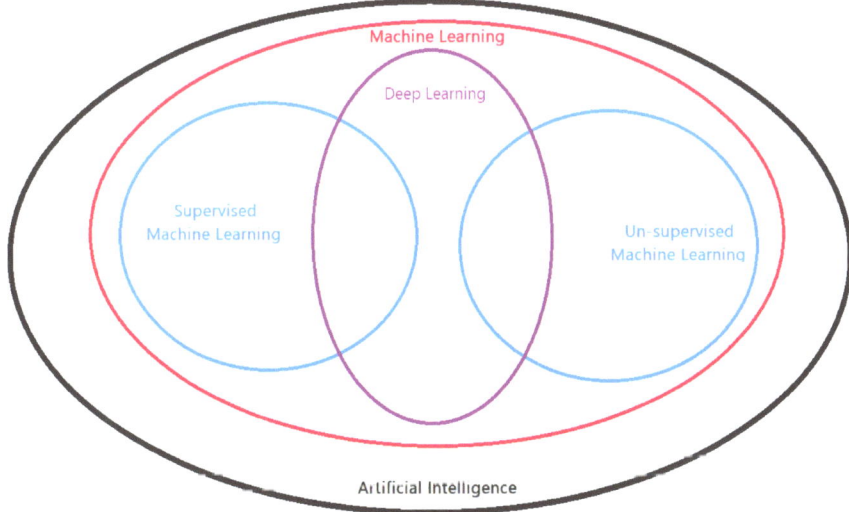

Figure 1. A Venn diagram visually explaining AI and machine learning relationship.

AI can become extremely useful for healthcare in the near future, as it is already becoming so for most other industries and our everyday lives. As healthcare is becoming more and more digitized and interconnected, productive integration of AI systems into standard hospital care is rapidly becoming inevitable. AI can improve many aspects of patient care like medical imaging quality, early diagnosis, prognosis prediction, risk stratification, patient data analysis, personalized treatments and more. For example, as compact devices and biosensors become more available and integrated in our lives, remote monitoring of vitals for the whole population or at least some specific risk groups will be discussed and this will only be feasible with AI shouldering the immense volume of data analysis necessary [7,8].

Additionally, physicians and other healthcare professionals are treating more and more cases per day as the population grows, life expectancy increases and as technology required to treat previously unmanageable diseases becomes more and more available. In order to alleviate their workload, which is already much higher than many other fields of work, and avoid related mistakes that are inevitable, AI assistance will become indispensable. Instead of losing precious time, energy and hospital budget on tasks that can be relegated to AI, physicians and other healthcare professionals can focus on their patients [9,10].

Purpose of this study is to review and highlight recent advances in diagnostic uses of artificial intelligence (AI) for cardiac diseases, in order to emphasize expected benefits to both patients and healthcare specialists, as the future of AI and machine learning (ML) is to be integrated in all aspects of our lives, especially in medicine.

Towards that goal, we will be highlighting some noteworthy challenges relevant to this topic like computing power limitations, data set availability in medical fields, inefficient research targets, and some future directions like ethical/legal considerations that may arise and the idea for a multi-national network of an integrated healthcare system.

2. Method

In this review, we focused on four key search terms (cardiac disease, diagnosis, artificial intelligence, machine learning) across three different databases (Pubmed, European Heart Journal, Science Direct). As per our aim, we limited our search to publications between 2017–2022 in order to reach relatively more recent developments in the field.

There were 346 results in total for original articles with keywords mentioned above, after review articles, case reports and meta-data analysis articles were filtered out. Looking into the content of each publication, we identified that some of the results were not related to cardiac diseases and/or artificial intelligence. Among those that were, some of the results were about disease/feature classification and predictive risk stratification, not diagnostic works, further reducing the number of diagnosis relevant publications. In the end, we identified 38 publications that are relevant to our review.

We elected to subcategorized these publications under the results section in relation to the disease it aims to diagnose in order to provide a more comprehensive comparison and a more coherent reading experience for readers.

A flowchart detailing the process of how relevant publications are obtained, classified and explored can be found below.

Although machine learning methods utilized in each publication will be mentioned, the primary focus of this review will be on medical resources utilized, diagnosed condition and resulting success rates.

3. Results

3.1. Structural Heart Diseases

Hsiang et al. published an article in 2022 about using chest X-rays in order to identify a left ventricular ejection fraction (LVEF) that is lower than 35%. They used 77,227 chest X-rays to train a deep learning model and another 13,320 for testing. The area under curve (AUC) for detection of LVEF < 35% was found to be 0.867. Furthermore, patients with higher than 50% LVEF that were marked by the AI model were found to be at high risk for developing low LVEF in the future according to currently accepted risk assessment guidelines [11].

Salte et al. investigated the possibility of using echocardiography to automatically measure global longitudinal strain (GLS) in 2021. A total of 200 patients were examined in this study and their data were used to train a deep learning ML model. The process of GLS measurement, which was reported to be underused in clinical practices for the amount of time it takes to perform, only took 15 s for each patient. The proposed system could perform the measurement on 89% of the patients, where GLS was $-12.0 \pm 4.1\%$ for the AI method and $-13.5 \pm 5.3\%$ for the reference method [12].

Bahado-Singh et al. were interested in analyzing cell-free DNA that is present in maternal blood in order to identify fetal congenital heart defects. In 2022, they published that by identifying altered gene pathways that result in congenital heart defects, with the help of AI, they can determine various heart defects that will develop with fetus. A total of 6 different AI systems, like random forest, support vector machine and deep learning were used for cross validation since data set size was small (12 cases and 26 controls). Using a combination of nucleotide markers, they achieved an AUC of 0.97, sensitivity of 98% and specificity of 94% [13].

Cheema et al. sought to combine AI with an integrated health system where 11 hospitals are, patient data-wise, interconnected. These data include lab results, demographics, prescription information, procedure codes and more. A total of 7346 patients were identified within the health system to have either stage C or stage D heart failure (HF), and 7500 patients were chosen to be the control group as a result of their normal echocardiography. Using a deep learning algorithm, they were able to classify each case as belonging to one of three categories (stage C, D, healthy) with an overall accuracy of 83% compared to 75% accuracy of physician assessment [14].

Shrivastava et al. discussed how it is possible to diagnose dilated cardiomyopathy using AI with 12-lead ECG instead of an echocardiography in their 2021 publication. In total, 421 dilated cardiomyopathy patients and 16,025 control patients with normal LVEF were used as the database with AUC 0.955, sensitivity of 98.8%, and specificity of 44.8%. The negative predictive value was at 100% while positive predictive value was 1.8% where the reported conclusion was that it is a cost-effective screening tool [15].

Kwon et al. investigated the use of ECG data in 2020 in order to diagnose mitral regurgitation in patients. With a database of 56,670 training ECGs, 3174 internal and 10,865 external test ECGs, proposed AI model identified the P-wave and T-wave as the high weight features. This study produced an AUC of 0.816 for internal testing and 0.877 for external testing [16].

Jentzer et al. used ECG signals in order to identify LV systolic dysfunction for ICU patients in 2021. A study involving 5680 patients, AI was used to obtain 0.83 AUC and overall accuracy of 76% [17].

Lee et al. published an article in 2022 about detection of cardiomyopathy in the peripartum period using ECG signals. Utilizing a deep learning model, AI first learned to identify LV systolic dysfunction using 122,733 ECG samples. For external validation, 271 ECGs of pregnant women were used, producing a result of AUC 0.877, sensitivity 0.833, specificity 0.809, PPV 0.352 and NPV 0.975 [18].

Thalappillil et al. were looking to replace CT aortic annulus measurements for TAVI procedures with AI backed echocardiography. A total of 47 patients implanted with a new heart valve were included in this study. Comparing AI measurements with CT measurements, there was a -4.62 to 1.26 mm difference for derived area and -4.51 to 1.45 mm for the derived perimeter value [19].

Liu et al. used ECG and transthoracic echocardiography (TTE) together in order to diagnose pulmonary hypertension. In their 2022 work, they utilized a deep learning model with 10-fold cross-validation neural network, taking advantage of 41,097 patient data. Results show that AUC was 0.88 with 81.0% sensitivity and 79.6% specificity [20].

Sun et al. used 12-lead ECG and TTE in order to identify patients with <50% LVEF in 2021. A total of 21,732 data pairs trained a CNN deep learning model, while 2530 were used for testing. The ML model produced an overall accuracy of 73.9%, sensitivity of 69.2%, specificity of 70.5%, positive predictive value of 70.1%, and negative predictive value of 69.9% [21].

Thompson et al. published an article in 2019 that demonstrated valvular or congenital heart disease diagnosis could be made using AI assisted auscultation of heart murmurs. In the database obtained from Johns Hopkins Cardiac Auscultatory Recording Database, they wanted to classify each case into either pathological murmur, innocent murmur or no murmur classes. Using 3180 heart sounds, they were able to achieve 93% sensitivity, 81% specificity and 88% accuracy [22].

Harmon et al. used 12-lead ECG in order to detect LV systolic dysfunction with a CNN deep learning model. In total, 44,986 patients, who had an echo pair for independent verification, were used in this study and testing phase was done with 52,870 patients. With a 0.93 AUC, the AI model could detect EF < 35% [23].

Makimoto et al. investigated the use of auscultatory data in diagnosing severe aortic valve stenosis in 2022. By using the sound data that were reported to be cheaper and faster to acquire, they hoped to reduce the percentage of patients that goes undiagnosed. Using three separate CNNs with five-fold cross-validation, they trained the AI models with three different hospital data first separately for each location and then all data together. Comparing each result in order to find the best ML system for the task, they later exported the system to a smart phone as an application where it achieved a 97.6% sensitivity, 94.4% specificity, 95.7% accuracy, and F1 value of 0.93. Compared with the consensus of cardiologists, these results were 81.0%, 93.3%, 89.4% and 0.829, respectively [24].

Attia et al. sought to use a digital stethoscope in order to detect patients with low EF in 2022. Their aim is to significantly reduce the asymptomatic low EF patient numbers that might cause serious health issues along the line, which currently stands at a reported 8% of population. The conceived value of this study lies at diagnosis using a relatively very simple device that obtains 1-lead ECG signals and sound recordings. To accomplish this, they used a CNN based ML model to classify EF < 35%, EF < 40%, EF < 50%. Results were AUC 0.91 for EF < 35%, 0.89 for EF < 40% and 0.84 for EF < 50% [25].

Ghanayim et al. developed an electronic stethoscope which was able to record infrasound. They used this device to obtain heart sounds from 100 patients. Using an undisclosed AI structure, they were able to differentiate mild or severe aortic stenosis and no aortic stenosis classes. Their declared results in 2022 were 86% sensitivity and 100% specificity in testing phase. Validation group scored 84% sensitivity and 92% specificity while additional testing group had 90% sensitivity and 84% specificity [26].

Ueda et al. used chest X-rays in 2021 in order to detect aortic stenosis. Training three different deep learning models with 10,433 chest X-rays, binary classification of aortic stenosis positive or negative classes was prepared as output. Instead of using the best performing DL model out of the three, all of them were used simultaneously via a voting-based ensemble as it produced the best results. Looking at the final performance 0.83 AUC, 0.78 sensitivity, 0.71 specificity, 0.71 accuracy, 0.18 positive predictive value and 0.97 negative predictive value were achieved [27].

3.2. Electrophysiological Heart Diseases

Nakamura et al. looked into identifying premature ventricular complex (PVC) origin locations using 12-lead ECG in 2021. They used ML with two different methods to train the model, first of it being a support vector machine (SVM), and the second was a convolutional neural network (CNN) in order to classify a PVC's location of origin. They used four basic class groups for the AI to consider, which were left, right, outflow tract and others. They wanted to compare their ML model with electrophysiologists and another algorithm in order to measure their success. They reported obtaining the following accuracies: SVM 0.85, CNN 0.80, electrophysiologists 0.73, and existing algorithm 0.86 [28].

Chen et al. were interested in investigating if a wearable monitoring device that can record photoplethysmographic (PPG) data and single-channel ECG data can be used in order to detect atrial fibrillation (AF) presence in a patient. Their 2020 publication shows that using a deep convolutional neural network, they were able to measure wristband PPG classification performance as 88% sensitivity, 96.41% specificity and 93.27% accuracy.

Wristband ECG performance was 87.33%, 99.20% and 94.76%, respectively. Comparing these results with how physicians performed, their sensitivity, specificity and accuracy were 96.67%, 98.01%, and 97.51%, respectively [29].

Sau et al. used a CNN deep learning model in 2022 in order to distinguish between atrial tachyarrhythmias that can be cured with a cavotricuspid isthmus ablation, namely atrial flutter (AFL), and others atrial tachyarrhythmias. In this binary classification endeavour, they used 5 s 12-lead ECG recordings for each patient and achieved an accuracy of 86% versus median electrophysiologist accuracy of 79% [30].

Jo et al. used 12-lead ECG recordings of patients in 2021 in order to identify paroxysmal supraventricular tachycardia during sinus rhythm. Using data from a total of 12,955 patients, the Deep learning ML model was trained and tested. At the end of the study, research group was able to show results of 0.970 accuracy, 0.868 sensitivity, 0.972 specificity, 0.255 positive predictive value and 0.998 negative predictive value [31].

Chang et al. used an ML model with a recurrent neural network structure in 2021 in order to classify 12-lead ECG data into 13 arrhythmia classes (ST-elevation MI, AF, AFL, Atrial premature beat, ventricular bigeminy, complete heart block, ectopic atrial rhythm, first-degree AV block, sinus rhythm, paroxysmal SVT, second-degree AV block, sinus tachycardia, PVC). A total of 60,537 ECG recordings from 35,981 patients were used and, as a result, achieved a performance of 0.987 accuracy and 0.997 area under curve [32].

Au-Yeung et al. published an article in 2021 that attempted to develop a heart rhythm monitoring and an alert system for ICU using a PhysioNet database. They utilized a random forest classifier based supervised ML model in order to evaluate ECG, blood pressure and PPG data and they found out that they could discriminate between eight classes (six arrhythmias) with a sensitivity of 81.54% [33].

Lee et al. proposed a deep learning model in 2022 that can diagnose enlarged atrium from exercise ECG recordings that can lead to AF. Using a convolutional recurrent neural network, they were able to perform a binary categorization with an unspecified performance [34].

Pandey et al. utilized an ensemble-based support vector machine classifier using the arrhythmia database of MIT-BIH. Their aim was to classify ECG recordings into one of four classes of normal rhythm or arrhythmia (SV ectopic beat, PVC, fusion) using only four features (wavelets, high order statistics, R-R intervals, morphological features). They were able to produce a result of 94.4% accuracy [35].

Zhu et al. published an article in 2020 where their aim was to diagnose a patient ECG using ML. They employed a CNN ML model using 12-lead ECG data in order to differentiate 21 rhythms (normal, sinus tachycardia, sinus bradycardia, premature atrial contraction, atrial rhythm, atrial tachycardia, atrial flutter, atrial fibrillation, premature junctional contraction, junctional rhythm, paroxysmal supraventricular tachycardia, premature ventricular contraction, idioventricular rhythm, ventricular tachycardia, artificial atrial pacing rhythm, artificial ventricular pacing rhythm, left bundle branch block, first-degree atrioventricular block, Mobitz type I second-degree atrioventricular block, Wolff–Parkinson–White syndrome type A, and Wolff–Parkinson–White syndrome type B). Training with 135,817 ECG recordings and testing with 17,955 ECGs, they were able to outperform most physicians with an F1 score of 0.887 compared to 0.789–0.831 mean F1 scores for physicians [36].

3.3. Coronary Artery Disease

Otaki et al. published an article in 2022 that seeks to identify coronary artery disease in a patient using data obtained from SPECT images. With a dataset of 3578 patients, they trained a deep learning model where stress myocardial perfusion, wall motion, and wall thickening map, left ventricular volume, age and sex were selected as model input features. After integrating their system to a general-purpose clinical workstation, they obtained an AUC of 0.83 which was significantly higher than their compared results (automatic stress total perfusion deficit 0.73, reader diagnosis 0.65) [37].

Braun et al. utilized a supervised ML model in order to detect clinically asymptomatic coronary artery disease in 2020. With five lead vectorcardiography and a 595-patient database, they achieved a sensitivity score of $90.2 \pm 4.2\%$ for female patients and $97.2 \pm 3.1\%$ for male patients, specificity of $74.4 \pm 9.8\%$ and $76.1 \pm 8.5\%$ for females and males, respectively. Overall accuracy was $82.5 \pm 6.4\%$ for female and $90.7 \pm 3.3\%$ for male patients [38].

Zhao et al. used ECG signals in order to automatically identify ST segment elevated MI and regain precious time lost between identification and treatment time delay. Published in 2020, 667 ST elevated MI patient ECG data and 7571 control ECG data were used in order to train the ML algorithm. The trained system showed AUC of 0.9954 with sensitivity of 96.75%, specificity of 99.20%, accuracy of 99.01%, precision of 90.86% and F1 score of 0.9372 [39].

Choi et al. proposed an inventive idea in 2022 where they used an image of ECG recordings in their dataset instead of the electronic signal recording in order to detect ST elevated MI. Their reasoning was that a mobile phone with a camera is extremely accessible for everyone. With an undisclosed image-based ML model, they completed the training phase with 187 patient recordings where 96 of patients were known to be diagnosed with ST elevated MI. The AUC of proposed ML model was 0.919 where for it was 0.843 for emergency physicians and 0.817 for cardiologists [40].

Cho et al. used intravascular ultrasound (IVUS) images with a deep learning model in 2021 with the aim of identifying and classifying plaque characteristics present in a cardiac blood vessel. A total of 598 IVUS image sets were used in this study with a total of three classes, which are calcified plaque, attenuated plaque and none. The proposed model was able to achieve attenuation sensitivity of 80%, specificity of 96%, accuracy of 93% and calcium sensitivity of 86%, specificity of 97% and accuracy of 96%. Compared to human performance, per-vessel analysis achieved similar results (0.95 human, 0.89 ML model), producing these results in 7.8 s [41].

Stuckey et al. developed a supervised ML model using linear regression in 2018 in order to assess coronary artery disease presence. They acquired phase signals from CT for a total of 606 patients, just before the planned coronary angiography, which was used to produce labels for the supervised training model. A total of 512 patient data points were used for training and 94 patient data points were used for testing stage. The study produced a result of 92% sensitivity, 62% specificity, 46% positive predictive value and negative predictive value of 96% [42].

Cho et al. published an article in 2019, aiming to assess fractional flow reserve (FFR) using coronary angiography. A supervised machine learning model that evaluates intermediate lesions was built in order to classify the data into FFR > 80 or FFR < 80. With a dataset of 1501 patients, achieved results were $78 \pm 4\%$ diagnostic accuracy and 0.84 ± 0.03 AUC. Out of 24 features used in ML model, 12 of them were found to be high ranking, including segment, body surface area, distal lumen diameter, minimum lumen diameter and length of lumen. Using only these 12 high ranking features, they were able to achieve $81 \pm 1\%$ diagnostic accuracy and 0.87 ± 0.01 AUC [43].

Lee et al. predicted that they can assess coronary artery disease presence using a treadmill exercise test (TET). In a 2021 publication, they discussed using 93 features with five different ML models (random forest, logistic regression, support vector machine, k-nearest neighbour, extreme gradient boosting). Among these features, exercise performance, hemodynamics and ST-segment changes, comorbidity, smoking, Framingham risk score, height and weight were present. Out of the five different ML models, random forest showed the best performance, AUC of 0.74, sensitivity of 85% and false positive rate of 55% compared to the 76.3% of conventional TET [44].

Lipkin et al. proposed that they could use coronary CT angiography (CCTA) with AI-based quantitative CT (QCT) in order to produce a better detection rate than myocardial perfusion imaging (MPI) for obstructive stenosis. Using a pre-built cloud based QCT software on acquired CCTA data, they were able to outperform MPI on obstructive stenosis detection across two classes with AI-QCT. AUC scores for stenosis > 50% showed 0.66 for

MPI vs. 0.88 for AI-QCT, stenosis > 70% showed 0.7 for MPI vs 0.90 for AI-QCT. Publication suggests that CCTA with AI-QCT outperforms MPI and thus it could reduce the number of patients undergoing invasive tests and reduce healthcare costs [45].

Kurata et al. utilized coronary computed tomography-derived computational fractional flow reserve (CT-FFR) in 2019 in order to detect coronary artery disease. With a dataset of 74 patients, they employed a prototype ML model (cFFR version 3.0.0, Siemens Healthcare, Tokyo, Japan) comparing CCTA and CT-FFR performance. Obtained results show that FFR < 0.8 CT-FFR had AUC of 0.907 where CTA stenosis > 50% had 0.595 and stenosis > 70% had 0.603. CT-FFR had an analysis time of 16.4 ± 7.5 min [46].

Tang et al. used CCTA derived FFR in 2019 in order to detect lesion-specific ischemia. They adopted an ML algorithm called $cFFR_{ML}$ and obtained CT-FFR values from 136 patients across four healthcare centers. Invasive FFR measurements were used as reference. Study revealed that $cFFR_{ML}$ had 0.85 sensitivity, 0.94 specificity and 0.90 accuracy versus 0.95 sensitivity, 0.28 specificity and 0.55 accuracy for CCTA [47].

Choi et al. published an article in 2021 where they compare coronary artery disease assessments made by an AI assisted CCTA with level 3 expert CCTA readers. In this multicenter international study, patient history data (BMI, age, sex, smoking history, diabetes, etc) were combined with a deep convolutional neural network AI (Cleerly) labelled CCTA images in order to estimate stenosis percentage, plaque volume, composition and presence of high-risk plaque. Results of this 232-patient study showed 99.7% accuracy, 90.9% sensitivity, 99.8% specificity, 93.3% positive predictive value and 99.9% negative predictive value for stenosis > 70%. When stenosis > 50% is considered, 94.8% accuracy, 80.0% sensitivity, 97.0% specificity, 80.0% positive predictive value and 97.0% negative predictive value was shown. When the expert reader comparison was performed for maximal diameter stenosis per vessel, -0.8% mean difference was found and for per patient comparison -2.3% mean difference was found. Reportedly, these excellent results show that the time-consuming expert reader evaluations could be processed much more quickly and cost-effectively by an AI [48].

Table 1 shows the detailed information about the outcomes of the reviewed publications which are applied for the diagnosis of the selected diseases with AI models and their performance summary.

Table 1. Method and performance summary of reviewed publications.

Authors (et al.)	Year	Disease Diagnosed	Data Source	Machine Learning Method	Reported Results (Accuracy, Sensitivity, Specificity, PPV, NPV, AUC, F1)					
Hsiang [11]	2022	Low EF	Chest X-ray	Deep Learning						0.867
Salte [12]	2021	LV dysfunction	Echocardiography	Deep Learning	GLS for: AI $-12.0 \pm 4.1\%$, Reference $-13.5 \pm 5.3\%$					
Bahado-Singh [13]	2022	Fetal congenital heart defects	Cell-free DNA	RF, SVM, DL	98%	94%				0.97
Cheema [14]	2022	Heart Failure	IHS Data	Deep Learning	83%					
Shrivastava [15]	2021	Dilated Cardiomyopathy	ECG	N/A		98.8%	44.8%	1.8%	100%	0.955
Kwon [16]	2020	Mitral Regurgitation	ECG	N/A						0.816
Jentzer [17]	2021	LV dysfunction	ECG	N/A	76%					0.83
Lee [18]	2022	LV dysfunction	ECG	Deep Learning	0.833	0.809		0.352	0.975	0.877

Table 1. Cont.

Authors (et al.)	Year	Disease Diagnosed	Data Source	Machine Learning Method	Reported Results (Accuracy, Sensitivity, Specificity, PPV, NPV, AUC, F1)
Thalappillil [19]	2020	Aortic Annulus Size	Echocardiography	N/A	−4.62 to 1.26 mm difference for derived area and −4.51 to 1.45 mm for derived perimeter value
Liu [20]	2022	Pulmonary Hypertension	ECG, TTE	Cross Validation DL	81% 79.6% 0.88
Sun [21]	2021	Low EF	ECG, TTE	CNN Deep Learning	73.9% 69.2% 70.50% 70.1% 69.9%
Thompson [22]	2019	Valvular, congenital	Digital Stethoscope	N/A	88% 93% 81%
Harmon [23]	2022	LV dysfunction	ECG	CNN Deep Learning	0.93
Makimoto [24]	2022	AV Stenosis	Digital Stethoscope	CNN Cross Validation	95.7% 97.6% 94.4% 0.93
Attia [25]	2022	Low EF	Digital Stethoscope	CNN	0.89
Ghanayim [26]	2022	AV Stenosis	Digital Stethoscope	N/A	84% 92%
Ueda [27]	2021	AV Stenosis	Chest X-ray	Deep Learning Ensemble	0.71 0.78 0.71 0.18 0.97 0.83
Nakamura [28]	2021	PVC Origin	ECG	SVM, CNN	0.85
Chen [29]	2020	AF	1-Lead ECG, PPG	CNN Deep Learning	93.27% 88% 96.41%
Sau [30]	2022	AFL/SVT	ECG	N/A	86%
Jo [31]	2021	Paroxisymal SVT	Sinus ECG	Deep Learning	0.97 0.868 0.972 0.255 0.998
Chang [32]	2021	Arrhythmia	ECG	Recurrent NN	0.987 0.997
Au-Yeung [33]	2021	Arrhythmia	ECG, BP, PPG	Random Forest	81.54%
Lee [34]	2022	AF	Exercise ECG	Deep Learning	N/A
Pandey [35]	2020	Arrhythmia	ECG	Ensemble SVM	94.4%
Zhu [36]	2020	Arrhythmia	ECG	CNN	0.887
Otaki [37]	2022	CAD	SPECT	Deep Learning	0.83
Braun [38]	2020	CAD	VCG	Supervised ML	82.5% 90.20% 74.4%
Zhao [39]	2020	ST elevated MI	ECG	N/A	99.01% 96.75% 99.2% 0.995 0.937
Choi [40]	2022	ST elevated MI	ECG Image	N/A	0.919
Cho [41]	2021	Plaque Type	IVUS	Deep Learning	96% 86% 97%
Stuckey [42]	2018	CAD	CT	Supervised ML	92% 62% 46% 96%

Table 1. Cont.

Authors (et al.)	Year	Disease Diagnosed	Data Source	Machine Learning Method	Reported Results (Accuracy, Sensitivity, Specificity, PPV, NPV, AUC, F1)					
Cho [43]	2019	CAD	C. Angiography FFR	Supervised ML	81%					0.87
Lee [44]	2021	CAD	Treadmill Test	RF, SVM, LR, K-NN, EGB	85%					0.74
Lipkin [45]	2022	CAD	AI CCTA	N/A						0.88
Kurata [46]	2019	CAD	CT FFR	N/A						0.907
Tang [47]	2019	CAD	CCTA FFR	N/A	0.9	0.85	0.94			
Choi [48]	2021	CAD	AI CCTA	CNN Deep Learning	94.80%	80%	97%	80%	97%	

4. Discussion

As it is evident from the number of articles reviewed above, overall publication of machine learning-related healthcare diagnosis research has been multiplicatively growing each year. By the same token, there is a good amount of research performed on structural heart diseases and especially on coronary artery disease. However, relatively, there are significantly less electrophysiology-based AI research publications on medical journal databases. Figure 2 shows the flowchart of the method design of this paper. The selected papers are limited to the years between 2017 and 2022. Figure 3 shows the yearly published heart-related AI/ML studies increased exponentially on Science Direct, Pubmed and European Heart Journal.

Similarly, a striking amount of machine learning research is being carried out that is focused on using echocardiograms and especially so with ECG signals. It is natural that one of the most useful pieces of data gathering tools in cardiology, ECG, is used as input in ML and especially in electrophysiology. However, usefulness of other forms of data, we believe, should not be underestimated. Hospitals with integrated patient health record systems have the ability to provide researchers with an immense amount of lab data containing a multitude of metabolic measurements, as well as patient profile and history records which is usually critical to how cardiologists normally perform their patient care routines. Although there are some studies that utilize these opportunities, we believe it has nowhere near reached its full capacity. On a similar note, the same is true for medical imaging as well, since one of the most routinely performed imaging tests is coronary angiography and there should be a well of untapped potential in that metaphorical alley.

It is clear that when looking at machine learning techniques, deep learning approach variations are much more preferred in general as opposed to classical single hidden layer supervised ML or unsupervised ML models. Convolutional neural networks, recurrent neural networks and cross-validation seems to be popular according to publications relevant to this review.

Overall level of success for reviewed AI diagnosis systems seems to indicate that they achieved noteworthy improvements on similar previous works or they are fresh and innovative ideas with a good starting performance. In some works, although negative predictive values were high, positive predictive values were comparatively very low, which indicates a need for further development and refinement.

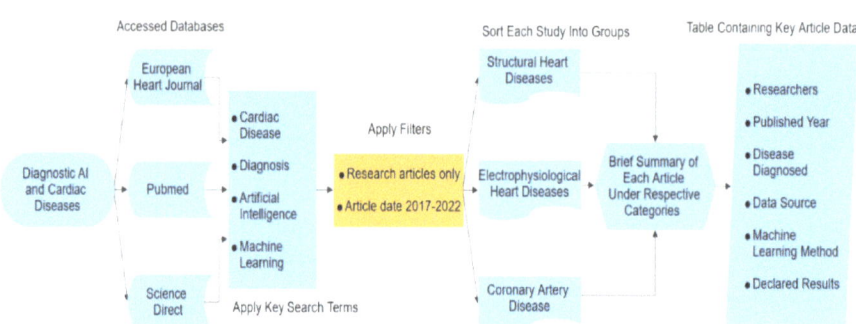

Figure 2. Flowchart of method design for this review.

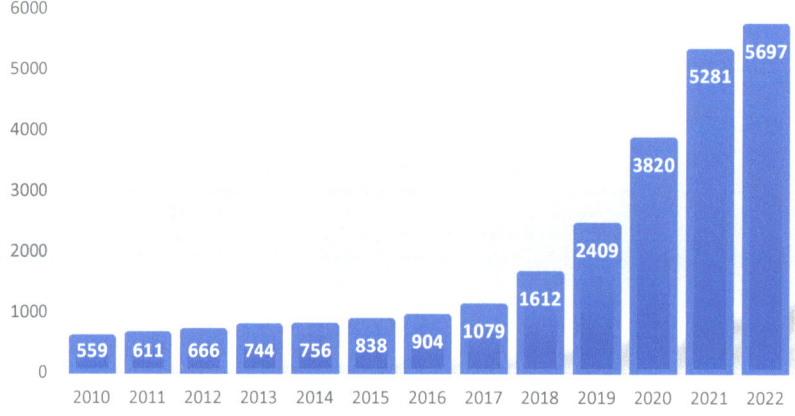

Figure 3. A bar chart showing the number of heart related AI/ML publications on Science Direct, Pubmed and European Heart Journal through years.

In our opinion, however, one of the most important factors of true success in modern technology research is being slightly overlooked. We believe that a stronger collaboration between doctors and AI engineers should be present. Any research team of engineers should have at least a few specialists that they consult and, similarly, any research hospital interested in AI technology should employ the skills of engineers more often. It is not useful for a remarkable ML model, from a technical stand point, to be created and yet end up not being used because it does not realistically fulfil a need in healthcare. In order to create profound technological advancements, we believe, experts in the field of healthcare should identify the areas to work on and then engineers can direct their research efforts accordingly in order to build innovative support systems that are desperately needed.

Finally, we wanted to briefly raise questions about some ethical and legal considerations. First of all, what safeguards should be put in place in order to protect patient confidentiality since AI will be able to reach all data of all patients? What should we do about early risk assessments when the AI can tell us that a patient might be diagnosed with an illness in 5–10 years time? Which organization decides that an AI diagnosis system is deemed safe to use for patients; individual hospitals or governments? Who should be investigated when a malpractice case is brought up that involves an AI; doctors, hospitals, tech companies or engineers? Finally, what happens if doctors become, in two generations time for example, overly reliant on AI for diagnosis and their own judgement standards get lowered, or how can we prevent such an occurrence? At some point, we believe these questions will need to be answered.

5. Conclusions

The future of diagnostic artificial intelligence looks very promising, especially for diagnosis of cardiac diseases. Each year there are more and better research publications in AI and machine learning. Every new publication gets us one step closer to improving our current diagnostic tools and systems, providing us with a powerful ally in researching new approaches to understanding disease mechanisms and innovating new treatments for them. However, there are some ethical and legal considerations, as mentioned in discussions section, that will need to be seriously debated by all parties involved in the near future.

As it has been for decades before, contemporary computing power available in order to facilitate ML is one of the most obvious and important limitations for AI in our time. Sophisticated ML models that could be designed, and datasets that could be much larger and much more detailed would result in better overall performance. However, they cannot be employed unless there are sufficient strides in making the commercially available computing power on the market on par with the requirements of AI researchers.

It is also important to note that predictions and classifications made by AI models are only as strong as the dataset quality and selected feature reliability. Therefore, it is paramount for any AI system to be tested rigorously before being implemented. Another issue is that medical data are much harder to acquire compared to other fields. This is a considerable limitation since machine learning in general uses large amounts of data to train a model. Deep learning, a very promising subset of ML, is especially affected by this limitation since it has to utilize massive data sets in order to learn in a way that is a closer approximation to how humans learn.

Despite this limitation, there are a decent number of publicly available datasets like "CardioNet" by Ahn et al. [49], "Cardiovascular Disease dataset" from Kaggle [50] and "Heart Disease Data Set" from UCI Machine Learning Repository [51] to give a few examples, which somewhat alleviates this problem at least for now. On the other hand, since more sophisticated ML methods tend to require exponentially larger and more detailed datasets, in order to achieve the full future potential of AI assisted diagnosis, a much more comprehensive and meticulous solution needs to be implemented. This is the point where, we believe, the need for a standardized multi-national network of integrated healthcare system arises.

Apart from some of the obvious benefits of using previously performed tests from a hospital in order to reliably and easily get healthcare services from another hospital, the amount of data that can be obtained with such a system would be profound for AI researchers. Digitized medical imaging data, lab results, patient information and medical background, resulting diagnosis and short/long term prognosis would be obtainable for each patient, of course excluding patient identifier data, which means that any dataset that could be needed for any research can be extracted from this emergent database. This type of undertaking, however, would bring a new set of issues to be handled by international organizations where they would need to enforce ethical conduct and patient privacy, mediate a common data format, facilitate data sharing infrastructure and provide end user training.

In the end, we believe AI based diagnosis will not, and should not aim to, replace specialists and their roles in healthcare. ML technology should be an additional tool assisting doctors' own judgement, save them and other healthcare professionals time on mundane and repeated tasks. Additionally, medical emergencies may benefit greatly from streamlined and fast decision-making processes where AI provides a lot of information to doctors with little data. Most importantly, AI end goal should be to provide better quality of healthcare, reduce hospital and administration costs to make getting medical help cheaper and more accessible, for everyone, everywhere.

Author Contributions: Conceptualization, D.U.O., O.B. and I.O.; methodology, C.O. and I.O.; validation, O.B., I.O. and D.U.O.; formal analysis C.O. and B.U.; investigations C.O. and O.B.; resources, C.O. and I.O.; data curation, C.O. and B.U.; writing—original draft preparation, C.O.; writing—review and editing D.U.O.; visualization, C.O.; supervision, D.U.O., I.O., O.B. and B.U.; project administration D.U.O., O.B., I.O. and B.U. All authors have read and agreed to the published version of the manuscript.

Funding: The research received no external funding.

Institutional Review Board Statement: Not applicable.

Informed Consent Statement: Not applicable.

Data Availability Statement: The data is provided within the manuscript.

Conflicts of Interest: The authors declare no conflict of interest.

Abbreviations

Abbreviations used in this article are listed below in alphabetical order.

AF	Atrial fibrillation
AFL	Atrial flutter
AI	Artificial intelligence
AUC	Area under curve
AV	Aortic valve
AV	Atrioventricular
BMI	Body mass index
BP	Blood pressure
CAD	Coronary artery disease
CCTA	Coronary computerized tomography angiography
CDC	Centers for Disease Control and Prevention
CNN	Convolutional neural network
CT	Computerized tomography
DL	Deep learning
ECG	Electrocardiogram
EF	Ejection Fraction
EGB	Extreme gradient boosting
FFR	Fractional flow reserve
GLS	Global longitudinal strain
HF	Heart failure
ICU	Intensive care unit
IHS	Integrated healthcare system
IVUS	Intravascular ultrasound
K-NN	K-nearest neighbor
LR	Logistic regression
LV	Left ventricule
LVEF	Left ventricular ejection fraction
MI	Myocardial infarction
ML	Machine learning
MPI	Myocardial perfusion imaging
NN	Neural network

NPV	Negative predictive value
PPG	Photoplethysmographic
PPV	Positive predictive value
PVC	Premature ventricular complex
QCT	Quantitative computerized tomography
RF	Random forest
SPECT	Single photon emission computerized tomography
SV	Supraventricular
SVM	Support vector machine
SVT	Supraventricular tachycardia
TAVI	Transcatheter aortic valve implantation
TET	Treadmill exercise test
TTE	Transthoracic echocardiography
VCG	Vectorcardiography

References

1. Heart Disease Statistics. Centers for Disease Control and Prevention (CDC). 2022. Available online: https://www.cdc.gov/nchs/fastats/heart-disease.htm (accessed on 5 October 2022).
2. Harnad, S. The Annotation Game: On Turing (1950) on Computing, Machinery and Intelligence Archived 18 October 2017 at the Wayback Machine. In *Parsing the Turing Test: Philosophical and Methodological Issues in the Quest for the Thinking Computer*; Epstein, R., Peters, G., Eds.; Springer: Cham, Switzerland, 2008.
3. Russell, S.J.; Norvig, P. *Artificial Intelligence: A Modern Approach*, 4th ed.; Pearson: Hoboken, NJ, USA, 2021; ISBN 9780134610993.
4. Mitchell, T.M. *Machine Learning*; McGraw-Hilll: New York, NY, USA, 1997. [CrossRef]
5. Bishop, C.M. *Pattern Recognition and Machine Learning*; Springer: New York, NY, USA, 2006; ISBN 978-1-4939-3843-8.
6. Mohri, M.; Rostamizadeh, A.; Talwalkar, A. *Foundations of Machine Learning*; The MIT Press: Cambridge, MA, USA, 2012; ISBN 9780262018258.
7. Nichols, J.A.; Chan, H.W.H.; Baker, M.A.B. Machine learning: Applications of artificial intelligence to imaging and diagnosis. *Biophys. Rev.* **2019**, *11*, 111–118. [CrossRef] [PubMed]
8. Quer, G.; Arnaout, R.; Henne, M.; Arnaout, R. Machine Learning and the Future of Cardiovascular Care: JACC State-of-the-Art Review. *J. Am. Coll. Cardiol.* **2021**, *77*, 300–313. [CrossRef]
9. Johnson, K.W.; Soto, J.T.; Glicksberg, B.S.; Shameer, K.; Miotto, R.; Ali, M.; Ashley, E.; Dudley, J.T. Artificial Intelligence in Cardiology. *J. Am. Coll. Cardiol.* **2018**, *71*, 2668–2679. [CrossRef] [PubMed]
10. Asselbergs, F.W.; Fraser, A.G. Artificial intelligence in cardiology: The debate continues. *Eur. Heart J. Digit. Health* **2021**, *2*, 721–726. [CrossRef]
11. Hsiang, C.-W.; Lin, C.; Liu, W.-C.; Chang, W.-C.; Hsu, H.-H.; Huang, G.-S.; Lou, Y.-S.; Lee, C.-C.; Wang, C.-H.; Fang, W.-H. Detection of Left Ventricular Systolic Dysfunction Using an Artificial Intelligence–Enabled Chest X-Ray. *Can. J. Cardiol.* **2022**, *38*, 763–773. [CrossRef] [PubMed]
12. Salte, I.M.; Østvik, A.; Smistad, E.; Melichova, D.; Nguyen, T.M.; Karlsen, S.; Brunvand, H.; Haugaa, K.H.; Edvardsen, T.; Lovstakken, L.; et al. Artificial Intelligence for Automatic Measurement of Left Ventricular Strain in Echocardiography. *JACC Cardiovasc. Imaging* **2021**, *14*, 1918–1928. [CrossRef]
13. Bahado-Singh, R.; Friedman, P.; Talbot, C.; Aydas, B.; Southekal, S.; Mishra, N.K.; Guda, C.; Yilmaz, A.; Radhakrishna, U.; Vishweswaraiah, S. cfDNA in maternal blood and Artificial Intelligence: Accurate Prenatal Detection of Fetal Congenital Heart Defects. *Am. J. Obstet. Gynecol.* **2022**, *2*, 721–726. [CrossRef]
14. Cheema, B.; Mutharasan, R.K.; Sharma, A.; Jacobs, M.; Powers, K.; Lehrer, S.; Wehbe, F.H.; Ronald, J.; Pifer, L.; Rich, J.D.; et al. Augmented Intelligence to Identify Patients With Advanced Heart Failure in an Integrated Health System. *JACC Adv.* **2022**, *1*, 100123. [CrossRef]
15. Shrivastava, S.; Cohen-Shelly, M.; Attia, Z.I.; Rosenbaum, A.N.; Wang, L.; Giudicessi, J.R.; Redfield, M.; Bailey, K.; Lopez-Jimenez, F.; Lin, G.; et al. Artificial Intelligence-Enabled Electrocardiography to Screen Patients with Dilated Cardiomyopathy. *Am. J. Cardiol.* **2021**, *155*, 121–127. [CrossRef]
16. Kwon, J.-M.; Kim, K.-H.; Akkus, Z.; Jeon, K.-H.; Park, J.; Oh, B.-H. Artificial intelligence for detecting mitral regurgitation using electrocardiography. *J. Electrocardiol.* **2020**, *59*, 151–157. [CrossRef]
17. Jentzer, J.C.; Kashou, A.H.; Attia, Z.I.; Lopez-Jimenez, F.; Kapa, S.; Friedman, P.A.; Noseworthy, P.A. Left ventricular systolic dysfunction identification using artificial intelligence-augmented electrocardiogram in cardiac intensive care unit patients. *Int. J. Cardiol.* **2021**, *326*, 114–123. [CrossRef]
18. Lee, Y.; Choi, B.; Lee, M.S.; Jin, U.; Yoon, S.; Jo, Y.-Y.; Kwon, J.-M. An artificial intelligence electrocardiogram analysis for detecting cardiomyopathy in the peripartum period. *Int. J. Cardiol.* **2022**, *352*, 72–77. [CrossRef]
19. Thalappillil, R.; Datta, P.; Datta, S.; Zhan, Y.; Wells, S.; Mahmood, F.; Cobey, F.C. Artificial Intelligence for the Measurement of the Aortic Valve Annulus. *J. Cardiothorac. Vasc. Anesthesia* **2020**, *34*, 65–71. [CrossRef] [PubMed]

20. Liu, C.-M.; Shih, E.S.; Chen, J.-Y.; Huang, C.-H.; Wu, I.-C.; Chen, P.-F.; Higa, S.; Yagi, N.; Hu, Y.-F.; Hwang, M.-J.; et al. Artificial Intelligence-Enabled Electrocardiogram Improves the Diagnosis and Prediction of Mortality in Patients With Pulmonary Hypertension. *JACC Asia* **2022**, *2*, 258–270. [CrossRef] [PubMed]
21. Sun, J.; Qiu, Y.; Guo, H.; Hua, Y.; Shao, B.; Qiao, Y.; Guo, J.; Ding, H.; Zhang, Z.; Miao, L.; et al. A method to screen left ventricular dysfunction through ECG based on convolutional neural network. *J. Cardiovasc. Electrophysiol.* **2021**, *32*, 1095–1102. [CrossRef]
22. Thompson, W.R.; Reinisch, A.J.; Unterberger, M.J.; Schriefl, A.J. Artificial Intelligence-Assisted Auscultation of Heart Murmurs: Validation by Virtual Clinical Trial. *Pediatr. Cardiol.* **2019**, *40*, 623–629. [CrossRef]
23. Harmon, D.M.; Carter, R.E.; Cohen-Shelly, M.; Svatikova, A.; Adedinsewo, D.A.; Noseworthy, P.A.; Kapa, S.; Lopez-Jimenez, F.; Friedman, P.A.; Attia, Z.I. Real-world performance, long-term efficacy, and absence of bias in the artificial intelligence enhanced electrocardiogram to detect left ventricular systolic dysfunction. *Eur. Heart J. Digit. Health* **2022**, *3*, 238–244. [CrossRef] [PubMed]
24. Makimoto, H.; Shiraga, T.; Kohlmann, B.; Magnisali, C.E.; Gerguri, S.; Motoyama, N.; Clasen, L.; Bejinariu, A.; Klein, K.; Makimoto, A.; et al. Efficient screening for severe aortic valve stenosis using understandable artificial intelligence: A prospective diagnostic accuracy study. *Eur. Heart J. Digit. Health* **2022**, *3*, 141–152. [CrossRef]
25. Attia, Z.I.; Dugan, J.; Rideout, A.; Maidens, J.N.; Venkatraman, S.; Guo, L.; Noseworthy, P.A.; Pellikka, P.A.; Pham, S.L.; Kapa, S.; et al. Automated Detection of Low Ejection Fraction from a One-lead Electrocardiogram: Application of an AI algorithm to an ECG-enabled Digital Stethoscope. *Eur. Heart J. Digit. Health* **2022**, *3*, 373–379. [CrossRef]
26. Ghanayim, T.; Lupu, L.; Naveh, S.; Bachner-Hinenzon, N.; Adler, D.; Adawi, S.; Banai, S.; Shiran, A. Artificial Intelligence-Based Stethoscope for the Diagnosis of Aortic Stenosis. *Am. J. Med.* **2022**, *135*, 1124–1133. [CrossRef]
27. Ueda, D.; Yamamoto, A.; Ehara, S.; Iwata, S.; Abo, K.; Walston, S.L.; Matsumoto, T.; Shimazaki, A.; Yoshiyama, M.; Miki, Y. Artificial intelligence-based detection of aortic stenosis from chest radiographs. *Eur. Heart J. Digit. Health* **2022**, *3*, 20–28. [CrossRef]
28. Nakamura, T.; Nagata, Y.; Nitta, G.; Okata, S.; Nagase, M.; Mitsui, K.; Watanabe, K.; Miyazaki, R.; Kaneko, M.; Nagamine, S.; et al. Prediction of premature ventricular complex origins using artificial intelligence–enabled algorithms. *Cardiovasc. Digit. Health J.* **2020**, *2*, 76–83. [CrossRef] [PubMed]
29. Chen, E.; Jiang, J.; Su, R.; Gao, M.; Zhu, S.; Zhou, J.; Huo, Y. A new smart wristband equipped with an artificial intelligence algorithm to detect atrial fibrillation. *Heart Rhythm* **2020**, *17*, 847–853. [CrossRef] [PubMed]
30. Sau, A.; Ibrahim, S.; Ahmed, A.; Handa, B.; Kramer, D.B.; Waks, J.W.; Arnold, A.D.; Howard, J.P.; Qureshi, N.; Koa-Wing, M.; et al. Artificial intelligence-enabled electrocardiogram to distinguish cavotricuspid isthmus dependence from other atrial tachycardia mechanisms. *Eur. Heart J. Digit. Health* **2022**, *3*, 405–414. [CrossRef]
31. Jo, Y.-Y.; Kwon, J.-M.; Jeon, K.-H.; Cho, Y.-H.; Shin, J.-H.; Lee, Y.-J.; Jung, M.-S.; Ban, J.-H.; Kim, K.-H.; Lee, S.Y.; et al. Artificial intelligence to diagnose paroxysmal supraventricular tachycardia using electrocardiography during normal sinus rhythm. *Eur. Heart J. Digit. Health* **2021**, *2*, 290–298. [CrossRef]
32. Chang, K.-C.; Hsieh, P.-H.; Wu, M.-Y.; Wang, Y.-C.; Wei, J.-T.; Shih, E.S.C.; Hwang, M.-J.; Lin, W.-Y.; Lee, K.-J.; Wang, T.-H. Usefulness of multi-labelling artificial intelligence in detecting rhythm disorders and acute ST-elevation myocardial infarction on 12-lead electrocardiogram. *Eur. Heart J. Digit. Health* **2021**, *2*, 299–310. [CrossRef]
33. Au-Yeung, W.-T.M.; Sevakula, R.K.; Sahani, A.K.; Kassab, M.; Boyer, R.; Isselbacher, E.M.; Armoundas, A.A. Real-time machine learning-based intensive care unit alarm classification without prior knowledge of the underlying rhythm. *Eur. Heart J. Digit. Health* **2021**, *2*, 437–445. [CrossRef]
34. Lee, H.-C.; Chen, C.-Y.; Lee, S.-J.; Lee, M.-C.; Tsai, C.-Y.; Chen, S.-T.; Li, Y.-J. Exploiting exercise electrocardiography to improve early diagnosis of atrial fibrillation with deep learning neural networks. *Comput. Biol. Med.* **2022**, *146*, 105584. [CrossRef] [PubMed]
35. Pandey, S.K.; Janghel, R.R.; Vani, V. Patient Specific Machine Learning Models for ECG Signal Classification. *Procedia Comput. Sci.* **2020**, *167*, 2181–2190. [CrossRef]
36. Zhu, H.; Cheng, C.; Yin, H.; Li, X.; Zuo, P.; Ding, J.; Lin, F.; Wang, J.; Zhou, B.; Li, Y.; et al. Automatic multilabel electrocardiogram diagnosis of heart rhythm or conduction abnormalities with deep learning: A cohort study. *Lancet Digit. Health* **2020**, *2*, e348–e357. [CrossRef]
37. Otaki, Y.; Singh, A.; Kavanagh, P.; Miller, R.J.; Parekh, T.; Tamarappoo, B.K.; Sharir, T.; Einstein, A.J.; Fish, M.B.; Ruddy, T.D.; et al. Clinical Deployment of Explainable Artificial Intelligence of SPECT for Diagnosis of Coronary Artery Disease. *JACC Cardiovasc. Imaging* **2022**, *15*, 1091–1102. [CrossRef]
38. Braun, T.; Spiliopoulos, S.; Veltman, C.; Hergesell, V.; Passow, A.; Tenderich, G.; Borggrefe, M.; Koerner, M.M. Detection of myocardial ischemia due to clinically asymptomatic coronary artery stenosis at rest using supervised artificial intelligence-enabled vectorcardiography—A five-fold cross validation of accuracy. *J. Electrocardiol.* **2020**, *59*, 100–105. [CrossRef]
39. Zhao, Y.; Xiong, J.; Hou, Y.; Zhu, M.; Lu, Y.; Xu, Y.; Teliewubai, J.; Liu, W.; Xu, X.; Li, X.; et al. Early detection of ST-segment elevated myocardial infarction by artificial intelligence with 12-lead electrocardiogram. *Int. J. Cardiol.* **2020**, *317*, 223–230. [CrossRef] [PubMed]
40. Choi, Y.J.; Park, M.J.; Ko, Y.; Soh, M.-S.; Kim, H.M.; Kim, C.H.; Lee, E.; Kim, J. Artificial intelligence versus physicians on interpretation of printed ECG images: Diagnostic performance of ST-elevation myocardial infarction on electrocardiography. *Int. J. Cardiol.* **2022**, *363*, 6–10. [CrossRef]

41. Cho, H.; Kang, S.-J.; Min, H.-S.; Lee, J.-G.; Kim, W.-J.; Kang, S.H.; Kang, D.-Y.; Lee, P.H.; Ahn, J.-M.; Park, D.-W.; et al. Intravascular ultrasound-based deep learning for plaque characterization in coronary artery disease. *Atherosclerosis* **2021**, *324*, 69–75. [CrossRef] [PubMed]
42. Stuckey, T.D.; Gammon, R.S.; Goswami, R.; Depta, J.P.; Steuter, J.A.; Iii, F.J.M.; Roberts, M.C.; Singh, N.; Ramchandani, S.; Burton, T.; et al. Cardiac Phase Space Tomography: A novel method of assessing coronary artery disease utilizing machine learning. *PLoS ONE* **2018**, *13*, e0198603. [CrossRef] [PubMed]
43. Cho, H.; Lee, J.-G.; Kang, S.-J.; Kim, W.-J.; Choi, S.-Y.; Ko, J.; Min, H.-S.; Choi, G.-H.; Kang, D.-Y.; Lee, P.H.; et al. Angiography-Based Machine Learning for Predicting Fractional Flow Reserve in Intermediate Coronary Artery Lesions. *J. Am. Heart Assoc.* **2019**, *8*, e011685. [CrossRef] [PubMed]
44. Lee, Y.-H.; Tsai, T.-H.; Chen, J.-H.; Huang, C.-J.; Chiang, C.-E.; Chen, C.-H.; Cheng, H.-M. Machine learning of treadmill exercise test to improve selection for testing for coronary artery disease. *Atherosclerosis* **2022**, *340*, 23–27. [CrossRef]
45. Lipkin, I.; Telluri, A.; Kim, Y.; Sidahmed, A.; Krepp, J.M.; Choi, B.G.; Jonas, R.; Marques, H.; Chang, H.-J.; Choi, J.H.; et al. Coronary CTA With AI-QCT Interpretation: Comparison with Myocardial Perfusion Imaging for Detection of Obstructive Stenosis Using Invasive Angiography as Reference Standard. *Am. J. Roentgenol.* **2022**, *219*, 407–419. [CrossRef]
46. Kurata, A.; Fukuyama, N.; Hirai, K.; Kawaguchi, N.; Tanabe, Y.; Okayama, H.; Shigemi, S.; Watanabe, K.; Uetani, T.; Ikeda, S.; et al. On-Site Computed Tomography-Derived Fractional Flow Reserve Using a Machine-Learning Algorithm—Clinical Effectiveness in a Retrospective Multicenter Cohort. *Circ. J.* **2019**, *83*, 1563–1571. [CrossRef]
47. Tang, C.X.; Wang, Y.N.; Zhou, F.; Schoepf, U.J.; van Assen, M.; Stroud, R.E.; Li, J.H.; Zhang, X.L.; Lu, M.J.; Zhou, C.S.; et al. Diagnostic performance of fractional flow reserve derived from coronary CT angiography for detection of lesion-specific ischemia: A multi-center study and meta-analysis. *Eur. J. Radiol.* **2019**, *116*, 90–97. [CrossRef] [PubMed]
48. Choi, A.D.; Marques, H.; Kumar, V.; Griffin, W.F.; Rahban, H.; Karlsberg, R.P.; Zeman, R.K.; Katz, R.J.; Earls, J.P. CT Evaluation by Artificial Intelligence for Atherosclerosis, Stenosis and Vascular Morphology (CLARIFY): A Multi-center, international study. *J. Cardiovasc. Comput. Tomogr.* **2021**, *15*, 470–476. [CrossRef] [PubMed]
49. Ahn, I.; Na, W.; Kwon, O.; Yang, D.H.; Park, G.-M.; Gwon, H.; Kang, H.J.; Jeong, Y.U.; Yoo, J.; Kim, Y.; et al. CardioNet: A manually curated database for artificial intelligence-based research on cardiovascular diseases. *BMC Med. Inform. Decis. Mak.* **2021**, *21*, 29. [CrossRef] [PubMed]
50. Cardiovascular Disease Dataset. Kaggle. 2022. Available online: https://www.kaggle.com/datasets/sulianova/cardiovascular-disease-dataset (accessed on 14 November 2022).
51. Heart Disease Data Set. UC Irvine Machine Learning Repository. 2022. Available online: https://archive.ics.uci.edu/ml/datasets/heart+disease (accessed on 14 November 2022).

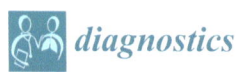

Systematic Review

Diagnostic Accuracy of Machine Learning AI Architectures in Detection and Classification of Lung Cancer: A Systematic Review

Alina Cornelia Pacurari [1], Sanket Bhattarai [2], Abdullah Muhammad [3], Claudiu Avram [4,*], Alexandru Ovidiu Mederle [5], Ovidiu Rosca [6], Felix Bratosin [4,6], Iulia Bogdan [4,6], Roxana Manuela Fericean [4,6], Marius Biris [7], Flavius Olaru [7], Catalin Dumitru [7], Gianina Tapalaga [8] and Adelina Mavrea [9]

[1] MedLife HyperClinic, Eroilor de la Tisa Boulevard 28, 300551 Timisoara, Romania; alina.pacurari@medlife.ro
[2] KIST Medical College, Faculty of General Medicine, Imadol Marg, Lalitpur 44700, Nepal; dr.sanketnep@gmail.com
[3] Islamic International Medical College, Faculty of General Medicine, 41 7th Ave, 46000 Islamabad, Pakistan; abdullahmuhammad65@gmail.com
[4] Doctoral School, "Victor Babes" University of Medicine and Pharmacy Timisoara, 300041 Timisoara, Romania; felix.bratosin@umft.ro (F.B.); iulia-georgiana.bogdan@umft.ro (I.B.); manuela.fericean@umft.ro (R.M.F.)
[5] Department of Surgery, "Victor Babes" University of Medicine and Pharmacy Timisoara, 300041 Timisoara, Romania; mederle.ovidiu@umft.ro
[6] Department of Infectious Diseases, "Victor Babes" University of Medicine and Pharmacy Timisoara, 300041 Timisoara, Romania; ovidiu.rosca@umft.ro
[7] Department of Obstetrics and Gynecology, "Victor Babes" University of Medicine and Pharmacy Timisoara, Eftimie Murgu Square 2, 300041 Timisoara, Romania; biris.marius@umft.ro (M.B.); olaru.flavius@umft.ro (F.O.); dumitru.catalin@umft.ro (C.D.)
[8] Department of Odontotherapy and Endodontics, Faculty of Dental Medicine, "Victor Babes" University of Medicine and Pharmacy Timisoara, Eftimie Murgu Square 2, 300041 Timisoara, Romania; tapalaga.gianina@umft.ro
[9] Department of Internal Medicine I, Cardiology Clinic, "Victor Babes" University of Medicine and Pharmacy Timisoara, Eftimie Murgu Square 2, 300041 Timisoara, Romania; mavrea.adelina@umft.ro
* Correspondence: avram.claudiu@umft.ro

Abstract: The application of artificial intelligence (AI) in diagnostic imaging has gained significant interest in recent years, particularly in lung cancer detection. This systematic review aims to assess the accuracy of machine learning (ML) AI algorithms in lung cancer detection, identify the ML architectures currently in use, and evaluate the clinical relevance of these diagnostic imaging methods. A systematic search of PubMed, Web of Science, Cochrane, and Scopus databases was conducted in February 2023, encompassing the literature published up until December 2022. The review included nine studies, comprising five case–control studies, three retrospective cohort studies, and one prospective cohort study. Various ML architectures were analyzed, including artificial neural network (ANN), entropy degradation method (EDM), probabilistic neural network (PNN), support vector machine (SVM), partially observable Markov decision process (POMDP), and random forest neural network (RFNN). The ML architectures demonstrated promising results in detecting and classifying lung cancer across different lesion types. The sensitivity of the ML algorithms ranged from 0.81 to 0.99, while the specificity varied from 0.46 to 1.00. The accuracy of the ML algorithms ranged from 77.8% to 100%. The AI architectures were successful in differentiating between malignant and benign lesions and detecting small-cell lung cancer (SCLC) and non-small-cell lung cancer (NSCLC). This systematic review highlights the potential of ML AI architectures in the detection and classification of lung cancer, with varying levels of diagnostic accuracy. Further studies are needed to optimize and validate these AI algorithms, as well as to determine their clinical relevance and applicability in routine practice.

Keywords: artificial intelligence; lung cancer; machine learning; diagnostic imaging

Citation: Pacurari, A.C.; Bhattarai, S.; Muhammad, A.; Avram, C.; Mederle, A.O.; Rosca, O.; Bratosin, F.; Bogdan, I.; Fericean, R.M.; Biris, M.; et al. Diagnostic Accuracy of Machine Learning AI Architectures in Detection and Classification of Lung Cancer: A Systematic Review. *Diagnostics* 2023, 13, 2145. https://doi.org/10.3390/diagnostics13132145

Academic Editors: Sameer Antani, Zhiyun Xue and Sivaramakrishnan Rajaraman

Received: 3 May 2023
Revised: 19 June 2023
Accepted: 21 June 2023
Published: 22 June 2023

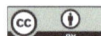

Copyright: © 2023 by the authors. Licensee MDPI, Basel, Switzerland. This article is an open access article distributed under the terms and conditions of the Creative Commons Attribution (CC BY) license (https://creativecommons.org/licenses/by/4.0/).

1. Introduction

Lung cancer accounts for the biggest proportion of mortality resulting from malignancy on the globe [1–3]. The majority of patients diagnosed with lung cancer are already in the advanced stages of the disease, which results in a dismal outlook for their future [4,5]. In addition to the advanced stages of diagnosis, the variability of imaging characteristics and histology of lung cancer makes it difficult for doctors to decide which treatment approach will be most effective for both curative and palliative purposes [6].

The imaging characteristics of lung cancer may range from a single microscopic nodule to a ground-glass opacity, several nodules, pleural effusion, lung collapse, and multiple opacities, of which simple and small lesions are exceedingly difficult to detect [7]. Histopathological characteristics include adenocarcinoma, squamous cell carcinoma, small-cell carcinoma, and a wide variety of other less common histological forms by each subgroup [8]. The clinical stage, histology, and genetic aspects of lung cancer all play a significant role in determining the treatment choices available. Nowadays, with the advancement of precision medicine, medical practitioners are required to compile a list of all the patient's characteristics and gather oncological decision-making teams before making a determination about whether or not to commence chemotherapy, targeted therapy, immunotherapy, and/or any combination of these treatments along with surgery or radiotherapy [9].

In clinical practice, the issue of whether or not the condition should be treated arises on a daily basis. One of the main goals is to identify a model for the detection, categorization, or prediction of lung cancer, although the medical, scientific understanding of the disease is based on the results of clinical tests and the experiences of medical professionals [10]. An important amount of time and energy is consumed for reviewing imaging studies, pathology slides, and reviewing patient documents in order to establish an appropriate diagnosis and identify the most appropriate therapy choices. A reliable prediction and classification model would make the whole process much easier to handle, the role of artificial intelligence (AI) being debatable since the most recent advancement of equipment and software [11].

Artificial intelligence (AI) is a broad term that can be difficult to define, but its applications may involve making predictions or classifications based on previously collected data, such as X-rays, computed tomography (CT), and magnetic resonance imaging (MRI) [12]. The primary components consist of a dataset that is used for training, a pretreatment technique, an algorithm that is used to construct the prediction model, and a pretrained model that is used to expedite the pace at which models are built and inherit past experience [13]. AI built its own logical method to recognize images quickly in order to fulfill its goal of acquiring information swiftly and without any gaps. Computer-aided detection (CAD) systems are neural networks backed by machine learning (ML) algorithms designed to mimic brain-like decisions used in order to ascertain the location of the target site in clinical images. The lesion areas may be marked by AI-based detection techniques, which also helps to eliminate observational oversights [14]. ML algorithms have been proven to facilitate diagnostic medical imaging by differentiating between bronchioles, lung wall, and parenchyma in a clear manner, all while indicating lesions that are abnormal in comparison to the healthy lung zones, helping clinicians to determine alterations with a low threshold for errors [15,16]. Computer-aided diagnostic methods, on the other hand, have given emphasis on identifying nodules as benign or malignant, even for dimensions that go lower than 3 mm in size [17].

In the 21st century, artificial intelligence has been more connected to human life, and this tendency can also be seen throughout all fields of medicine. In oncology, particularly for lung cancer, the goal of AI is to provide individualized solutions for each individual patient by taking into account the tumor's texture, character, stage, and invasion region [18]. Because of the many existing subtypes, lung cancer is the ideal subject for the use of AI. A significant number of studies have indicated the application's potential use in the identification of lung nodules, as well as diagnostic applications in histology, disease risk stratification, the creation of drugs, and even the prediction of prognosis. Therefore, this systematic review is primarily focused on analyzing and assessing the diagnostic accuracy of existing machine learning AI architectures in the detection and classification of lung cancer, thus providing a comprehensive evaluation of the current state of AI applications in this field.

2. Materials and Methods

2.1. Review Protocol

This systematic review was conducted in February 2023, utilizing four online databases: PubMed, Web of Science, Cochrane, and Scopus. The review encompassed the literature published up until December 2022. The investigation covered the following medical subject heading (MeSH) [19] keywords: "lung cancer", "pulmonary nodule", "pulmonary cancer", "lung neoplasms", "thoracic neoplasms", "AI", "artificial intelligence", "machine learning", "cancer screening", "neural network", and "diagnostic imaging". The search was restricted to English-language journal articles.

The study used a structured and systematic search strategy in compliance with the Preferred Reporting Items for Systematic Reviews and Meta-Analyses (PRISMA) [20] criteria and the International Prospective Register of Systematic Reviews (PROSPERO) [21] guidelines. All pertinent scientific papers examining the accuracy of machine learning AI algorithms in lung cancer detection were incorporated into the analysis. This systematic review was registered on the Open Science Framework (OSF) platform [22].

The primary objective of this systematic review was to address the following research questions:

- What is the accuracy of machine learning AI algorithms in lung cancer detection?
- What machine learning architectures are currently in use?
- What is the clinical relevance of these diagnostic imaging methods?

2.2. Data Extraction

The main sources of information for the gathered material included the text, tables, figures, and additional web resources present in the articles. The initial stage of the selection process involved the elimination of duplicate submissions, followed by a thorough examination of each abstract and, ultimately, a complete review of the entire text. Additionally, the reference lists of the collected papers were meticulously inspected to identify relevant content.

In the context of our review, we considered the following variables to be considered for reporting: (1) study characteristics: study number and author, country of the study, the year of study development, study design, and quality assessment; (2) summary of findings: number of patients, AI architecture, the reference group for the ML architecture, and type of lesions identified; (3) performance of the ML architecture: total positive, total negative, false positive, false negative value, and the type of images used for testing; (4) other particularities of the ML architecture: sensitivity, specificity, accuracy, and study particularities.

We included studies involving adults who were screened for lung cancer incidentally or by screening. The index evaluations included machine learning AI algorithms for analyzing medical images for lung cancer detection. The ML architectures considered for inclusion in the study comprised neural networks and CADs that are built on machine learning models [23,24]. The ML algorithms used radiological parameters to determine the presence of lung cancer and classify the nodules. We excluded the studies employing phantom, histopathology, or microscopic images, non-imaging modalities, and those investigating the accuracy of image segmentation without the augmentation of machine learning architectures. Similarly, studies that assessed other AI algorithms, such as deep learning methods, were excluded in order to allow for a proper standardization of ML algorithms. Other excluded studies were those that assessed other forms of pulmonary disease. Commentaries, editorials, abstract-only assessments, and critiques were also not included in this systematic review. Estimates of diagnostic accuracy, such as true negative

(TN), true positive (TP), false negative (FN), and false positive (FP), or sufficient information from which estimates could be computed were required for inclusion.

The diagnostic test accuracy (DTA) measurements comprised sensitivity and specificity, which showed the proportion of individuals with the target condition who had positive test findings and the percentage of those without the disease who had negative test results, respectively. A diagnostic test that was both sensitive and specific was considered to be ideal.

2.3. Study Selection and Quality Assessment

The preliminary search results yielded a total of 5894 articles, out of which 517 were identified as duplicates. After excluding 5062 papers based on their abstracts, 315 full-text articles were assessed for eligibility. Ultimately, nine articles were selected for inclusion in the systematic review, as presented in Figure 1. Based on the Study Quality Assessment Tools provided by the National Heart, Lung, and Blood Institute (NHLBI) [25], two investigators independently evaluated the published material and documented their findings. These tools are tailored to specific study designs, enabling the detection of methodological or design concerns.

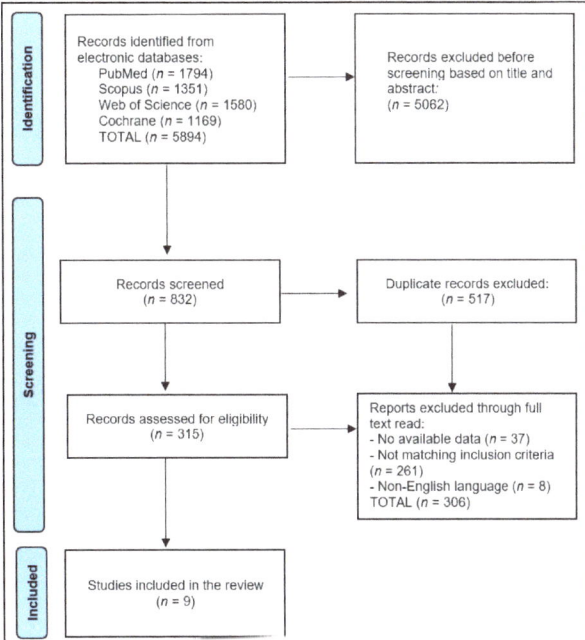

Figure 1. PRISMA flow diagram.

For the remaining studies, the Quality Assessment Tool for Observational Cohort and Cross-Sectional Investigations was employed. Each question within the tool received a score of 1 point for "Yes" answers and 0 points for "No" and "Other" responses. Subsequently, the final performance score was calculated. Accordingly, studies with scores ranging from 0 to 4 were considered to be of fair quality, those with scores between 5 and 9 were deemed to be of good quality, and those with a score of 10 or higher were classified as excellent quality. To mitigate inherent biases in the included studies, two researchers were assigned to evaluate the quality of the chosen articles. This approach minimized the risks associated with selection bias, missing data, and measurement bias.

3. Results

3.1. Overview

Data from nine studies [26–34] were analyzed to determine the diagnostic accuracy of machine learning AI architecture in the detection and classification of lung cancer. The studies were conducted in various countries, including Turkey, the United States, Poland, Pakistan, Italy, Bangladesh, and India, and were published between 2014 and 2022. The study designs varied among the selected articles, with five case–control studies [28–31,33], three retrospective cohort studies [26,27,34], and one prospective cohort study [32]. The quality of the included studies ranged from excellent to fair, with one study deemed excellent [26], three rated as good [29,30,32], and five considered fair [27,28,31,33,34].

A summary of the study characteristics is presented in Table 1. Dandil et al. [26] conducted the earliest study in 2014, which was a retrospective cohort study in Turkey and was the only one rated as excellent in quality. Wu et al. [27] and Kumar et al. [34] also utilized retrospective cohort study designs conducted in the United States and India, respectively, with both being rated as fair in quality. Chauvie et al. [32] carried out a prospective cohort study in Italy, which was rated as good in quality. The remaining five studies were case–control studies conducted in various countries, including Poland [28,31], Pakistan [29], the United States [30], and Bangladesh [33]. The quality of these studies was mixed, with two rated as good [29,30] and three considered fair [28,31,33].

Table 1. Study characteristics.

Study and Author	Country	Study Year	Study Design	Study Quality
1 [26] Dandil et al.	Turkey	2014	Retrospective cohort	Excellent
2 [27] Wu et al.	USA	2017	Retrospective cohort	Fair
3 [28] Wozniak et al.	Poland	2018	Case–control	Fair
4 [29] Khan et al.	Pakistan	2019	Case–control	Good
5 [30] Petousis et al.	USA	2019	Case–control	Good
6 [31] Capizzi et al.	Poland	2020	Case–control	Fair
7 [32] Chauvie et al.	Italy	2020	Prospective cohort	Good
8 [33] Hoque et al.	Bangladesh	2020	Case–control	Fair
9 [34] Kumar et al.	India	2022	Retrospective cohort	Fair

The studies employed various machine learning architectures, including artificial neural network (ANN) [26], entropy degradation method (EDM) [27], probabilistic neural network (PNN) [28,31], support vector machine (SVM) [29,33,34], partially observable Markov decision process (POMDP) [30], and random forest neural network (RFNN) [32]. The type of lesions analyzed in the studies included small-cell lung cancer (SCLC) [26,27], non-small-cell lung cancer (NSCLC) [34], and comparisons of malignant and benign lesions [28–33].

The patient population in the studies ranged from as few as 32 patients [34] to as many as 5402 patients [30]. Comparison groups varied among the studies, with some employing microscopic analysis [26,32], expert radiologists' opinions [29,30,34], random X-rays [28,31], and random slices from healthy lung scans [27,33] as the benchmark for assessing the AI architecture's performance.

The AI architectures demonstrated promising results in detecting and classifying lung cancer across different lesion types. ANN [26], EDM [27], and SVM [34] showed effectiveness in detecting SCLC and NSCLC, respectively, while PNN [28,31], SVM [29,33], POMDP [30], and RFNN [32] were successful in differentiating between malignant and benign lesions, as described in Table 2.

Table 2. Summary of findings.

Study	Number of Patients	AI Architecture	Comparison Group	Type of Lesions
1 [26] Dandil et al.	47	ANN	Microscopic analysis	SCLC
2 [27] Wu et al.	72	EDM	Random slices from healthy lung scans	SCLC
3 [28] Wozniak et al.	404 for training, 100 for testing	PNN	Random X-rays	Malignant vs. benign
4 [29] Khan et al.	84	SVM	Expert radiologists	Malignant vs. benign
5 [30] Petousis et al.	5402	POMDP	Expert radiologists	Malignant vs. benign
6 [31] Capizzi et al.	320 for training, 120 for testing	PNN	Random X-rays	Malignant vs. benign
7 [32] Chauvie et al.	1594	RFNN	Microscopic analysis	Malignant vs. benign
8 [33] Hoque et al.	78	SVM	Random slices from healthy lung scans	Malignant vs. benign
9 [34] Kumar et al.	32	SVM	Expert radiologists	NSCLC

AI—artificial intelligence; ANN—artificial neural network; NR—not reported; PNN—probabilistic neural network; EDM—entropy degradation method; SCLC—small-cell lung cancer; PNN—probabilistic neural network; SVM—support vector machine; POMDP—partially observable Markov decision process; RFNN—random forest neural network; NSCLC—non-small-cell lung cancer.

3.2. Performance Evaluation

The performance analysis of the ML architectures focused on true positives (TP), true negatives (TN), false positives (FP), and false negatives (FN) for each study, as well as the type and number of images used for testing. The studies demonstrated varying degrees of success in the diagnostic accuracy of ML algorithms. Dandil et al. [26] reported a high overall accuracy, with 24 TP, 34 TN, 4 FP, and 2 FN using 128 CT scans. In contrast, Wu et al. [27] reported a slightly higher number of false results, with 30 TP, 26 TN, 10 FP, and 6 FN using 12 high-resolution computed tomography (HRCT) scans, each containing 100–500 slices. Wozniak et al. [28] achieved a balanced performance with 40 TP, 52 TN, 6 FP, and 2 FN using 100 X-rays, of which 80 were from healthy individuals. Khan et al. [29] showed high overall accuracy with 383 TP, 389 TN, 4 FP, and 10 FN using CT scans.

Petousis et al. [30] reported a relatively high number of false positives with 31 TP, 482 TN, 565 FP, and 1 FN using low-dose computed tomography (LDCT) images. Capizzi et al. [31] demonstrated a balanced performance with 43 TP, 68 TN, 7 FP, and 2 FN using X-ray images. Chauvie et al. [32] showed an impressive performance with 18 TP, 1573 TN, 1 FP, and 2 FN using Lung CT Screening Reporting & Data System (RADS) images. Hoque et al. [33] reported a high true positive rate but a low true negative rate with 71 TP, 3 TN, 3 FP, and 1 FN using CT scans. Lastly, Kumar et al. [34] achieved a high true positive rate and low false results with 32 TP, 6 TN, 2 FP, and 2 FN using CT scans, as presented in Table 3.

Table 3. Performance of the ML architecture.

Study	TP	TN	FP	FN	Images Used for Testing
1 [26] Dandil et al.	24	34	4	2	128 CTs
2 [27] Wu et al.	30	26	10	6	12 HRCTs (100–500 slices)
3 [28] Wozniak et al.	40	52	6	2	100 X-rays (80 healthy)
4 [29] Khan et al.	383	389	4	10	CT scans
5 [30] Petousis et al.	31	482	565	1	LDCT
6 [31] Capizzi et al.	43	68	7	2	X-rays
7 [32] Chauvie et al.	18	1573	1	2	RADS
8 [33] Hoque et al.	71	3	3	1	CT scans
9 [34] Kumar et al.	32	6	2	2	CT scans

ML—machine learning; TP—total positive; TN—total negative; FP—false positive; FN—false negative; CT—computed tomography; HRCT—high-resolution computed tomography; LDCT—low-dose computed tomography; RADS—Lung CT Screening Reporting & Data System.

The findings from Table 4 provide insight into the sensitivity, specificity, accuracy, and particularities of the machine learning architectures used in the nine studies. The sensitivity ranged from 0.81 [34] to 0.99 [29], while the specificity varied from 0.46 [30] to 1.00 [32]. The accuracy of the ML algorithms ranged from 77.8% [27] to 100% [32].

Table 4. Other particularities of the machine learning architectures.

Study	Sensitivity	Specificity	Accuracy	Particularities
1 [26] Dandil et al.	0.92	0.89	92.3%	The designed CAD system provides the segmentation of nodules on the lobes with a neural networks model of SOM and ensures classification between benign and malignant nodules with the help of ANN.
2 [27] Wu et al.	0.83	0.72	77.8%	The algorithm makes 10 false positive predictions among 36 tests and misses 6 cases.
3 [28] Wozniak et al.	0.95	0.90	92.0%	This method starts with the localization and extraction of the lung nodules by computing, for each pixel of the original image, the local variance obtaining an output image with the same size as the original image. The PNN architecture has a lower computational complexity, and it can detect low-contrast nodules.
4 [29] Khan et al.	0.97	0.99	98.0%	The ML architecture consists of multiple phases that include image contrast enhancement, segmentation, and optimal feature extraction, followed by the employment of these features for training and testing of SVM.
5 [30] Petousis et al.	0.97	0.46	NR	The ML algorithm reduced the rate of false positives yet preserved a high rate of true positives comparable to that of human experts and identified lung malignancies earlier.
6 [31] Capizzi et al.	0.96	0.91	92.5%	The algorithm can identify nodules with a diameter ≤ 20 mm and minimal contrast.
7 [32] Chauvie et al.	0.90	1.00	100%	Given the various radiological characteristics of nodules on CT and DTS, the lung-RADS category did not improve the diagnostic accuracy of visual examination. The neural network was the only technique to achieve a high PPV without sacrificing sensitivity, as compared with binary visual analysis, logistic regression, and random forest algorithm.
8 [33] Hoque et al.	0.99	0.50	95.0%	The improved SVM model achieved higher accuracy in identifying regions of interest in the lung area where the cancer was localized.
9 [34] Kumar et al.	0.81	0.82	98.8%	The SVM model achieved higher precision than KNN, naïve Bayes, and J48 classifier, with or without SMOTE.

ML—machine learning; CAD—computer-aided diagnosis; SOM—self-organizing maps; ANN—artificial neural network; SVM—support vector machine; NR—not reported; CT—computed tomography; DTS—digital tomosynthesis; RADS—Lung CT Screening Reporting & Data System; PPV—positive predictive value; KNN—K-nearest neighbors; SMOTE—synthetic minority oversampling technique.

Dandil et al. [26] reported a sensitivity of 0.92, a specificity of 0.89, and 92.3% accuracy. The computer-aided diagnosis (CAD) system they designed involved a combination of self-organizing maps (SOM) and artificial neural networks (ANN). Wu et al. [27] reported lower sensitivity (0.83), specificity (0.72), and accuracy (77.8%) compared to Dandil et al., with their algorithm making 10 false positive predictions and missing 6 cases. Wozniak et al. [28] achieved high sensitivity (0.95), specificity (0.90), and accuracy (92.0%), with their probabilistic neural network (PNN) architecture demonstrating lower computational complexity and the ability to detect low-contrast nodules.

Khan et al. [29] reported impressive results, with a sensitivity of 0.97, specificity of 0.99, and 98.0% accuracy. Their support vector machine (SVM) ML architecture included image contrast enhancement, segmentation, and optimal feature extraction. Petousis et al. [30] achieved high sensitivity (0.97) but relatively low specificity (0.46), and the algorithm was noted to reduce the rate of false positives while maintaining a high rate of true positives. Capizzi et al. [31] reported high sensitivity (0.96), specificity (0.91), and 92.5% accuracy, with their algorithm capable of identifying nodules with a diameter ≤ 20 mm and minimal contrast.

Chauvie et al. [32] achieved a sensitivity of 0.90, a specificity of 1.00, and a remarkable 100% accuracy. Their neural network was the only technique to achieve a high positive predictive value (PPV) without sacrificing sensitivity. Hoque et al. [33] reported a high sensitivity of 0.99 and a specificity of 0.50, with an accuracy of 95.0%. Their improved SVM model effectively identified regions of interest in the lung area where the cancer was localized. Lastly, Kumar et al. [34] reported a sensitivity of 0.81, a specificity of 0.82, and 98.8% accuracy. Their SVM model outperformed other classifiers, such as K-nearest neighbors (KNN), naïve Bayes, and J48, even when using the synthetic minority oversampling technique (SMOTE).

4. Discussion

4.1. Summary and Contributions

The present study aimed to analyze the diagnostic accuracy of machine learning AI architectures in detecting and classifying lung cancer. Various machine learning AI architectures have the potential to improve the diagnostic accuracy of lung cancer detection and classification. The analyzed studies [26–34] demonstrated that AI-based methods could be effective alternatives or supplementary tools to conventional diagnostic approaches, such as microscopic analysis or expert radiologists' assessments. Moreover, our results, based on data from the nine studies conducted between 2014 and 2022, demonstrated that AI architectures show promise in accurately detecting and classifying lung cancer across different lesion types. These findings are consistent with previous research, which has similarly found AI-based systems to be effective in diagnosing lung cancer [35–37].

The analysis of the data collected from the nine studies highlighted the potential of machine learning AI architecture for detecting and classifying lung cancer. While the study designs and quality varied, the findings demonstrated a consistent trend toward improved diagnostic accuracy using AI-based methods. Nevertheless, the variations in study design, patient population, AI architecture, and comparison groups highlight the need for further research to establish the most effective AI algorithms and techniques for lung cancer detection and classification.

Comparing and contrasting the results from the nine studies, it is evident that the ML architectures demonstrated promising results in the detection and classification of lung cancer, with generally high true positive and true negative rates and low false positive and false negative rates. However, the performance varied across studies, with some achieving higher overall accuracy than others. The studies employed various types of imaging, including CT, HRCT, LDCT, X-rays, and RADS, indicating that ML architectures can potentially be effective across a range of imaging modalities.

In our analysis, the performance of AI architectures varied between studies, with the highest accuracy reported by Chauvie et al. [32] at 100% and the lowest by Wu et al. [27] at 77.8%. These variations may be attributed to differences in study design, quality, AI architecture, and patient populations. A possible explanation for the high accuracy achieved by Chauvie et al. [32] is the use of a random forest neural network (RFNN) in combination with Lung CT Screening Reporting & Data System (RADS) images, which may have improved the detection of malignant and benign lesions.

In comparing our findings with other studies, Narshullah et al. [35] reported an overall accuracy of 94.7% using a deep learning model for lung cancer diagnosis. This is consistent with the high accuracy results reported by Khan et al. [29] and Kumar et al. [34] in our analysis, both of which used support vector machine (SVM) models. Additionally, Ardila et al. [36] found that a deep learning model outperformed expert radiologists in detecting lung cancer, achieving an area under the curve (AUC) of 0.94 compared to 0.88 for human experts. This supports the findings of Petousis et al. [30], who reported a high true positive rate for their AI architecture, despite the relatively low specificity.

The selected studies were conducted in different countries and employed a range of ML architectures, including ANN, EDM, PNN, SVM, POMDP, and RFNN. The findings from these studies were generally promising, demonstrating the potential of AI as a tool for lung cancer diagnosis. Our results are consistent with the growing body of evidence that supports the use of AI for lung cancer detection and classification. For instance, Ardila et al. reported a deep learning algorithm that achieved an area under the curve (AUC) of 94.4% for lung cancer detection on low-dose computed tomography (LDCT) scans [36]. Similarly, a study by Nam et al. showed that a deep-learning-based nodule detection model had a sensitivity of 93.8% and a specificity of 87.4% [37]. These findings indicate that AI architectures have the potential to achieve high diagnostic accuracy in lung cancer detection.

The sensitivity and specificity of the ML architectures in our analysis ranged from 81% [34] to 99% [29] and 46% [30] to 100% [32], respectively. This variation may be attributed to differences in study design, data quality, and the type of ML architecture used. For example, Chauvie et al. [32] achieved a high specificity of 1.00 and an impressive 100% accuracy using the RFNN architecture, while Petousis et al. [30] reported a relatively low specificity of 0.46 using the POMDP architecture. These results suggest that the choice of ML architecture may impact the diagnostic performance of AI systems.

Another study compared the diagnostic performance of two AI methods and found that machine learning was superior to deep learning in early lung cancer detection from medical imaging. The results of deep learning had a sensitivity of 83.7% and a specificity of 82.6%, consistent with previous findings [38]. Deep learning requires large datasets for optimal performance, but some studies used smaller datasets [39,40], reducing statistical power. In cases with insufficient data, traditional machine learning was preferable for accurately detecting lung cancer, although deep learning still held potential for clinical applications with comparable diagnostic accuracy [41].

Deep learning algorithms have been of high interest lately, and various studies attempted to determine their utility as diagnostic tools. In one study [42], the authors compared a deep learning model with an SVM model, which had been widely used in disease prediction, as well as in three of the studies included in our systematic review [29,33,34]. The SVM performed poorly on high-dimensional gene expression datasets, resulting in low prediction accuracy. However, their deep learning model achieved higher accuracy and AUC scores than SVM, as it could automatically learn direct interactions and nonlinear relationships. The results confirmed deep learning's ability to fit complex relationships without manual intervention, suggesting its increasing importance in disease diagnosis and potential for further development.

Wang et al. [43] utilized a deep learning model to predict EGFR mutation status in lung adenocarcinoma using CT images. Their model achieved an accuracy of 85.4%. In comparison to these studies that focus on deep learning AI algorithms, their findings also show the potential of deep learning AI in lung cancer detection and classification. However, our findings highlight the superiority of traditional ML when dealing with smaller and insufficient datasets. In such cases, ML architectures may be more suitable for accurately detecting lung cancer in different imaging modalities. While deep learning has demonstrated considerable potential in clinical applications, it requires larger and high-dimensional datasets for optimal diagnostic performance. Therefore, both deep learning and machine learning approaches have their merits and can be complementary depending on the available data and specific use cases.

Our findings also highlight the importance of careful evaluation and validation of AI algorithms for lung cancer diagnosis. In some studies, the ML architectures demonstrated high true positive rates but relatively low true negative rates [33], which may lead to unnecessary follow-up procedures or interventions for patients with benign lesions. Moreover, the studies used various comparison groups, such as microscopic analysis, expert radiologists' opinions, random X-rays, and random slices from healthy lung scans, which could influence the performance evaluation of the AI systems.

The results of this systematic review not only offer an overview of the current state of machine learning AI architectures used in lung cancer detection, but also provide insights for future research directions. For AI researchers and data scientists, the performance metrics we present here could guide the selection and optimization of models in further studies. For clinicians, understanding the capabilities of these AI tools may open up new possibilities for early lung cancer detection and timely treatment, potentially improving patient outcomes. Moreover, policymakers and healthcare administrators might use this information to inform decisions about incorporating AI diagnostics into routine healthcare, potentially reducing the workload of radiologists and pathologists and improving overall healthcare efficiency.

4.2. Study Limitations and Future Directions

Our study has several limitations that should be acknowledged. First, the included studies were heterogeneous in terms of patient populations, imaging techniques, lesion types, and ML architectures used. This heterogeneity may have affected the pooled diagnostic accuracy measures, limiting the generalizability of our findings. Second, the number of studies included in our analysis was relatively small. As a result, our findings should be interpreted with caution, and further research is needed to confirm these results. Moreover, publication bias may have influenced our findings, as studies with positive results are more likely to be published than those with negative results. Additionally, the quality of the included studies varied, with some studies having a relatively small sample size or lacking clear methodological details that may have affected the reliability of our results. Although pooled data analysis can provide more robust and statistically significant insights, the current variability in methodologies, AI architectures, and evaluation metrics among the reviewed studies may limit the applicability and reliability of a pooled analysis. Finally, our study focused on the diagnostic accuracy of AI in detecting and classifying lung cancer but did not explore other important aspects, such as the impact of AI on clinical decision making, patient outcomes, or cost-effectiveness.

The potential of AI for lung cancer detection and classification is evident; however, further research is needed to optimize ML architectures and evaluate their performance in diverse patient populations. Some future research directions should include the development and validation of AI algorithms in large, multi-center studies that include diverse patient populations to ensure the generalizability of the results. Another important topic is the investigation of the optimal combination of imaging modalities, such as CT, PET, and MRI, and their integration with AI algorithms for improved lung cancer diagnosis. Other possible study hypotheses include the exploration of AI's role in predicting treatment response, prognosis, and patient outcomes; evaluation of the cost-effectiveness of AI-based lung cancer diagnosis, including the potential reduction in unnecessary follow-up procedures or interventions for patients with benign lesions; and the assessment of the impact of AI on clinical decision making and patient–physician communication, which may lead to better patient-centered care.

5. Conclusions

This systematic review has provided a thorough evaluation of the diagnostic accuracy of machine learning AI architectures in lung cancer detection and classification with varying degrees of success, demonstrating their potential and areas for improvement. The study designs and quality varied, while the algorithms employed included ANN, EDM, PNN, SVM, POMDP, and RFNN. The AI architectures were effective in differentiating malignant from benign lesions and identifying small-cell lung cancer and non-small-cell lung cancer. Although the sensitivity, specificity, and accuracy of the AI architectures varied, promising results were demonstrated in many cases, indicating the potential of machine learning algorithms to improve lung cancer detection and classification. However, further research and optimization are needed to enhance the performance and reliability of these AI techniques in real-world settings.

Author Contributions: Conceptualization, A.C.P., S.B. and A.M. (Abdullah Muhammad); methodology, A.C.P., S.B. and A.M. (Abdullah Muhammad); software, C.A., I.B. and A.O.M.; validation, C.A., I.B. and A.O.M.; formal analysis, O.R. and F.B.; investigation, O.R. and F.B.; resources, C.D. and R.M.F.; data curation, C.D. and R.M.F.; writing—original draft preparation, A.C.P. and F.B.; writing—review and editing, S.B. and A.M. (Abdullah Muhammad); visualization, G.T., F.O. and M.B.; supervision, G.T., F.O. and A.M. (Adelina Mavrea); project administration, A.M. (Adelina Mavrea) and M.B. All authors have read and agreed to the published version of the manuscript.

Funding: This research received no external funding.

Institutional Review Board Statement: Not applicable.

Informed Consent Statement: Not applicable.

Data Availability Statement: Not applicable.

Conflicts of Interest: The authors declare no conflict of interest.

References

1. Thandra, K.C.; Barsouk, A.; Saginala, K.; Aluru, J.S.; Barsouk, A. Epidemiology of lung cancer. *Contemp. Oncol.* **2021**, *25*, 45–52. [CrossRef]
2. Septimiu-Radu, S.; Gadela, T.; Gabriela, D.; Oancea, C.; Rosca, O.; Lazureanu, V.E.; Fericean, R.M.; Bratosin, F.; Dumitrescu, A.; Stoicescu, E.R.; et al. A Systematic Review of Lung Autopsy Findings in Elderly Patients after SARS-CoV-2 Infection. *J. Clin. Med.* **2023**, *12*, 2070. [CrossRef]
3. Toma, A.-O.; Boeriu, E.; Decean, L.; Bloanca, V.; Bratosin, F.; Levai, M.C.; Vasamsetti, N.G.; Alambaram, S.; Oprisoni, A.L.; Miutescu, B.; et al. The Effects of Lack of Awareness in Age-Related Quality of Life, Coping with Stress, and Depression among Patients with Malignant Melanoma. *Curr. Oncol.* **2023**, *30*, 1516–1528. [CrossRef]
4. Knight, S.B.; Phil, A.; Crosbie, P.A.; Balata, H.; Chudziak, J.; Hussell, T.; Dive, C. Progress and prospects of early detection in lung cancer. *Open Biol.* **2017**, *7*, 170070. [CrossRef]
5. Tudorache, E.; Motoc, N.S.; Pescaru, C.; Crisan, A.; Ciumarnean, L. Impact of pulmonary rehabilitation programs in improving health status in COPD patients. *Balneo Res. J.* **2019**, *10*, 472–477. [CrossRef]
6. Lee, S.-H.; Cho, H.-H.; Lee, H.Y.; Park, H. Clinical impact of variability on CT radiomics and suggestions for suitable feature selection: A focus on lung cancer. *Cancer Imaging* **2019**, *19*, 54. [CrossRef]
7. Panunzio, A.; Sartori, P. Lung Cancer and Radiological Imaging. *Curr. Radiopharm.* **2020**, *13*, 238–242. [CrossRef]
8. Albasri, A.M. A histopathological analysis of lung cancers. An 11-year retrospective study from Al-Madinah Al-Munawwarah, Saudi Arabia. *Saudi Med. J.* **2019**, *40*, 503–506. [CrossRef]
9. Mambetsariev, I.; Pharaon, R.; Nam, A.; Knopf, K.; Djulbegovic, B.; Villaflor, V.M.; Vokes, E.E.; Salgia, R. Heuristic value-based framework for lung cancer decision-making. *Oncotarget* **2018**, *9*, 29877–29891. [CrossRef]
10. Wu, J.; Zan, X.; Gao, L.; Zhao, J.; Fan, J.; Shi, H.; Wan, Y.; Yu, E.; Li, S.; Xie, X. A Machine Learning Method for Identifying Lung Cancer Based on Routine Blood Indices: Qualitative Feasibility Study. *JMIR Public Health Surveill.* **2019**, *7*, e13476. [CrossRef]
11. Mathew, C.J.; David, A.M.; Mathew, C.M.J. Artificial Intelligence and its future potential in lung cancer screening. *EXCLI J.* **2020**, *19*, 1552–1562. [CrossRef]
12. Waller, J.; O'connor, A.; Raafat, E.; Amireh, A.; Dempsey, J.; Martin, C.; Umair, M. Applications and challenges of artificial intelligence in diagnostic and interventional radiology. *Pol. J. Radiol.* **2022**, *87*, 113–117. [CrossRef]
13. Sarker, I.H. AI-Based Modeling: Techniques, Applications and Research Issues Towards Automation, Intelligent and Smart Systems. *SN Comput. Sci.* **2022**, *3*, 158. [CrossRef]
14. Chan, H.P.; Hadjiiski, L.M.; Samala, R.K. Computer-aided diagnosis in the era of deep learning. *Med. Phys.* **2020**, *47*, e218–e227. [CrossRef]
15. Firmino, M.; Angelo, G.; Morais, H.; Dantas, M.R.; Valentim, R. Computer-aided detection (CADe) and diagnosis (CADx) system for lung cancer with likelihood of malignancy. *Biomed. Eng. Online* **2016**, *15*, 2. [CrossRef]
16. Neelakantan, S.; Xin, Y.; Gaver, D.P.; Cereda, M.; Rizi, R.; Smith, B.J.; Avazmohammadi, R. Computational lung modelling in respiratory medicine. *J. R. Soc. Interface* **2022**, *19*, 20220062. [CrossRef]
17. Wang, H.; Li, Y.; Liu, S.; Yue, X. Design Computer-Aided Diagnosis System Based on Chest CT Evaluation of Pulmonary Nodules. *Comput. Math. Methods Med.* **2022**, *2022*, 7729524. [CrossRef]
18. Zhang, H.; Meng, D.; Cai, S.; Guo, H.; Chen, P.; Zheng, Z.; Zhu, J.; Zhao, W.; Wang, H.; Zhao, S.; et al. The application of artificial intelligence in lung cancer: A narrative review. *Transl. Cancer Res.* **2021**, *10*, 2478–2487. [CrossRef]
19. Dhammi, I.K.; Kumar, S. Medical subject headings (MeSH) terms. *Indian J. Orthop.* **2014**, *48*, 443–444. [CrossRef]
20. Moher, D.; Liberati, M.; Tetzlaff, J.; Altman, D.G.; PRISMA Group. Preferred reporting items for systematic reviews and meta-analyses: The PRISMA statement. *PLoS Med.* **2009**, *6*, e1000097. [CrossRef]
21. Schiavo, J.H. PROSPERO: An International Register of Systematic Review Protocols. *Med. Ref. Serv. Q.* **2019**, *38*, 171–180. [CrossRef]
22. Foster, M.E.D.; Deardorff, M.A. Open Science Framework (OSF). *J. Med. Libr. Assoc.* **2017**, *105*, 203–206. [CrossRef]
23. Santos, M.K.; Júnior, J.R.F.; Wada, D.T.; Tenório, A.P.M.; Nogueira-Barbosa, M.H.; Marques, P.M.D.A. Artificial intelligence, machine learning, computer-aided diagnosis, and radiomics: Advances in imaging towards to precision medicine. *Radiol. Bras.* **2019**, *52*, 387–396. [CrossRef]
24. Prisciandaro, E.; Sedda, G.; Cara, A.; Diotti, C.; Spaggiari, L.; Bertolaccini, L. Artificial Neural Networks in Lung Cancer Research: A Narrative Review. *J. Clin. Med.* **2023**, *12*, 880. [CrossRef]
25. Farrah, K.; Young, K.; Tunis, M.C.; Zhao, L. Risk of bias tools in systematic reviews of health interventions: An analysis of PROSPERO-registered protocols. *Syst. Rev.* **2019**, *8*, 280. [CrossRef]
26. Dandil, E.; Cakiroglu, M.; Eksi, Z.; Ozkan, M.; Kurt, O.K.; Canan, A. Artificial neural network-based classification system for lung nodules on computed tomography scans. In Proceedings of the 2014 6th International Conference of Soft Computing and Pattern Recognition (SoCPaR), Tunis, Tunisia, 11–14 August 2014. [CrossRef]

27. Wu, Q.; Zhao, W. Small-Cell Lung Cancer Detection Using a Supervised Machine Learning Algorithm. In Proceedings of the 2017 International Symposium on Computer Science and Intelligent Controls (ISCSIC), Budapest, Hungary, 20–22 October 2017. [CrossRef]
28. Woźniak, M.; Połap, D.; Capizzi, G.; Sciuto, G.L.; Kośmider, L.; Frankiewicz, K. Small lung nodules detection based on local variance analysis and probabilistic neural network. *Comput. Methods Programs Biomed.* **2018**, *161*, 173–180. [CrossRef]
29. Khan, S.A.; Hussain, S.; Yang, S.; Iqbal, K. Effective and Reliable Framework for Lung Nodules Detection from CT Scan Images. *Sci. Rep.* **2019**, *9*, 4989. [CrossRef]
30. Petousis, P.; Winter, A.; Speier, W.; Aberle, D.R.; Hsu, W.; Bui, A.A.T. Using Sequential Decision Making to Improve Lung Cancer Screening Performance. *IEEE Access* **2019**, *7*, 119403–119419. [CrossRef]
31. Capizzi, G.; Sciuto, G.L.; Napoli, C.; Połap, D.; Wozniak, M. Small Lung Nodules Detection Based on Fuzzy-Logic and Probabilistic Neural Network With Bioinspired Reinforcement Learning. *IEEE Trans. Fuzzy Syst.* **2019**, *28*, 1178–1189. [CrossRef]
32. Chauvie, S.; SOS Study Team; De Maggi, A.; Baralis, I.; Dalmasso, F.; Berchialla, P.; Priotto, R.; Violino, P.; Mazza, F.; Melloni, G.; et al. Artificial intelligence and radiomics enhance the positive predictive value of digital chest tomosynthesis for lung cancer detection within SOS clinical trial. *Eur. Radiol.* **2020**, *30*, 4134–4140. [CrossRef]
33. Hoque, A.; Farabi, A.A.; Ahmed, F.; Islam, Z. Automated Detection of Lung Cancer Using CT Scan Images. In Proceedings of the 2020 IEEE Region 10 Symposium (TENSYMP), Dhaka, Bangladesh, 5–7 June 2020; pp. 1030–1033. [CrossRef]
34. Kumar, C.A.; Harish, S.; Ravi, P.; Svn, M.; Kumar, B.P.P.; Mohanavel, V.; Alyami, N.M.; Priya, S.S.; Asfaw, A.K. Lung Cancer Prediction from Text Datasets Using Machine Learning. *BioMed Res. Int.* **2022**, *2022*, 6254177. [CrossRef]
35. Nasrullah, N.; Sang, J.; Alam, M.S.; Mateen, M.; Cai, B.; Hu, H. Automated Lung Nodule Detection and Classification Using Deep Learning Combined with Multiple Strategies. *Sensors* **2019**, *19*, 3722. [CrossRef]
36. Ardila, D.; Kiraly, A.P.; Bharadwaj, S.; Choi, B.; Reicher, J.J.; Peng, L.; Tse, D.; Etemadi, M.; Ye, W.; Corrado, G.; et al. End-to-end lung cancer screening with three-dimensional deep learning on low-dose chest computed tomography. *Nat. Med.* **2019**, *25*, 954–961. [CrossRef]
37. Nam, J.G.; Park, S.; Hwang, E.J.; Lee, J.H.; Jin, K.-N.; Lim, K.Y.; Vu, T.H.; Sohn, J.H.; Hwang, S.; Goo, J.M.; et al. Development and Validation of Deep Learning–based Automatic Detection Algorithm for Malignant Pulmonary Nodules on Chest Radiographs. *Radiology* **2019**, *290*, 218–228. [CrossRef]
38. Aggarwal, R.; Sounderajah, V.; Martin, G.; Ting, D.S.W.; Karthikesalingam, A.; King, D.; Ashrafian, H.; Darzi, A. Diagnostic accuracy of deep learning in medical imaging: A systematic review and meta-analysis. *NPJ Digit. Med.* **2021**, *4*, 65. [CrossRef]
39. Nakaura, T.; Higaki, T.; Awai, K.; Ikeda, O.; Yamashita, Y. A primer for understanding radiology articles about machine learning and deep learning. *Diagn. Interv. Imaging* **2020**, *101*, 765–770. [CrossRef]
40. Elaziz, M.A.; Dahou, A.; Mabrouk, A.; Ibrahim, R.A.; Aseeri, A.O. Medical Image Classifications for 6G IoT-Enabled Smart Health Systems. *Diagnostics* **2023**, *13*, 834. [CrossRef]
41. Manco, L.; Maffei, N.; Strolin, S.; Vichi, S.; Bottazzi, L.; Strigari, L. Basic of machine learning and deep learning in imaging for medical physicists. *Phys. Med.* **2021**, *83*, 194–205. [CrossRef]
42. Liu, S.; Yao, W. Prediction of lung cancer using gene expression and deep learning with KL divergence gene selection. *BMC Bioinform.* **2022**, *23*, 175. [CrossRef]
43. Wang, S.; Shi, J.; Ye, Z.; Dong, D.; Yu, D.; Zhou, M.; Liu, Y.; Gevaert, O.; Wang, K.; Zhu, Y.; et al. Predicting EGFR mutation status in lung adenocarcinoma on computed tomography image using deep learning. *Eur. Respir. J.* **2019**, *53*, 1800986. [CrossRef]

Disclaimer/Publisher's Note: The statements, opinions and data contained in all publications are solely those of the individual author(s) and contributor(s) and not of MDPI and/or the editor(s). MDPI and/or the editor(s) disclaim responsibility for any injury to people or property resulting from any ideas, methods, instructions or products referred to in the content.

MDPI AG
Grosspeteranlage 5
4052 Basel
Switzerland
Tel.: +41 61 683 77 34

Diagnostics Editorial Office
E-mail: diagnostics@mdpi.com
www.mdpi.com/journal/diagnostics

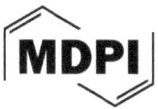

Disclaimer/Publisher's Note: The title and front matter of this reprint are at the discretion of the Guest Editors. The publisher is not responsible for their content or any associated concerns. The statements, opinions and data contained in all individual articles are solely those of the individual Editors and contributors and not of MDPI. MDPI disclaims responsibility for any injury to people or property resulting from any ideas, methods, instructions or products referred to in the content.

www.ingramcontent.com/pod-product-compliance
Lightning Source LLC
LaVergne TN
LVHW072326090526
838202LV00019B/2362